Child Health Nursing
Nursing Process Approach

Child Health Nursing
Nursing Process Approach

Second Edition

A Padmaja MA (Psy) MSc (N) PhD
Ex-Professor and Vice-Principal (Administration)
College of Nursing
Sri Venkateswara Institute of Medical Sciences
Tirupati, Andhra Pradesh, India

Forewords
K Rajalakshmi
Saradha Suresh

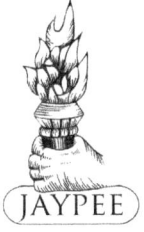

JAYPEE BROTHERS MEDICAL PUBLISHERS
The Health Sciences Publisher
New Delhi | London

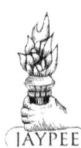 **Jaypee Brothers Medical Publishers (P) Ltd**

Headquarters
Jaypee Brothers Medical Publishers (P) Ltd
EMCA House, 23/23-B
Ansari Road, Daryaganj
New Delhi 110 002, India
Landline: +91-11-23272143, +91-11-23272703
+91-11-23282021, +91-11-23245672
Email: jaypee@jaypeebrothers.com

Overseas Office
J.P. Medical Ltd
83 Victoria Street, London
SW1H 0HW (UK)
Phone: +44 20 3170 8910
Email: info@jpmedpub.com

Corporate Office
Jaypee Brothers Medical Publishers (P) Ltd
4838/24, Ansari Road, Daryaganj
New Delhi 110 002, India
Phone: +91-11-43574357
Fax: +91-11-43574314
Email: jaypee@jaypeebrothers.com

EU GPSR Authorised Representative
Logos Europe, 9 rue Nicolas Poussin
17000, La Rochelle, France
Phone: +33 (0) 6 67 93 73 78
E-mail: Contact@logoseurope.eu

Website: www.jaypeebrothers.com
Website: www.jaypeedigital.com

© 2024, Jaypee Brothers Medical Publishers

The views and opinions expressed in this book are solely those of the original contributor(s)/author(s) and do not necessarily represent those of editor(s) and publisher of the book.

All rights reserved. No part of this publication may be reproduced, stored or transmitted in any form or by any means, electronic, mechanical, photocopying, recording or otherwise, without the prior permission in writing of the publishers.

All brand names and product names used in this book are trade names, service marks, trademarks or registered trademarks of their respective owners. The publisher is not associated with any product or vendor mentioned in this book.

Medical knowledge and practice change constantly. This book is designed to provide accurate, authoritative information about the subject matter in question. However, readers are advised to check the most current information available on procedures included and check information from the manufacturer of each product to be administered, to verify the recommended dose, formula, method and duration of administration, adverse effects and contraindications. It is the responsibility of the practitioner to take all appropriate safety precautions. Neither the publisher nor the author(s)/editor(s) assume any liability for any injury and/or damage to persons or property arising from or related to use of material in this book.

This book is sold on the understanding that the publisher is not engaged in providing professional medical services. If such advice or services are required, the services of a competent medical professional should be sought.

Every effort has been made where necessary to contact holders of copyright to obtain permission to reproduce copyright material. If any have been inadvertently overlooked, the publisher will be pleased to make the necessary arrangements at the first opportunity.

Inquiries for bulk sales may be solicited at: jaypee@jaypeebrothers.com

Child Health Nursing: Nursing Process Approach

First Edition: 2015

Second Edition: **2024**

ISBN: 978-93-5696-324-5

Dedication

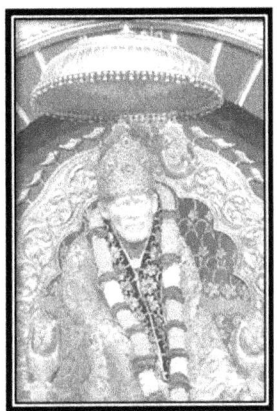

I am heartfully dedicating my work to "Sri Shirdi Sainath", who strengthens me by helping me each and every second in all my deeds by showering his blessings abundantly through various resources, which helped me in the accomplishment of all the tasks in my life.

This book is also dedicated to my incredible family, without whom I could never have accomplished this monumental task. In loving memory of my father Late A Adinarayana, for his eternal blessings and my mother Smt A Kausalyamma, and my mother-in-law Smt K Chengamma, for rendering emotional support. My husband Dr K Munuswamy, SMO, Causality, Sri Venkateswara Institute of Medical Sciences (SVIMS), has unfailingly stood by my side, providing continuous positive affirmation and infinite support for this project. My brothers S Somprakash, founder President of Viswadharma Peetam (Center for Universal Philosophy), A Venkata Ramanaiah, founder of Sri Shirdi Sai Industries, Avilala, for their motivation and moral support, my sister A Nagaraja Kumari and my son K Prabhat Kiran, for their patience and tireless efforts to help me in computer work.

Foreword

This is yet another unique and very important book *Child Health Nursing: Nursing Process Approach* written by Professor Dr A Padmaja, College of Nursing, Sri Venkateswara Institute of Medical Sciences, Tirupati, Andhra Pradesh, India.

In the multifaceted world of healthcare, nursing is no longer separate in practice and education. It is a team work and at the same time to work independently in areas assigned. Each profession brings it's own knowledge base and nature of practice. In nursing, nursing is a scientific and client-oriented approach and an evidence-based practice. It is designed to give standard, quality, holistic customer care/patient in any area of specialties whether in hospital, outpatient department, community or home care. It may be surgical nursing intervention or in medical.

Now this book is based on advanced technology with scientific approach to provide nursing process for clinical nursing diagnosis and management. It is well focused and compiled with critical thinking on the steps of nursing process start from assessment phase of child, pathophysiology flow sheet, diagnosis phase by using NANDA Taxonomy for clinical judgment, planning, implementation, and valuation.

There is so much advancement in child health care but there is a dearth of well-written books on practical approach to child health nursing with disease mechanism. She has tried to bring an inspiring clinical climate where quality nurses will rise up. Let us take pride of her contribution and achievement for the benefit of nursing world.

It requires a high level of competence to deal with children of all age groups. The author has succeeded with her distinction and insight to cover all important systems including ENT, congenital anomalies and discusses the intervention to carry out with rationale. This is a very handy book in specialties of child health, ready reckoner, simple language to follow with more detailed presentation to follow, very useful to solve the problems in circuital subjects for graduates and postgraduates of nursing as well as medical students. The students preparing for examination may face a dilemma. But, following this book will be a boost of courage to right method of approach.

The author has endeavored and integrated extensive contents for better understanding for prevention and relieving suffering. It is, therefore, for timely opportune that this standard book by Indian author to meet the requirements of graduates, undergraduates, and postgraduates.

I congratulate the author for accepting this challenging task to present for nursing world. I am confident that her contribution to this book will be a great value for professionals and will have more editions and wish her to bring many books in child health nursing, education, administration, and research.

K Rajalakshmi MSc (N) PhD
Professor, Pediatric (N) and Research Guide
CSI Jeyaraj Annapackiam College of Nursing
Madurai, Tamil Nadu, India

Foreword

The book *Child Health Nursing: Nursing Process Approach* is the first of its kind in our country that deals with the management of various illnesses in children for nurses. In the recent times, specialization in the various specialties and subspecialties has been the norm as it helps in improving and fine tuning the skills that are specifically required for care of the patients in those departments. In this context, this book will be a great help to all those involved in the nursing care of sick children.

This book not only deals with general pediatric illnesses but also with various illnesses in the different systems of pediatrics namely, cardiovascular, renal, orthopedics, etc. to name a few. Such detailed descriptions will be very helpful to all the nurses working in those departments as a ready reckoner and to refresh their knowledge when needed.

The categorization into five steps is a very welcome approach as it lends clarity and objective care. This will also help to identify the areas where there are gaps in skill or knowledge, so that those issues can be addressed specifically. In this way, this book will be a great help to nursing students and teachers in their practical teaching and assessment.

As teachers, we all know good books are hard to come by as it takes enormous effort to write one. I really congratulate Dr A Padmaja for her enthusiasm and hard work in writing and bringing out this book which I am sure will be found useful to each and every working nurse not to mention teachers and other medical faculties involved in teaching and care of sick children. It is with great pleasure and a sense of honor that I am writing the Foreword for this book and not hoping but very sure that this book will go into several edition and prints as it readily deserves. Once again, I express my appreciation to Dr A Padmaja and her Guru Professor Dr K Rajalakshmi who had been instrumental in inspiring her to write this book.

Saradha Suresh MD PhD FRCP (Glas)
Former Director and Superintendent
Institute of Child Health and Hospital for Children, Egmore
Head
Department of Pediatrics
Madras Medical College
Chennai, Tamil Nadu, India

Preface to the Second Edition

It gives me immense pleasure to present the Second Edition of this textbook titled, *Child Health Nursing: Nursing Process Approach*, to Nursing students, educators, and practitioners in the field of Child Health Nursing.

A reasonable time has been spent on the revision of this book. The nursing process chapter has been elaborated as per the components of the nursing process and also added application of nursing theories.

The whole book is updated and some of the topics such as Nursing Process for Normal Newborn and Family to Adolescent, Hospitalized Child, Genetic Disorders, Neoplastic Disorders, Communicable Diseases and Mental Disorders (including Behavioral Disorders) are included.

Practice questions are given at the end of each chapter which will help the students to evaluate their understanding of the matter and ability to recall the information. This textbook is going to be a valuable companion to all nursing students and personnel.

I sincerely invite suggestions, constructive criticism, and comments from the readers about this book, so that acceptable changes can be made in the forthcoming edition. Kindly mail me at raajinaidu@rocketmail.com.

I wish all the readers success in nursing career.

A Padmaja

Preface to the First Edition

I am very much delighted to present this textbook titled *Child Health Nursing: Nursing Process Approach* to the nursing students of India. The primary objective of this book is to prepare nurses who combine the highest level of scientific knowledge and rationale with responsible caring practice.

Pediatric nursing promotes, restores, and maintains the health of children and the nursing process is a written tool that identifies problem areas, and documents nursing activities in an individual manner to facilitate an ill child's journey to wellness or comfort a child's journey during a life-threatening illness leading to death. The nursing process covers common acute and chronic illnesses associated with the general age group of infants, toddler, preschoolers, and school-age children. Conditions specific to the neonatal and adolescents have been excluded although some conditions with onset during the neonatal period and those continuing into adolescence are included. Emergency conditions and illnesses requiring acute care in an intensive care unit are also excluded.

Each condition within the system includes an introductory paragraph that provides information about the condition in relation to the infant and child; a pathophysiological flowchart illustrated with diagrams, depicting causative factors, pathology, resultant signs and symptoms, complications; nursing process that includes the essential nursing diagnoses with specific related factors or risks and defining characteristics as they relate to the condition and taken from the system that includes the essential diagnoses and process used (these are referenced so that developed plan may be used in this condition), followed by specific nursing diagnoses and their related or risk factors, defining characteristics followed by the same format as the essential diagnose and nursing process.

Since it is not uncommon for an infant or child to develop complications to an illness, more than one nursing process may be used or combined with the plan for presenting illness, more than one nursing care plan may be used or combined with the plan for the illness if appropriate. It is hoped that the practitioners will find these processes to be flexible enough to accomplish this interrelationship among the nursing diagnoses and their related care options.

Since it is prepared according to the syllabus of Indian Nursing Council, the undergraduate and postgraduate nursing students will find it as a textbook for their studies. The nursing educators will find it easy to teach their students and prepare them for the examinations.

This book will also bring a uniform standard of the nursing education in India. It also serves as a reference book for the practicing nurses.

I will be much appreciated, if readers send their criticisms, suggestions, corrections, if any for further improvement of this book.

A Padmaja

Acknowledgments

I am most grateful to my teacher Professor Dr K Rajalakshmi and Professor Dr Saradha Suresh who have kindly honored me by writing the foreword.

I would like to have the opportunity to thank Professor Dr B Vengamma, Director; Professor Dr D Rajasekhar, Head and Dean, Department of Cardiology, and Professor Dr PV Ramasubba Reddy, Registrar, Sri Venkateswara Institute of Medical Sciences (SVIMS), and other administrators for permitting me to publish this book.

I extend my special thanks to Professor Dr Alladi Mohan, Head, Department of Medicine, SVIMS and all my colleagues, friends, and well-wishers who have cooperated directly or indirectly on completion of the task. I am thankful to all my past and present students who have insisted me to accept this work.

My special acknowledgment to Mrs Samhita and other MSc (N) students for designing the diagrams and reviewing of whole text for their requirements and encouragement in their own way.

I am very grateful to the whole team of M/s Jaypee Brothers Medical Publishers (P) Ltd, New Delhi, India, who helped and guided me, Shri Jitendar P Vij (Group Chairman), Mr Ankit Vij (Managing Director), Mr MS Mani (Group President), Dr Madhu Choudhary (Director-Educational Publishing), Ms Pooja Bhandari [Director-Production (Books and Journals)], Ms Sunita Katla (Executive Assistant to Group Chairman and Publishing Manager), Mr Ajay Kumar Sharma (Deputy General Manager), Ms Samina Khan (Executive Assistant to Director-Educational Publishing), Mr Rajesh Sharma (Production Coordinator), Ms Seema Dogra (Cover Visualizer), Mr Rahul Jadli and Mr Anil Singh (Proofreader), Mr Dinesh Bhardwaj (Typesetter), Mr Nitin Bhardwaj (Graphic Designer) and their team members, for all their support to work in this project and make it a success. Without their cooperation, I could not have completed this project.

I express my heartfelt gratitude to Ms Teresa Lamniang (Development Editor), for her constant support and continuous follow-up to complete the task in revising the book for second edition, and especially Mr Venugopal (Regional Manager, Bengaluru) and Mr Shanta Raj for publishing this book.

Contents

1. **Nursing Process** — 1
   - Nursing Process Overview — 1
   - Components of Nursing Process — 1

2. **Application of Nursing Theories** — 11
   - Katharine Kolcaba Comfort Theory in Postoperative Child — 11
   - Theory of Interpersonal Relations — 11
   - Neuman's System Model — 21

3. **Nursing Care of Newborn and Family** — 30
   - Nursing Process for the Newborn and Family — 30

4. **Nursing Care for an Infant** — 35
   - Nursing Process for an Infant — 35

5. **Nursing Care for a Toddler** — 38
   - Nursing Process for the Toddler — 38

6. **Nursing Care for a Preschool Child** — 41
   - Nursing Process for a Preschool Child — 41

7. **Nursing Care for School-Age Child** — 45
   - Nursing Process for the School-Age Child — 45

8. **Nursing Care for an Adolescent Child** — 48
   - Nursing Process for an Adolescent Child — 48

9. **Nursing Process for a Hospitalized Child** — 51
   - Nursing Process for a Hospitalized Child — 52

10. **Nursing Process for the Child with Genetic Disorder** — 62
    - Nursing Process for the Child with Genetic Disorder — 62

11. **Nursing Process for the Child with Respiratory Disorder** — 65
    - Nursing Process for the Child with Respiratory Disorder (In General) — 65
    - Nursing Process for Respiratory Disorders (Specific Conditions) — 68

12. **Nursing Process for the Child with Neurological Disorder** — 95
    - Nursing Process for the Child with Neurological Disorder (In General) — 95
    - Nursing Process for Specific Neurological Disorders — 101

Contents

13. Nursing Process of the Child with Gastrointestinal Disorder — 142
- Nursing Process of the Child with Gastrointestinal Disorder (In General) — 142
- Nursing Process for Specific Gastrointestinal Disorder — 146

14. Nursing Process for the Child with Cardiovascular Disorder — 177
- Nursing Process for the Child with Cardiovascular Disorder (In General) — 177
- Nursing Process for Specific Cardiovascular Disorders — 181

15. Nursing Process for the Child with Renal Disorder — 213
- Nursing Process for the Child with Renal Disorder — 213
- Nursing Process for Specific Renal Disorders — 217

16. Nursing Process for the Child with a Neoplastic Disorder — 253
- Nursing Process for the Child with a Neoplastic Disorder — 253

17. Nursing Process for the Child with Communicable Diseases — 259
- Nursing Process for the Child with Communicable Diseases — 259

18. Nursing Process for the Child with Hematologic Disorder — 263
- Nursing Process for the Child with Hematologic Disorder (In General) — 263
- Nursing Process for Specific Hematological Disorders — 266

19. Nursing Process for the Child with Endocrine Disorders — 293
- Nursing Process for the Child with Endocrine Disorders (In General) — 293
- Nursing Process for Specific Endocrine Disorders — 297

20. Nursing Process for the Child with Disorder of Eyes, Ears, Nose and Throat — 306
- Nursing Process for the Child with Disorder of Eyes, Ears, Nose and Throat — 306
- Nursing Process for Specific Eye, Ear, Nose and Throat Disorders — 309

21. Nursing Process for the Child with Integumentary Disorder — 324
- Nursing Process for the Child with Integumentary Disorder (In General) — 324
- Nursing Process for Specific Integumentary Disorders — 326

22. Nursing Process for the Child with Musculoskeletal Disorder — 336
- Nursing Process for the Child with Musculoskeletal Disorder (In General) — 336
- Nursing Process for Specific Musculoskeletal Disorders — 339

23. Nursing Management of Child with Mental Health Disorders (Including Behavioral Disorders) — 378
- Nursing Management of Child with Mental Health Disorders (Including Behavioral Disorders) in General — 378
- Nursing Process for Specific Mental Health Disorders — 381

Index — 391

CHAPTER 1

Nursing Process

LEARNING OBJECTIVES
- To identify a client health status.
- To identify his/her actual/present and potential/possible health problems or needs.
- To establish a plan of care to meet identified needs.
- To provide nursing interventions to meet those needs.
- To evaluate the interventions.

NURSING PROCESS OVERVIEW

A systematic problem-solving approach is used to identify, prevent and treat actual or potential health problems and promote wellness. A systematic way to plan, implement and evaluate care for individuals, families, groups and communities.

COMPONENTS OF NURSING PROCESS

The nursing process consists of five dynamic and interrelated phases:
1. **Assessment:** Collecting subjective and objective data.
2. **Diagnosis:** Analysis subjective and objective data to make nursing diagnosis.
3. **Planning:** Determining outcome criteria and developing a plan.
4. **Implementation:** Carrying out a plan.
5. **Evaluation:** Assessing whether outcome criteria have been met and revising the plan as necessary.

Health Assessment

Introduction
- It is a systematic and continuous collection, validation and communication of client data as compared to what is standard/norm.
- It includes the client's perceived needs, health problems, related experiences, health practices, values and lifestyles.

Purpose
To establish a data base (all the information about the client):
- Nursing health history.
- Physical assessment.
- The physician's history and physical examination.
- Results of laboratory and diagnostic tests.
- Material from other health personnel.

Steps of Assessment

1. **Collection of data**
   - Subjective data collection
   - Objective data collection
2. **Validation of data**
3. **Organization of data**
4. **Recording/documentation of data**

1. Collection of Data

- Gathering information about the client
- Includes physical, psychological, emotional, sociocultural, spiritual factors that may affect client's health status.
- Includes past health history of client (allergies, past surgeries, chronic diseases, use of folk healing methods).
- Includes current/present problems of client (pain, nausea, sleep pattern, religious practices, medications or treatment the client is taking now).

Types of data

a. **Subjective data:**
   - Also referred to as symptom or sensations.
   - Information from the client's point of view or are described by the person experiencing it.
   - Information supplied by the family members, significant others; others health professionals are considered subjective data.

   Example: Pain, dizziness, ringing of ears/tinnitus

b. **Objective data:**
   - Also referred to as sign.
   - These that can be detected, observed or measured/tested using accepted standard or norm
   - Mainly collected by general observation and by using the four physical examination techniques:
     1. Inspection
     2. Percussion
     3. Palpation
     4. Auscultation.

   Example: Pallor, diaphoresis, BP = 150/100, yellow discoloration of skin.

2. Validation of Data

The act of "Double Checking" or verifying data to confirm that it is accurate and complete. Validation of data is the process of confirming or verifying that the subjective and objective data collected are reliable and accurate. The steps of validation include deciding whether the data require validation, determining ways to validate the data, and identifying areas where data are missing. Failure to validate data may result in premature closure of the assessment or collection of inaccurate data.

Purposes of data validation:

- Ensure that data collection is complete.
- Ensure that objective and subjective data agree.

- Obtain additional data that may have been overlooked.
- Avoid jumping to conclusion.
- Differentiate cues and inferences.

3. Organization of Data

Uses a written or computerized format that organizes assessment data systematically

4. Communicate/Record/Document Data

- Nurse records all data collected about the client's health status.
- Data are recorded in a factual manner not as interpreted by the nurse.
- Record subjective data in client's word; restating in other words what client says might change its original meaning.

Purposes of documentation:

- Provides a chronological source of client assessment data and a progressive record of assessment findings that outline the client's course of care.
- Ensure that information about client and family is easily accessible to members of the healthcare team; provides a vehicle for communication; and prevents fragmentation, repetition, and delays in carrying out the plan of care.
- Establishes a basis for screening or validation of proposed diagnoses.
- Acts as source of information to help diagnose new problems.
- Offers a basis for determining the educational needs of the client, family, and significant others.
- Provides a basis for determining eligibility for care and reimbursement. Careful recording of data can support financial reimbursement or gain additional reimbursement for transitional or skilled care needed by the client.
- Constitutes a permanent legal record of the care that was or was not give to the client.
- Provides access to significant epidemiological data for future investigation and research and educational endeavors.

Guidelines for documentation:

- Document legibly or print neatly in unerasable ink
- Use correct grammar and spelling
- Avoid wordiness that creates redundancy
- Use phrases instead of sentences to record data
- Record data findings, not how they were obtained
- Write entries objectively without making premature judgements or diagnosis
- Record complete information and details for all client symptoms or experiences
- Include additional assessment content when applicable
- Support objective data with specific observations obtained during the physical examination.

Nursing Diagnosis

Standards developed by the Joint Commission on the Accreditation of Healthcare Organization (JCAHO) mandate that each client's nursing care be based on identified nursing diagnosis or client care needs (1996). Nurse continue to develop new nursing diagnosis, refine the existing diagnosis and organize them into a classification system useful to practicing nurses. NANDA has been the leader in nursing diagnosis classification and has been endorsed by the ANA as having the responsibility to do so. To date 50 conferences have been held to refine the classification system for nursing diagnosis (**Table 1.1**).

Definition

A nursing diagnosis is a statement that describes the client's actual or potential responses to a health problem that the nurse is licensed and competent to treat. For example, **impaired skin integrity related to decreased mobility and risk for infection related to poor nutritional intake**.

Nursing diagnosis provides the basis for selection of nursing intervention to achieve outcome for which the nurse is accountable. Outcomes and interventions are selected in relationship to particular nursing diagnosis. The reason for formulating a nursing diagnosis after analyzing assessment data are to identify the health problems involving the client and family and to provide direction for nursing care.

Table 1.1: List of the NANDA nursing diagnosis.

- Activity planning
- Activity tolerance
- Acute substance withdrawal syndrome
- Adaptive capacity
- Adverse reaction to iodinated contrast media
- Airway clearance
- Allergy reaction
- Anxiety
- Aspiration
- Attachment
- Autonomic dysreflexia
- Balanced energy field
- Balanced fluid volume
- Balanced nutrition
- Bathing self-care
- Bleeding
- Blood glucose level
- Body image
- Breasting feeding
- Breast milk production
- Breathing pattern
- Cardiac out put
- Child bearing process
- Chronic pain syndrome
- Comfort
- Communication
- Confusion
- Constipation
- Contamination
- Coping
- Death anxiety
- Decisional conflict
- Labour pain
- Latex allergy reaction
- Life style
- Liver function
- Loneliness
- Maternal fetal dyad
- Memory
- Metabolic imbalance syndrome
- Mobility
- Mood regulation
- Moral distress
- Mucous membrane integrity
- Nausea
- Neonatal abstinence syndrome
- Neurovascular function
- Nutrition
- Obesity
- Occupational injury
- Organized behavior
- Other directed violence
- Pain
- Parenting
- Perioperative hypothermia
- Perioperative positioning injury
- Personal identity
- Physical trauma
- Poisoning
- Post-trauma syndrome
- Power
- Pressure ulcer
- Protection
- Rape-trauma syndrome

Contd...

Contd...

- Decision making
- Denial
- Dentition
- Development
- Diarrhea
- Disuse syndrome
- Diversional activity engagement
- Dressing self-care
- Dry eye
- Dry mouth
- Dysfunctional gastrointestinal motility
- Eating dynamics
- Electrolyte balance
- Elimination
- Emancipated decision making
- Emotional control
- Falls
- Family process
- Fatigue
- Fear
- Feeding dynamics
- Feeding pattern
- Feeding self care
- Female genital mutilation
- Fluid volume
- Frail elderly syndrome
- Functional constipation
- Gas exchange
- Grieving
- Health
- Health behavior
- Health literacy
- Health maintenance
- Health management
- Home maintenance
- Hope
- Human dignity
- Hyperbilirubinemia
- Hyperthermia
- Hypothermia
- Imbalanced nutrition more than body requirements
- Immigration transition
- Impulse control
- Incontinence
- Infection
- Injury
- Insomnia
- Knowledge
- Relationship
- Religiosity
- Relocation stress syndrome
- Resilience
- Retention
- Role conflict
- Role performance
- Role strain
- Self-care
- Self-concept
- Self-directed violence
- Self-esteem
- Self-mutilation
- Self-neglect
- Sexual function
- Sexuality pattern shock
- Sitting
- Skin integrity
- Sleep
- Sleep pattern
- Social interaction
- Social isolation
- Sorrow
- Spiritual distress
- Spiritual well being
- Spontaneous ventilation
- Stable blood pressure
- Standing
- Stress
- Sudden death
- Suffocation
- Suicide
- Surgical recovery
- Surgical site infection
- Swallowing
- Thermal injury
- Thermoregulation
- Tissue integrity
- Tissue perfusion
- Toileting self-care
- Transfer ability
- Trauma
- Unilateral neglect
- Venous thromboembolism
- Ventilator weaning response
- Walking
- Wandering

Table 1.2: Types of diagnostic statements.

Type	Construction	Example
Actual nursing diagnosis	Three-part statement includes: • Diagnostic label • Related factors • Defining characteristics	Acute pain related to surgical trauma and inflammation, as evidenced by grimacing and verbal reports of pain
Risk nursing diagnosis	Two-part statement includes: • Diagnostic label • Risk factors	Risk for infection related to surgery and immune suppression
Possible nursing diagnosis	Two-part statement includes: • Diagnostic label • Related factors (unknown)	Possible self-esteem disturbance related to unknown etiology
Wellness diagnosis	One-part statement include: Diagnostic label	Readiness for enhanced spiritual wellbeing

What is not a nursing diagnosis? The nursing diagnosis statement is written in terms of a client problem, alteration in health state for which the nursing provides the primary therapy **(Table 1.2)**. The following are not nursing diagnosis:
- Medical diagnosis
- Medical pathology
- Diagnostic tests
- Treatments
- Equipment

Propose Possible Nursing Diagnosis

If the situation requires primarily nursing intervention, then the nursing diagnosis may be wellness diagnosis, risk diagnosis or actual diagnosis **(Table 1.3)**. A wellness diagnosis indicates that the client has the opportunity for enhancement of a health state. A risk diagnose indicates the client does not currently have the problem but is at high-risk for developing it. An actual

Table 1.3: Comparison of wellness, risk and actual nursing diagnosis.

	Wellness diagnosis	Risk diagnosis	Actual diagnosis
Client status	State of harmony and balance	State of risk for identified diagnosis	State of health problems
Format for stating	Opportunity to enhance		Nursing diagnosis
Examples	• Opportunity to enhance body image • Opportunity to enhance effective breast feeding • Opportunity to enhance skin integrity	• Risk for altered body image • Risk for altered family process • Risk for ineffective breast feeding • Risk for impaired skin Integrity	• Altered body image related to hand wound that is not healing • Altered family process related to hospitalization • Ineffective breast feeding related to poor mother infant attachment • Impaired skin integrity related to immobility

nursing diagnosis indicates the client is currently experiencing the stated problem or has a dysfunctional pattern.

Document Conclusions

Be sure to document all your professional judgements and the data that supports those judgments. Nursing diagnosis can be documented and worded in different formats like: Wellness diagnosis, risk diagnosis, and actual nursing diagnosis.

Nursing Diagnosis Application to Care Planning

The use of nursing diagnosis is a mechanism for identifying the domain of nursing:
- The formulated nursing diagnosis provides direction for the planning process and the selection of nursing interventions to achieve the desired outcome. The care plan is a mechanism for demonstrating accountability.
- In addition, the nursing diagnosis and subsequent care plan assist in communicating to other professionals the client centered problems through the nursing care plan, consultations, and discharge planning and client care conferences.
- Making accurate nursing diagnosis helps to ensure that clients receive quality nursing care.
- Nursing diagnosis helps to increase the specificity of nursing interventions for each client.
- Coding of nursing diagnosis in computerized systems allows direct reimbursement for nurses.
- Studies of specific nursing diagnosis improve understanding of nursing diagnostic process and contribute to examination of nurse's role in healthcare.
- The development of taxonomy of nursing diagnosis should significantly affect practice, education, research, legislation, and nursing as a profession.
- A nursing diagnosis will help to bridge a gap between knowledge and practice and will articulate the scope of nursing practice, essential to developing nursing professional role in healthcare.

Advantages of Nursing Diagnosis

Nursing diagnosis is advantageous for both nurses and clients:
- They facilitate communication among nurses about the clients level of wellness and assist in discharge planning.
- Nursing diagnosis helps in prioritizing the clients needs.
- Nursing diagnosis are also used for charting in the progress notes, writing referrals and providing effective transition of care from one unit to another, from one clinic to another or from the hospital to community.
- Nursing diagnosis can also serve as focus for quality improvement. When focusing the nursing diagnosis, the reviewer can determine whether nursing care was correct and delivered according to standards of practice.
- Nursing diagnosis is beneficial for the client and family.

Limitations of Nursing Diagnosis

Nursing diagnosis has limitations and the beginning practitioner should be aware of their existence. Because of the continuous evolution of the terms and use of nursing diagnosis, the language can occasionally be verbose and contain jargon. This may limit the use of nursing diagnosis to only nursing professionals and result is confusion among other members of health team.

Planning

Once you have listed the nursing diagnosis you have to plan the care. This step consists of goal setting and nursing strategies. The major activity in planning is the development of the nursing care plan that provides basis for intervention. The pediatric client, the family and the nurse must be involved. The nurse's plan of action must be structured to include all the identified nursing diagnosis, actual or potential and should be based on principles and sound rationale. With this concept of planning, we shall now define nursing care plan.

Nursing care plan is a written document that states specific nursing interventions planned for a particular client.

Practical Points in Preparation of Nursing Care Plan

- You first review the nursing diagnosis, then assign this priority or the order in which these are to be met.
- Along with client and family develop goals specific to the client's individual needs.
- These goals may be designated (by the client/family) as high, medium or low priority.
- Your nursing strategies should be client centered.
- Each strategy that you consider should be based on a specific reason.
- Document or write down nursing diagnosis, goals with time periods and nursing strategies. This information is to be written in a systematic and concise manner so that other nursing personnel can understand and use it.
- Remember that nursing care plan focuses on nursing problems and have a nursing approach.
- Write nursing care plan in clear and specific terms.
- Take time to sit down and write out a plan of care that will help you to organize your mental thoughts to think through what you hope to accomplish by nursing care
- Take into account potential problems as well as those which are actually resent. Review the possibilities of alternative nursing interventions and develop a plan of care that can be followed through by all nursing personnel concerned with the client.

Advantages of Written Plan of Care

It helps to ensure:
- Continuity
- Completeness of care
- That everyone is using the same approach with the client
- That nothing is let out in care.

Implementation

Definition

Implementation refers to the action phase of the nursing process in which nursing care is provided. It is the actual initiation of the plan and recording of nursing actions. Its purpose is to provide technical and therapeutic nursing care required to help the client achieve an optimal level of health.

Implementation Skills

The implementation phase of the nursing process draws heavily on the intellectual, interpersonal, and technical skills of the nurse. These are also known as cognitive, affective and conative skills. Decision-making, observation, and communication are significant skills, enhancing the success of action. These skills are utilized with the client, the nurse, nursing team members, and health team members. Competence in intellectual, interpersonal and technical skills is required to carry out the implementation phase.

Implementation Activities

The activities of implementation include the following:
- Reassessing
- Setting priorities
- Performing nursing intervention
- Recording nursing actions.

Responsibilities in Implementation of Nursing Care

It is the professional responsibility to carry out the nursing care as the primary nurse, delegate certain interventions to appropriate nursing or allied health professionals and carry out physician orders, thereby integrating medical therapy into overall care plan. Nursing care is implemented to assist people in achieving the outcomes established in the plan of care, to prevent disease and illness by promoting wellness, to restore functioning and to facilitate coping with illness.

Evaluation

Definition

Evaluation is defined as the judgment of the effectiveness of nursing care to meet client goals based on the client's behavioral responses.

Types

There are three types of evaluation:
  i. **Structure evaluation:** Structure evaluation focuses on the attributes of the setting or surroundings where healthcare is provided. It deals with the environmental aspects that directly or indirectly influence the quality of care provided. Availability of equipment, layout of physical facilities, nurse-client ratios, administrative support, and maintenance of nursing staff competence are some areas of concern for structure evaluation.
  ii. **Process evaluation:** Process evaluation focuses on the nurse's performance and whether the nursing care provided was appropriate and competent. The phases of the nursing process are used as the framework for the evaluation of nursing care. Areas of concern for

this type of evaluation include the type of information obtained by interview and physical assessment, the validity of the nursing diagnostic statements, and the nurse's technical competence.

iii. **Outcome evaluation:** Outcome evaluation, which focuses on the client and the client's function. Outcome evaluation determines the extent to which the client's behavioral response to nursing intervention reflects the desired client goal and outcome criteria. Outcome evaluation can take place only after standards have been developed. An example of an outcome evaluation is to establish standards of care for a specific diagnosis and then compare actual client outcome with that standard.

PRACTICE QUESTIONS

1. Write the process of collecting data.
2. Define nursing diagnosis. Frame 5 nursing diagnosis for a child with 30% burns.

CHAPTER 2

Application of Nursing Theories

LEARNING OBJECTIVES
- To explain phenomena important to clinical practice.
- To guide nursing practice.
- To understand and analyze patient data.
- To make appropriate decisions related to nursing interventions.

INTRODUCTION

Nursing science is an identifiable discrete body of knowledge comprising paradigms, frameworks and theories. The integration of nursing theories practice demonstrates an evolutionary pathway for introducing a paradigm shift in the essence of the science of nursing.

KATHARINE KOLCABA COMFORT THEORY IN POSTOPERATIVE CHILD

Hospitalization is one of the most stressful events that children and adults can experience. Not only are the physical surroundings different, but the procedures that children encounter for the first time are new. Anxiety, fear, withdrawal, depression, regression and defiance are a few reactions shown by children as well as adults, and they can be more severe than their reaction to illness.

Definition

Comfort theory is a middle range nursing theory in which comfort is defined by Katharine Kolcaba as "Immediate state of being strengthened by having the needs for relief, ease, and transcendence (types of comfort) addressed in the four contexts of holistic human experience: physical, psychospiritual, sociocultural and environmental".

Taxonomic structure of comfort needs of child in postoperative setting is given in **Table 2.1**.

Application of Katharine Kolcaba comfort theory of nursing for a 6-year-old child with laparotomy is given in **Table 2.2**.

THEORY OF INTERPERSONAL RELATIONS

Hildegard E. Peplau

Application of Interpersonal Theory in Nursing Practice

Peplau's theory focuses on the interpersonal processes and therapeutic relationship that develops between the nurse and client. The interpersonal focus of Peplau's theory requires

Application of Nursing Theories

Table 2.1: Taxonomic structure of comfort needs of child in postoperative setting.

Need	Relief	Ease	Transcendence
Physical	Pain, Thirst, Fever, Dehydration	By comfortable position, application of wetcotton over lip to reduce thirst, fluid administration, administering medication	• Motivating the child to tolerate pain by diverting mind with bubble blowing • Motivating the child to tolerate thirst by positive talk
Psychospiritual	Anxiety, Fever	Listening, emotional support, positive talk, hand holding. Ease the child by allowing parents to stay with child. Psychological support and preparation before any procedure	Motivating the child to indulge in play, e.g., bubble blowing
Sociocultural	Separation anxiety	Providing reassurance and developmentally appropriate information. Asking mother to stay with child, story telling as per child interest to ease the child and induce sleep	Need for socialization, indulging the child in coloring picture book, help the child to rise above separation if necessary
Environmental	Noise of instruments, crying of other children, visitors disturbance	Minimize crying of other children by indulging them with other play activity by nursing students and staff. Ask mother only to stay and avoid frequent disturbance by visitors	Need for calm and familiar environment

that the nurse attend to the interpersonal process that occurs between the nurse and client. Interpersonal process is maturing force for personality. Interpersonal processes include the nurse client relationship, communication pattern integration and the roles of the nurse. Psychodynamic nursing is being able to understand one's own behavior to help others identify felt difficulties and to apply principles of human relations to the problems that arise at all levels of experience. This theory stressed the importance of nurse's ability to understand own behavior to help others identify perceived difficulties.

The four phases of nurse-patient relationships are:
1. Orientation
2. Identification
3. Exploitation
4. Resolution

Orientation
During this phase, the individual has a felt need and seeks professional assistance. The nurse helps the individual to recognize and understand his/her problem and determine the need for help **(Fig. 2.1)**.

Application of Nursing Theories

Table 2.2: Delivering of integrative comfort care interventions to a 6-year-old child with laparotomy by using Katharine Kolcaba comfort theory of nursing.

Type of comfort	Assessment of comfort need (Assessed separately)	Goal	Planning (Planned separately)	Implementation (Implemented in integrated way)	Evaluation
Relief Often meet by standard nursing interventions	Assessment of comfort by using • Observational checklist comfort score—47, moderate discomfort • Comfort daises feeling—sort of bad • Taxonomy structure of comfort grid • Physical – Pain – Thirst – Fever – Dehydration – Distressing symptoms	Goal: The child will experience comfort in the relief sense as evidence by patient observation and expression	Standard nursing care • Assessment of patient • Recording vitals • Care of wound • Maintain intake and output chart • Provision of comfortable bed comfort positioning • Administering medication and fluid as prescribed by the doctor • Use of comfortable device • Consoling child • Reducing unnecessary noise • Blowing water soap bubble • Patient was thirsty due to NPO status so soaked cotton swab in water and apply over the lip to reduce feeling of thirst.	• Standard nursing care delivered with the help of staff assigned for patient care • Comfortable bed provided • Semi-fowler position given as per child comfort • Extra comfort measures, pillow provided • Wound care given by assigned staff, during wound care patient mind diverted by blowing water soap bubble • Analgesic administered to reduce pain. • While administering medication child mind diverted by indulging child in blowing water soap bubble • Cotton swab soaked in water applied over lip • Explained all procedure or things before carrying out on the child • Child consoled after crying episode • Developmentally appropriate information provided in order to reduce stress and anxiety • Explained reason for parent separation child consoled by proper explanation of parent separation • Surrounded noise minimized • Bright light avoided by use of curtain, switching off unnecessary lights disturbing child • Heater used to stable environmental temperature • Blanket provided to give warmth	Relief in the sense of pain anxiety, stress, separation anxiety and environment disturbance as evidenced by patient verbalization and increased comfort level as observed by observational checklist

Contd...

Contd...

Type of comfort	Assessment of comfort need (Assessed separately)	Goal	Planning (Planned separately)	Implementation (Implemented in integrated way)	Evaluation
	Psychospiritual ▪ Anxiety ▪ Fear		▪ Explanation to child before carrying out procedure ▪ Consoling child and providing developmentally appropriate information to relieve anxiety		
	Sociological Relief from separation anxiety		▪ Explanation ▪ Consoling		
	Environmental Relief from environmental stressors		Minimize/eliminate environmental stressors		
Ease Often meet by emotional oriented comfort care intervention	▪ Physical ▪ Ease in pain ▪ Ease from distressing symptoms	The child will experience state of contentment (pleasure) by comfort care interventions as evidenced by patient observation and expression	Emotional oriented comfort care interventions ▪ Ease the child by asking parents to stay with child ▪ For providing sense of security hold child hand ▪ Listen child concern and remove fear and anxiety by providing development appropriate information ▪ Emotional support provided by positive talk	Emotional oriented comfort care interventions used to ease the child ▪ Parents remained with the child and separation limited ▪ For providing sense of security hold child hand ▪ Listen child concern and remove fear and anxiety by providing development appropriate information ▪ Emotional support provided by positive talk ▪ Listening carefully about child concern ▪ Unnecessary articles and instruments which create fear removed from child proximity ▪ Unnecessary disturbances in environment avoided ▪ Parents were instructed to avoid unnecessary visitors in order to comfort the child ▪ Recitation of story as per child interest	Child contended or eased as evidence by patient verbalization, content talk, lack of fear, reduced anxious behavior

Contd...

Contd...

Type of comfort	Assessment of comfort need (Assessed separately)	Goal	Planning (Planned separately)	Implementation (Implemented in integrated way)	Evaluation
	Psychospiritual • Ease in anxiety • Ease in fear		• Listening carefully about child concern and fear • Psychological support and preparation before any procedure • Removing unnecessary fear		
	Environmental Ease from environmental stressors, i.e., noise, light		• Creating objects • Minimize crying of other children by including them with other play activity by student nurses and staff		
	Sociological Ease in separation anxiety		• Ask mother only to stay and avoid frequent disturbance by visitors • Nurse caring activity must be planned for avoiding frequent disturbances • Reduce surrounding noise to ease the child • Story telling as per child interest to ease the child and induce sleep		

Contd...

Contd...

Type of comfort	Assessment of comfort need (Assessed separately)	Goal	Planning (Planned separately)	Implementation (Implemented in integrated way)	Evaluation
Transcendence emotional oriented Cognitive and functional oriented comfort care interventions	**Physical** Rise above pain and distressing symptoms **Psychospiritual** • Crying • Fear • Separation anxiety **Sociological** • Need for raising above separation • Need for support from family or significant other **Environment** Need for rising above the level of environmental stressors	The child will experience state of transcendence (child is able to rise above their challenges) by using following comfort care interventions as evidence by patient observation and expression	• Motivating the child to tolerate pain by diverting mind with bubble blowing • Motivating the child to tolerate thirst by positive talk • Motivating the child to indulge in play, e.g., bubble blowing • Indulging the child in coloring picture book; help the child to rise above separation • Calm and familiar environment will motivate the child to indulge in other activity	• Carting team members were mutually instructed to avoid unnecessary disturbances to child • Child blowed bubble with water soap bubble blower • While blowing bubble child was motivated by positive talk regarding recovery treatment discharge and other issues raised by the child • To reduce separation anxiety child was indulged in coloring picture book as per child interest • Child mind diverted from separation anxiety by recitation story from story book as per child interest • Calm and familiar environment provided by asking the parents to bring favorite and familiar things of child from home.	Level of discomfort reduced child was comfortable comfort observation checklist comfort score -107. Comfort daisies feeling – very good. Child was motivated as raised above the problems and child indulged in participation of ADL, cooperated while doing procedures. Child adjusted with parental separation. Child was relaxed with calm and familiar environment

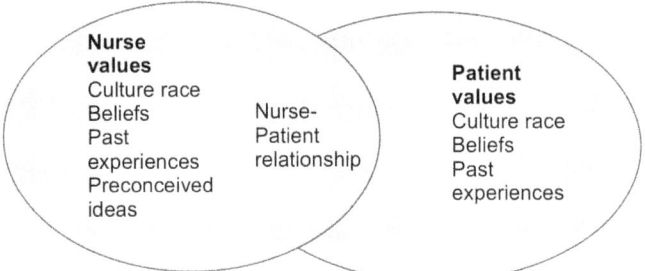

Fig. 2.1: Factors influencing: Orientation phase.

Identification

The patient identifies with those who can help him/her. The nurse permits exploration of feelings to aid the patient in undergoing illness as an experience that reorients feelings and strengthens positive forces in the personality and provides needed satisfaction.

Exploitation

During this phase, the patient attempts to receive full value from what he/she is offered through the relationship. The nurse can project new goals to be achieved through personal effort and power shifts from the nurse to the patient as the patient delays gratification to achieve the newly formed goals. Patient actively seeks and draws knowledge and expertise those who can help.

Resolution

Occurs after other phases are completed successfully. This leads to termination of relationship. In nursing process, the orientations phase parallels were assessment phase where both the patient and nurse are strangers; meeting initiated by patient who expresses a felt need. Conjointly, the nurse and patient work together, clarifies and gathers important information. Based on this assessment the nursing diagnoses are formulated, outcome and goal set. The interventions are planned, carried out and evaluation done based on mutually established expected behaviors.

Peplau's Theory Application, Nursing Process (Table 2.3)

The nursing process for Mr. Anand based on Peplau's theory is as follows:

Mr. Anand

15 Years/Male

Summary

1. **Orientation phase:**
   - Client is initially reluctant to talk due to pain
   - Client is expressing that while standing he is having much pain
   - Client expressed without movement and supine position gave him relief from pain.
2. **Identification:**
   - The client participates and interdependent with the nurse
   - Expresses the need for measure to get relief from pain

Table 2.3: Diagnosis: Intervertebral disc prolapse.

Assessment (Orientation phase)	Nursing diagnosis	Planning (Identification phase)	Implementation (Exploitation phase)	Evaluation (Resolution phase)
Anand is on pelvic traction and he is restricted to bed. The need for bed rest and restriction was discussed	Impaired physical mobility related to the presence of pelvic traction	<ul><li>Goal setting was done along with patient.</li><li>Patient will have improved physical mobility as evidenced by participating in self-care within the limits</li><li>Provide active and passive exercises to all the extremities to improve the muscle tone and strength</li><li>Make the patient perform the breathing exercises which will strengthen the respiratory muscle</li><li>Massage the upper and lower extremities which help to improve the circulation</li><li>Provide articles near to the patient and encourage doing activities within limits</li><li>Provide positive reinforcement for even a small improvement to increase the frequency of the desired activity</li></ul>	<ul><li>Carried out plans mutually agreed upon.</li><li>Provided active and passive exercises to all the extremities</li><li>Made the patient to perform breathing exercises</li><li>Massaged the upper and lower extremities.</li><li>Provided articles within the reach of the patient.</li><li>Provided positive reinforcement to the patient</li></ul>	<ul><li>Anand was free to express problems regarding difficulty in mobilizing</li><li>He expressed satisfaction when able to move without difficulty</li></ul>
Anand expresses pain in the low back region	Pain related to the degenerative changes in the lumbar region	<ul><li>Goal setting was done along with patient.</li><li>Anand will have reduction in pain as evidenced by his verbalization of reduction in pain responses</li><li>Provide non-pharmacological measures for pain relief such as divisional activity which diverts the patients mind</li></ul>	<ul><li>Carried out plans mutually agreed upon</li><li>Provided non-pharmacological measures like diversion, massaging and pelvic traction</li></ul>	Anand was free to express problems of pain

Contd...

Contd...

Assessment (Orientation phase)	Nursing diagnosis	Planning (Identification phase)	Implementation (Exploitation phase)	Evaluation (Resolution phase)
Regarding pain, discussion was made to assess the severity and the type and duration of pain. Also, the measures to reduce pain were discussed		• Give the client a neutral position. • Always use back support while turning the patient that reduces the strain on the back • Support the areas with extra pillow to allow the normal alignment and to prevent strain • Administer analgesics as prescribed by the physician • Provide pelvic traction to the patient	• Provided supine position to the client. • Supported the back during position change • Used pillows to support the back. • Administered analgesics as prescribed • Given pelvic traction and explained the need for traction	Anand expressed that he got slight relief from pain
Anand expresses that he need assistance to get down from bed. Regarding self-care discussion was done and discussed regarding the measures to solve the problems	Self-care deficit related to the presence of pelvic traction	• Goal setting was done along with patient • Client will achieve and maintain self-care activities with assistance of caregiver or within his limits • Keep all the articles within the reach of the patient • Provide a call bell to the patient to call in an emergency • Frequently visit the patient and enquire for any needs • Assist the patient in doing his self-care activities • Remove the weight of the traction as needed by the patient	• Carried out plans mutually agreed upon • Kept the articles within the reach of the client • Frequently visited the patient and enquired for any needs • Assisted the client in doing his self-care activities • Removed the weight of the traction as and when needed	• Anand was free to express problems of self-care • Assistance and all he needs were met appropriately • He achieved and maintained self-care activities within his limits

Contd...

Contd...

Assessment (Orientation phase)	Nursing diagnosis	Planning (Identification phase)	Implementation (Exploitation phase)	Evaluation (Resolution phase)
Anand is enquiring about the disease condition, its outcome and need for surgery. Discussed with the client regarding the disease process and the finding the in the client.	Anxiety related to hospital admission as evidenced by verbalization and client and family appearing withdrawn	• Goal setting was done along with patient • Client will have reduced feeling of anxiety as evidenced by asking fewer questions • Teach the family and client regarding the disease process • Explain in simple understandable language of the client • Allow and encourage the client and family to ask questions. • Allow the client and family to verbalize anxiety • Stress that frequent assessment are routine and do not necessarily imply a deteriorating condition • Allow the family member to visit the client frequently	• Carried out plans mutually agreed upon • Taught the family regarding the disease process in simple language • Allowed the client and family members to ask questions, she and his wife expressed their anxiety • Allowed the family members to frequently visit the client	• Anand was free to express problems of self-care • He asked his doubts regarding the illness and the diagnostic procedures • He verbalized that his anxiety has reduced to some extent
Anand is enquiring about the disease condition, its outcome and need for surgery. Discussed with the client regarding the disease process and the need for follow-up	Deficient knowledge related to the treatment measures to be continued even after the discharge	• Goal setting was done along with patient • Patient will acquire adequate knowledge regarding the treatment and home care • Explain the treatment measures to the patient and their benefits • Explain to the client the signs of aggravation of illness • Use simple and understandable terms • Clarify all the doubts of the patient if important • Repeat the information whenever necessary to reinforce learning	• Carried out plans mutually agreed upon • Explained treatment measures and the need for follow up • Explained regarding the signs of aggravation of disease • Use simple and understandable terms for explaining • Clarified her doubts and repeat the information if necessary.	• Anand was free to express problems of self-care • He expressed acquisition of knowledge regarding the disease and the signs of aggravation of illness

Contd...

Assessment (Orientation phase)	Nursing diagnosis	Planning (Identification phase)	Implementation (Exploitation phase)	Evaluation (Resolution phase)
Regarding pain, discussion was made to assess the severity and the type and duration of pain. Also, the measures to reduce pain were discussed		• Give the client a neutral position. • Always use back support while turning the patient that reduces the strain on the back • Support the areas with extra pillow to allow the normal alignment and to prevent strain • Administer analgesics as prescribed by the physician • Provide pelvic traction to the patient	• Provided supine position to the client. • Supported the back during position change • Used pillows to support the back. • Administered analgesics as prescribed • Given pelvic traction and explained the need for traction	Anand expressed that he got slight relief from pain
Anand expresses that he need assistance to get down from bed. Regarding self-care discussion was done and discussed regarding the measures to solve the problems	Self-care deficit related to the presence of pelvic traction	• Goal setting was done along with patient • Client will achieve and maintain self-care activities with assistance of caregiver or within his limits • Keep all the articles within the reach of the patient • Provide a call bell to the patient to call in an emergency • Frequently visit the patient and enquire for any needs • Assist the patient in doing his self-care activities • Remove the weight of the traction as needed by the patient	• Carried out plans mutually agreed upon • Kept the articles within the reach of the client • Frequently visited the patient and enquired for any needs • Assisted the client in doing his self-care activities • Removed the weight of the traction as and when needed	• Anand was free to express problems of self-care • Assistance and all he needs were met appropriately • He achieved and maintained self-care activities within his limits

Contd...

Contd...

Assessment (Orientation phase)	Nursing diagnosis	Planning (Identification phase)	Implementation (Exploitation phase)	Evaluation (Resolution phase)
Anand is enquiring about the disease condition, its outcome and need for surgery. Discussed with the client regarding the disease process and the finding the in the client.	Anxiety related to hospital admission as evidenced by verbalization and client and family appearing withdrawn	• Goal setting was done along with patient • Client will have reduced feeling of anxiety as evidenced by asking fewer questions • Teach the family and client regarding the disease process • Explain in simple understandable language of the client • Allow and encourage the client and family to ask questions. • Allow the client and family to verbalize anxiety • Stress that frequent assessment are routine and do not necessarily imply a deteriorating condition • Allow the family member to visit the client frequently	• Carried out plans mutually agreed upon • Taught the family regarding the disease process in simple language • Allowed the client and family members to ask questions, she and his wife expressed their anxiety • Allowed the family members to frequently visit the client	• Anand was free to express problems of self-care • He asked his doubts regarding the illness and the diagnostic procedures • He verbalized that his anxiety has reduced to some extent
Anand is enquiring about the disease condition, its outcome and need for surgery. Discussed with the client regarding the disease process and the need for follow-up	Deficient knowledge related to the treatment measures to be continued even after the discharge	• Goal setting was done along with patient • Patient will acquire adequate knowledge regarding the treatment and home care • Explain the treatment measures to the patient and their benefits • Explain to the client the signs of aggravation of illness • Use simple and understandable terms • Clarify all the doubts of the patient if important • Repeat the information whenever necessary to reinforce learning	• Carried out plans mutually agreed upon • Explained treatment measures and the need for follow up • Explained regarding the signs of aggravation of disease • Use simple and understandable terms for explaining • Clarified her doubts and repeat the information if necessary.	• Anand was free to express problems of self-care • He expressed acquisition of knowledge regarding the disease and the signs of aggravation of illness

- Expresses need for improving the mobility
- Expresses need to know more about prognosis, discharge and home care and follow up.

3. **Exploitation:**
   - Client explains that he gets relief of pain when lying down supine
   - Cooperates and participates actively in performing exercises
   - Client mobilizes changes position and cooperates during position changes.

4. **Resolution:**
   - Client expressed that pain has reduced a lot and he is able to tolerate it now
   - He was agreed upon to continue the exercises at home
   - He also expressed that he would come for regular follow up after discharge.

Evaluation of the Theory of Interpersonal Relations by Peplau

With the help of the theory of interpersonal relations, the clients need could be assessed. It helped him to achieve them within her limits. This theory application helped in providing comprehensive care to the client.

NEUMAN'S SYSTEM MODEL

- Betty Neuman's system model provides a comprehensive flexible holistic and system-based perspective for nursing
- It focuses attention on the response of the client system to actual or potential environmental stressors
- And the use of primary, secondary and tertiary nursing prevention intervention for retention, attainment, and maintenance of optimal client system wellness.

Concepts

- **Content:** The variables of the person in interaction with the internal and external environment comprise the whole client system
- **Basic structure/Central core:** Common client survival factors in unique individual characteristics representing basic system energy resources.
  The basic structure, or central core, is made up of the basic survival factors that are common to the species
- **These factors include:** Normal temperature range, genetic structure response pattern. Organ strength or weakness, Ego structure
  - Stability or homeostasis, occurs when the amount of energy that is available exceeds that being used by the system
  - A homeostatic body system is constantly in a dynamic process of input, output, feedback and compensation, which leads to a state of balance.
- **Degree to reaction:** The amount of system instability resulting from stressor invasion of the normal line of defense.
- **Entropy:** A process of energy depletion and disorganization moving the system toward illness or possible death.
- **Flexible line of defense:** A protective, accordion-like mechanism that surrounds and protects the normal line of defense from invasion by stressors.

- **Normal line of defense:** It represents what the client has become over time, or the usual state of wellness. It is considered dynamic because it can expand or contract over time.
- **Lines of resistance:** The series of concentric circles that surrounds the basic structure. Protection factors activated when stressors have penetrated the normal LOD, causing a reaction symptomatology, e.g., mobilization of WBC and activation of immune system mechanism
- **Input-output:** The matter, energy, and information exchanged between client and environment that is entering or leaving the system at any point in time.
- **Negentropy:** A process of energy conservation that increase organization and complexity, moving the system towards stability or a higher degree of wellness.
- **Open system:** A system in which there is continuous flow of input and process, output and feedback. It is a system of organized complexity where all elements are in interaction.
- **Prevention as intervention:** Interventions modes for nursing action and determinants for entry of both client and nurse into healthcare system.
- **Reconstitution:** The return and maintenance of system stability, following treatment for stressor reaction, which may result in a higher or lower level of wellness.
- **Stability:** A state of balance of harmony requiring energy exchanges as the client adequately copes with stressors to retain, attain or maintain an optimal level of health thus preserving system integrity.
- **Stressors:** Environment factors, intra- (emotion, feeling), inter- (role expectation), and extrapersonal (job or finance pressure) in nature that have potential for disrupting system stability.
  A stressor is any phenomenon that might penetrate both the flexible and normal line of defense, resulting in either a positive or negative outcome. Stressors can be intrapersonal, interpersonal and extrapersonal.
- **Wellness/Illness:** Wellness is the condition in which all system parts and subparts are in harmony with the whole system of the client.
  - Illness is a state of insufficiency with disrupting needs unsatisfied
  - Illness is an excessive expenditure of energy when more energy is used by the system in its state of disorganization than is built and stored, the outcome may be death.

Prevention

According to the Neuman's model, prevention is the primary nursing intervention. Prevention focuses on keeping stressors and the stress response from having a detrimental effect on the body.

Primary Prevention

- Primary prevention occurs before the system reaches a stressor. On one hand, it strengthens the person (primary the flexible line of defense) to enable him to better deal with stressors.
- On the other hand manipulates the environment to reduce or weaken stressors.
- Primary prevention includes health promotion and maintenance of wellness.

Secondary Prevention
- Secondary prevention occurs after the system reaches a stressor and is provided in terms of existing system.
- Secondary prevention focuses on prevention damage to the central core by strengthening the lines of resistance and/or removing the stressor.

Tertiary Prevention
- Tertiary prevention occurs after the system has been treated through secondary prevention states.
- Tertiary prevention offers support to the client and attempts to add energy to the system or reduce energy needed in order to facilitate reconstitution.

Four Major Concepts

Person
- The focus of the Neuman model is based on the philosophy that each human being is a total person as a client system and the person is a layer multidimensional being.
- Each layer consists of five-person variable subsystems:
    - *Physiological:* Refers to the physicochemical structure and function of the body
    - *Psychological:* Refers to mental processes and emotions
    - *Sociocultural:* Refers to relationship; and social/cultural expectations and activities
    - *Spiritual:* Refers to the influence of spiritual beliefs
    - *Developmental:* Refers to those processes related to development over the lifespan.

Environment
- Its environment is seen to be the totality of the internal and external forces which surround a person and with which they interact at any given time.
- These forces include the intrapersonal, interpersonal and extrapersonal stressors which can affect the person's normal line of defense and so can affect the stability of the system.
- The **internal environment** exists within the client system.
- The **external environment** exists outside the client system.
- Neuman also identified a created environment which is an environment that is created and developed unconsciously by the client and is symbolic of system wholeness.

Health
- Neuman sees health as being equated with wellness. She defines health/wellness as "the condition in which all parts and subparts (variables) are in harmony with the whole of the client".
- The client system moves toward illness and death when more energy is needed than is available. The client system moved toward wellness when more energy is available than is needed.

Nursing
- Neuman sees nursing as a unique profession that is concerned with all the variables which influence that response a person might have to a stressor.

- The person is seen as a whole, and it is the task of nursing to address the whole person.
- Neuman defines nursing as "action which assists individuals, families and group to maintain a maximum level of wellness, and the primary aim is stability of the patient/client system through nursing interventions to reduce stressors".
- Neuman states that, because the nurse's perception will influence the care given, then not only must the patient/client perception be assessed, but so must those of the caregiver (nurse).
- The role of the nurse is seen in terms of degree of reaction to stressors and the use of primary, secondary and tertiary interventions (Refer **Table 2.4** for application of Betty Neuman systems model in the nursing care).

Neuman's System Model Format (Fig. 2.2)

Neuman's nursing process format designates the following categories of data about the client system as the major areas of assessment.

Assessment

- Potential and actual stressors
- Condition and strength of basic structure factors and energy sources
- Characteristics of flexible and normal line of defenses, lines of resistance, degree of reaction and potential for reconstitution
- Interaction between client and environment
- Life process and coping factors (past, present and future) actual and potential stressors (internal and external) for optimal wellness external
- Perceptual difference between caregiver and the client.

Nursing Diagnosis

- The data collected are then interpreted to condition and formulate the nursing diagnosis
- Health seeking behaviors
- Activity intolerance
- Ineffective coping
- Ineffective thermoregulation.

Goal

In Neuman's systems model, the goal is to keep the client system stable.

Planning

Planning is focused on strengthening the lines of defense and resistance.

Implementation

The goal of stabilizing the client system is achieved through three modes of prevention:
1. **Primary prevention:** Actions taken to retain stability
2. **Secondary prevention:** Actions taken to attain stability
3. **Tertiary prevention:** Actions taken to maintain stability.

Table 2.4: Application of the Betty Neuman systems model in the nursing care of child with multiple sclerosis.

Example: 15 year old male child admitted with multiple sclerosis

Type of patient/client variable	Nursing diagnoses	Aim	Level of prevention	Interventions
Physi-ological	Not tolerating any activity associated with weakness, fatigue, and irritability	Helping the patient/client carry out activities without depending on others	Secondary	■ Avoiding exposure to environments with high temperatures, taking hot shower, eating heavy foods, too many activities, hunger and stress, which exacerbate fatigue ■ Exercise and sports, such as swimming and simple gestures, as much as tolerated ■ Reduction in ambient noise ■ Avoiding too much work, resting between work periods, and getting adequate sleep ■ Compliance with energy saving techniques, such as sitting while showering, and brushing teeth ■ Cold shower sucking ice, using ice packs or wet towel, when feeling hot.
Physi-ological	Eating disorder, eating less than what the body needs, anorexia and nausea	Improving the quality of the patient/client's appetite, nutrition, and proper diet	Secondary	■ Avoidance of irritant materials and odors ■ Resting before each meal to minimize weakness ■ Eating in a quiet and clean environment and devoting enough time to it ■ Eating frequent meals in small amounts ■ Gentle position-changing to avoid nausea ■ Avoiding fatty foods, like butter, sauces, and nuts ■ Avoiding fluid intake during food intake to prevent early satiety ■ Avoiding foods that contain caffeine, such as tea, coffee, and spicy food
Physi-ological	Risk of trauma and falls in association with visual and movement disorders, weakness and dizziness	Avoiding trauma, injury and controlling the situation during weakness and dizziness	Primary	■ Availability of necessary supplies and avoiding disorganization and chaos ■ Using appropriate shoes and slippers ■ Sufficient ambient light ■ Keeping calm and avoiding rush during work ■ Avoiding abrupt changes in a situation to avoid dizziness ■ Sitting during dizziness

Contd...

Application of Nursing Theories

Contd...

Type of patient/ client variable	Nursing diagnoses	Aim	Level of prevention	Interventions
Physiological	Disturbance in bowel habits associated with illness, weakness, and disability	Improving the patient/client's defecation pattern	Secondary	• Assigning regular hours for defecation, preferably an hour after meal • Encouraging to eat high-fiber foods such as bran, bread, fruits, and fresh herbs • Increasing fluid intake during the day • Activity as much as possible
Physiological	Disorders in sleep pattern, associated with an urge for urination, headache, and flushing	Improving the status and quality of sleep and rest	Secondary	• Reducing fluid intake in the evening to avoid waking up at night • Refraining from beverages containing caffeine • Creating a quiet and peaceful environment • Using cooling devices • Using proper cover
Physiological	Disorder in reading and writing associated with visual disturbances, and vertigo	Encouraging the patient/client to use the remaining abilities and prevent the progression of weakness and faintness	Secondary and tertiary	• Protecting eyes from sunlight • Emphasizing and encouraging the patient/client to regularly have a visual check-up • Resting the eyes and preventing eye fatigue • Avoiding exposure to severe light
Physiological	Impaired skin integrity in association with drugs, and associated complications	Maintaining tissue integrity	Secondary and tertiary	• Avoiding exposure to severe sunlight • Encouraging the use of protective clothing, such as hats, and gloves • Recommending the use of gloves when working with detergent • Recommending brushing hair gently and not using rough combs • Avoiding the use of chemical hair colors • Cold showers to stop itching

Contd...

Application of Nursing Theories

Contd...

Type of patient/client variable	Nursing diagnoses	Aim	Level of prevention	Interventions
Physi-ological	Urinary dysfunction, associated with the disease and bladder nerve damage	Improving the patient/client's defecation pattern	Secondary and tertiary	<ul><li>Avoiding beverages containing caffeine</li><li>Not limiting fluid intake due to damage to the kidneys</li><li>Reducing fluid intake after sunset</li><li>Pouring hot water on the perineal area to stimulate urination.</li><li>Encouraging to consume at least eight glasses of fluids during the day and reduce it before sunset</li><li>Encouraging good hygiene to prevent urinary tract infections.</li></ul>
Physi-ological	Disruption of the concept of self-associated with disease, decreased muscle strength, power, and weakness	<ul><li>Encouraging the patient/client to talk about beliefs and parameter, such as the concept of "self", power and self-efficacy</li><li>Helping the patient/client find incentives to continue with life and activities despite limitations of power and energy</li></ul>	Secondary and tertiary	<ul><li>Allowing the patient/client to express feelings, moods and behavior</li><li>Encouraging her to talk to other patient/clients with MS and participate in meetings conducted by the Centre for Special Diseases (MS)</li><li>Meeting children</li><li>Encouraging physical activity as much as muscle strength allowed</li></ul>
Physi-ological	Avoiding loneliness, associated with being away from children and family	Promoting patient/client's support and getting rid of loneliness	Secondary	<ul><li>Encouraging phone calls with siblings during their absence</li><li>Encouraging the patient/client to continue participating in religious activities, sports, and art classes</li><li>Encouraging the patient/client to interact and communicate with neighbors to get rid of loneliness</li></ul>

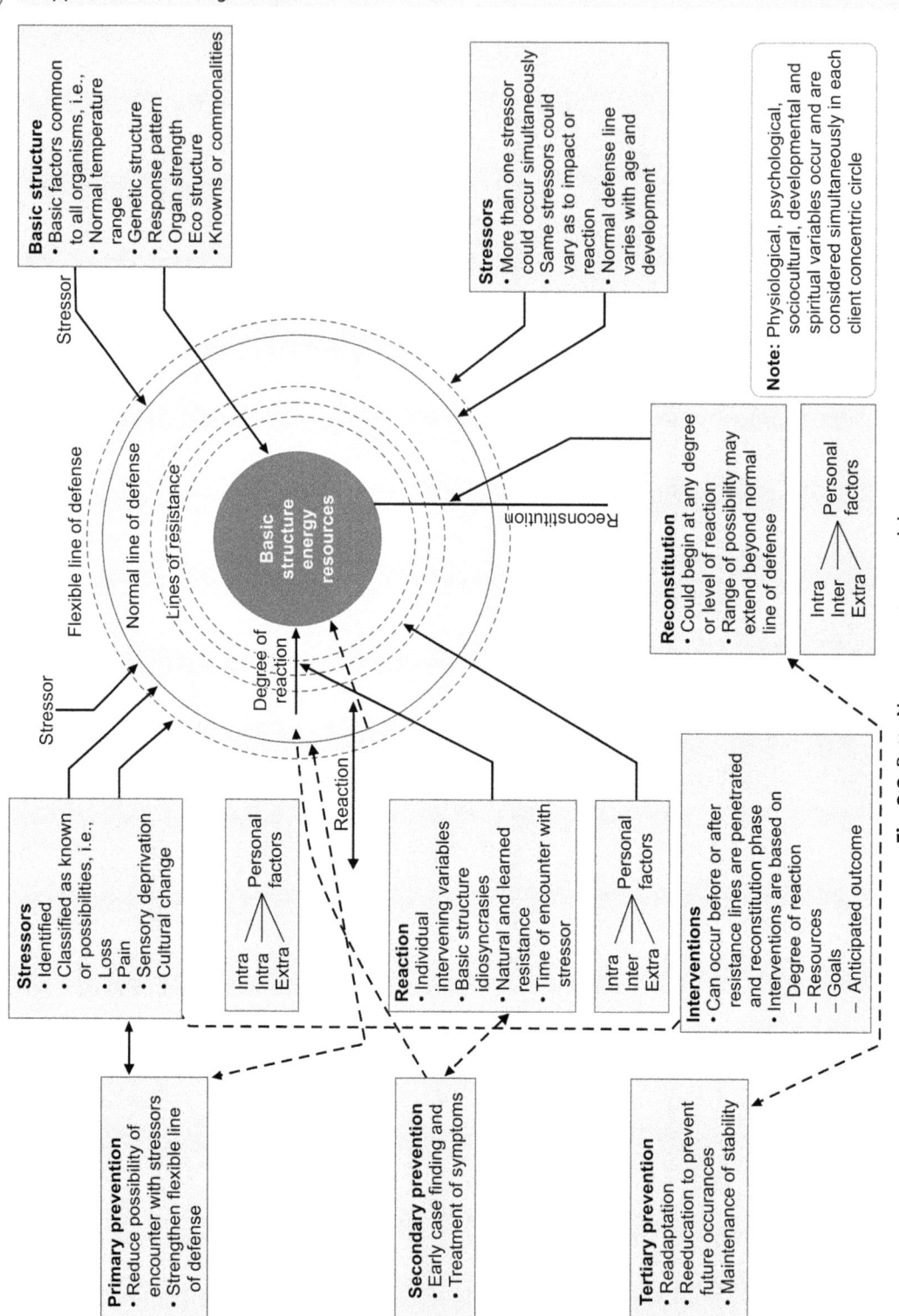

Fig. 2.2: Betty Neuman system model.

Evaluation

The nursing process is evaluated to determine whether equilibrium is restored and a steady state maintained.

PRACTICE QUESTIONS

1. Write the nursing process for a 5-year-old child with appendectomy by applying theory.
2. Write the nursing process for a 7-year-old child admitted with typhoid fever by applying theory.

CHAPTER 3

Nursing Care of Newborn and Family

LEARNING OBJECTIVES
- To observe the baby general condition including color, breathing, behavior, activity, posture and cry.
- To understand the delivery of care to the healthy newborn immediately after birth.
- To understand the importance of communicating with parents to convey information, provide support and counseling.

NURSING PROCESS FOR THE NEWBORN AND FAMILY

1. **Nursing diagnosis:** Ineffective airway clearance related to excess mucus, improper positioning.
   Goal: Patient will maintain a patent airway.
   Nursing interventions/rationales:
   - Suction mouth and nasopharynx with bulb syringe as needed, compress bulb before insertion and aspirate pharynx, then nose, to prevent aspiration of fluid mechanical suction, limit each suctioning attempt to 5 seconds with sufficient time between attempts to allow reoxygenation
   - Position infant on right side after feeding to prevent aspiration
   - Position infant supine or on side during sleep as recommended by American Academy of Pediatrics
   - Perform as few procedures as possible on infant during 1st hour and have oxygen ready for use if respiratory distress should develop
   - Take vital signs according to institutional policy and more frequently if necessary
   - Observe for signs of respiratory distress and report any of the following immediately:
     - Tachypnea
     - Grunting, stridor
     - Abnormal breath sounds flaring alae nasi
     - Cyanosis or pallor.
   - Keep diapers, clothing, and blankets loose enough to allow maximum lung (abdominal) expansion and to avoid overheating
   - Clean nares for any crusted secretions during bath or when necessary
   - Check for patent nares.

   Expected outcomes:
   - Airway remains patent
   - Breathing is regular and unlabored
   - Respiratory rate is within normal limits.

2. **Nursing diagnosis:** High risk for altered body temperature related to immature temperature control, change in environmental temperature.
   Goal: Will maintain a stable body temperature.

Nursing Care of Newborn and Family

Nursing interventions/rationales:
- Wrap infant snugly in a warmed blanket
- Place infant in a preheated environment (under radiant warmer or next to mother)
- Place infant on a padded, covered surface
- Take infant's temperature on arrival at nursery or mother's room; proceed according to hospital policy regarding method and frequency of monitoring
- Maintain room temperature between 24°C and 25.5°C (75° and 78°F) and humidity about 40–50%
- Give initial bath according to hospital policy:
  - Prevent chilling of infant during bath
  - Postpone bath if there is any question regarding stabilization of body temperature
  - Dress infant in a shirt and diaper and swaddle in a blanket or cover with blanket
  - Provide infant with a head covering if heat loss is a problem, since large surface area of head favors heat loss
  - Keep infant away from drafts, air conditioning vents, or fans
  - Place infant in a recessed cubicle with high-enough walls to shield from cross-ventilation
  - Warm all objects used to examine or cover infant (e.g., place them under radiant warmer)
  - Uncover only one area of body for examination or procedures
  - Postpone circumcision until after temperature stabilizes or use radiant warmer during procedure
  - Be alert to signs of hypothermia or hyperthermia.

Expected outcome: Infant's temperature remains at optimum level (36.5–37.5°C) (97.7–99.5°F)

3. **Nursing diagnosis:** High risk for infection or inflammation related to deficient immunologic defenses, environmental factors, maternal disease.
   Goal: Will exhibit no evidence of infection.
   Nursing interventions/rationale:
   - Wash hands before and after caring for each infant
   - Wear gloves when in contact with body secretions
   - Keep infant from potential sources of infection (e.g., persons with respiratory or skin infections, improperly prepared food sources, other unclean items)
   - Clean in posterior direction to prevent contamination of vagina or urethra; stress this to cleaning penis, do not retract foreskin.
   - Maintain asepsis during circumcision
   - If infant has been circumcised, cover area with a petrolatum jelly gauze (if ordered)
   - Check for voiding after circumcision; disposable diaper may feel dry when wet, but crotch area of diaper will feel 'clumpy' or 'doughy' and heavy. Keep umbilical stump clean and dry
   - Place diapers below umbilical stump
   - Assess cord daily for odor, color and drainage
   - Apply antibacterial agent and/or alcohol to cord as ordered
   - Administer HBV in vastus lateralis.

Expected outcomes:
- Infant exhibits no evidence of infection or inflammation
- Eyes remain clear with no evidence of irritation
- General area is free of irritation; appears dry, surrounding area free of infection; infant receives HBV vaccine.

4. **Nursing diagnosis:** High risk for trauma related to physical helplessness.
   Goal 1: Will be clearly and correctly identified.
   Nursing interventions/rationales:
   - Make certain infant is properly identified for placement with correct mother
   - Ensure that identification (ID) band (s) are properly and securely placed
   - Check infant's ID band often to ensure correct infant identify
   - Discuss safety issues with parents, especially mother, to present 'switching' of infants and possible kidnapping. Observe staff's ID badge and give infant only to properly identified personnel
   - Never leave infant alone in crib or room.

   Expected outcomes:
   - Infant is clearly and correctly identified
   - Observe safety practices and remains in place.

   Goal 2: Will have no physical injury.
   Nursing interventions/rationales:
   - Avoid using rectal thermometer because of risk of rectal perforations
   - Never leave infant unsupervised on a raised surface without rails; Nappies' close diaper pins (if used) and place them away from infant's body
   - Keep top pointed or sharp objects away from infant
   - Keep own fingernails short and trimmed; avoid jewelry that can scratch infant
   - Employ appropriate methods of handling and transporting infant.

   Expected outcome:
   Infant remains free of physical injury.

   Goal 3: Will exhibit no evidence of bleeding.
   Nursing interventions/rationales:
   Administer vitamin K intramuscularly, using vastus lateralis muscle as site of injection; check circumcision site; assess for any oozing that may indicate bleeding tendencies.
   Expected outcome: Infant exhibits no evidence of bleeding.

5. **Nursing diagnosis:** Altered nutrition, less than body requirements (high risk) related to immaturity, parental knowledge deficit.
   Goal: Will receive optimum nutrition.
   Nursing interventions/rationales:
   - Assess strength of suck and coordination with swallowing to identify possible problem affecting feeding. Offer initial intake according to parent's preference, hospital policy, and practitioner's protocol
   - Prepare for demand feeding of breastfed infants; night feedings determined by condition and preferences of mother; offer bottle-fed infants 2-3 ounces of formula every 3-4 hours or on demand
   - Support and assist breastfeeding mothers during initial feedings and more frequently, if necessary

- Avoid routine water or supplemental feedings for breastfeeding infants because they may decrease the desire to suck and cause nipple preference
- Encourage father or other support person to remain with mother to help her and infant with positioning, relaxation and reinforcement
- Encourage father or other support person to participate in bottle-feeding. Place infant on right side after feeding to prevent aspiration
- Observe stool pattern.

Expected outcomes:
- Infant demonstrates strong suck.
- Infant retains feedings.
- Infant receives an adequate amount of nutrients (specify amount and frequency of feedings).
- Infant loses <10% of birth weight.

6. **Nursing diagnosis:** Altered family processes related to maturational crisis, birth of term infant, change in family unit.
   Goal 1 (Family): Will exhibit parent-infant attachment behaviors.
   Nursing interventions/rationales:
   - As soon after delivery as possible encourage parents to see and hold infant, place newborn close to face of parents to establish physical contact.
   - Ideally, perform eye care after initial meeting of infant and parents, within 1 hour after birth when infant is alert and must likely to visually relate to parent.
   - Identify for parents specific behaviors manifested by infant (e.g., alertness, ability to see, vigorous suck, rooting behavior and attention to human voice).
   - Discuss with parents their expectations of fantasy child versus real child if indicated
   - Encourage parents to 'talk out' their labor and delivery experience; identify any events that signify loss of control to either parent, especially mother. Identify behavioral steps in attachment process and evaluate those aspects that could be considered positive and those that may represent inadequate or delayed parenting.
   - Encourage family to call for infant frequently if not rooming-in. Observe and assess reciprocity of cues between infant and parent to identify behaviors that may need strengthening.
   - Assist parents in recognizing attention, no attention cycles and in understanding their significance.
   - Assess variables affecting development of attachment through observing infant and parent, and interviewing each parent or other significant caregiver.

   Expected outcomes:
   - Parents establish contact with infant immediately or soon after birth.
   - Parents demonstrate attachment behaviors such as touch, eye contact, naming and calling infant by name, talking to infant, participating in care giving activities.
   - Parents recognize attention, no attention cycles.

   Goal 2: Will demonstrate adjustment/attachment behaviors toward newborn.
   Nursing interventions/rationales:
   - Allow to visit and touch newborns when feasible.
   - Explain physical differences in newborns, such as bald head, umbilical stump and clamp, circumcision, to lessen any fear siblings might have.

- Explain to siblings realistic expectations regarding newborn's abilities and needs requires complete care.
- Encourage siblings to participate in care at home to make them feel part of the experience.
- Encourage parents to spend individual time with other children at home to reduce feelings of jealousy toward new sibling.

Expected outcome: Siblings express interest in newborn and realistic expectations for their age.

Patient (Family) Goal 3: Will be prepared for discharge and home care.

Nursing interventions/rationales:
- Discuss with parents correct preparation of formula: Stress that proportions must not be altered to dilute or concentrate the formula.
- Discourage microwaving of bottles to avoid burns
- Instruct in other aspects of newborn care:
  - Bathing
  - Umbilical and circumcision care
- Recognize states of activity for optimum interaction. Advocate on immunization.
- Discuss the importance of IMNCI program.
- Advise for follow-up.

Expected outcomes:
- Family demonstrates the ability to provide care for infant.
- Family keeps appointments for follow-up care.
- Family members avail themselves of needed services.

PRACTICE QUESTION

1. Write nursing care plan for a newborn baby by applying nursing process.

CHAPTER 4

Nursing Care for an Infant

> **LEARNING OBJECTIVES**
> - To understand the age specific needs of the infant.
> - To establish nursing diagnosis based on the needs of the infant.
> - To plan the nursing interventions for an infant.
> - To evaluate the nursing interventions.

NURSING PROCESS FOR AN INFANT

1. **Nursing diagnosis:** Breastfeeding, ineffective, related to lack of exposure, misconceptions or knowledge deficit as evidenced by first baby, mother's verbalization, or nursing observations.
   Outcome identification and evaluation: Mother/infant both will experience successful breastfeeding; infant will latch on, suck and swallow at the breast; mother will not experience sore nipples.
   Interventions: Promoting effective breastfeeding.
   - Educate mother on recognition of and response to infant hunger cues to promote on-cue breastfeeding, which will establish milk supply
   - Educate mother on appropriate diet and fluid intake to ensure ability to manufacture adequate supply of breastmilk
   - Demonstrate breastfeeding position with infant at the breast (appropriate positioning increases probability of successful latch)
   - Assess infant's latch technique, sucking motion, and audible swallowing (an appropriately latch infant will take most of the areola in the mouth, suck in spurts, and demonstrate audible swallowing)
   - Assess infant voiding/stool patterns; at least six voids per day and passage of stool ranging from one or more day to one every several days is a normal pattern for breastfed infants
   - Assess infant weight gain; gain of 15–30 g per day after the second week of life indicates infant is receiving appropriate nutrition
   - Assess mother's nipples for redness or soreness; if infant appropriately leaches on nipples will not become sore.

2. **Nursing diagnosis:** Risk for altered growth pattern (risk factors: caregiver knowledge deficit, first infant, premature infant, maladaptive feeding behaviors).
   Outcome identification and evaluation: Infant will demonstrate adequate growth and appropriate feeding behaviors; steady increases in weight, length, and head circumference; infant feeds appropriately for age.
   Interventions: Promoting adequate growth.
   - Observe mother/infant dyad breastfeeding or bottle-feeding to determine need for further education or identify infant difficulties with feeding
   - Educate mother about appropriate breastfeeding or bottle-feeding, so that mother is aware of what to expect in normal feeding pattern

- When infant is old enough, provide education about addition of solid foods, spoon and cup feeding; after 6 months of age, breast milk or formula, needs to be supplemented with a variety of foods
- Determine need for additional caloric intake if necessary (premature infants and infants with chronic illnesses or metabolic disorders often need adjustments in caloric intake to demonstrate adequate or catch-up growth)
- Obtain daily weights (if hospitalized, weekly if outpatient) and weekly length and head circumference to determine whether feeding pattern is sufficient to promote adequate growth.

3. **Nursing diagnosis:** Nutrition, altered, less than body requirements, related to possible ineffective feeding pattern or inadequate caloric intake as evidenced by failure to gain weight or by inadequate increases in weight, length, and head circumference over time.
Outcome identification and evaluation: Infant will take adequate nutrients using effective feeding pattern; infant will demonstrate adequate weight gain (15–30 g per day) and steady increases in length and head circumference.
Intervention: Promoting adequate nutritional intake.
   - Assess current feeding pattern and daily intake to determine area of bottle-feeding if needed to meet caloric needs
   - Increase frequency of breastfeeding or volume of bottle feeding if needed to meet caloric needs
   - Introduce solid foods on age-appropriate schedule; introducing solids at the right time improves the chances will learn to take solid foods
   - Limit juice intake or discontinue altogether (juice has little value and displaces nutrients from breast milk or formula)
   - Use human milk fortifier (if order) to increase caloric density of breast milk
   - Increase caloric density of formula (if ordered), by mixing to a more concentrated level or with additive (facts or carbohydrates) to provide increased calories need to support adequate growth
   - If an infant is taking solids already, choose high-calorie foods to maximize nutrient intake.

4. **Nursing diagnosis:** Parent/infant attachment, altered, risk for (risk factors such as premature infant with difficult temperament or medical problems).
Outcome identification and evaluation: Parent and infant will demonstrate attachment via eye contact, parental response to infant cues, parental verbalization of caring for infant, infant response to parent's caretaking behaviors.
Interventions: Encouraging appropriate parent-infant attachment.
   - Assess parent's response to infant cues to determine of attachment and level of parent's knowledge about infant care
   - Assess infant's response to parent's caretaking behaviors to determine degree of attachment
   - Determine infant's temperament to counsel parent effectively about responses appropriate for that type of temperament
   - Encourage face positioning for holding or feeding the young infant to encourage give-and-take response between infant and parent
   - Encourage parent to meet infant's needs promptly and with affection to promote sense of trust in the infant

- Reinforce parent's attempts at improving attachment with infant (positive reinforcement naturally encourages appropriate behaviors).

5. **Nursing diagnosis:** Growth and development, altered, related to speech, motor, psychosocial or cognitive concerns as evidenced by delay in meeting expected milestones.
   Outcome identification and evaluation: Development will be maximized; infant will make continued. Progress toward attainment of development milestones.
   Interventions: Maximizing development.
   - Perform development evolution of the infant to determine infant's current level of functioning
   - Offer age-appropriate play, activates and toys to encourage further development
   - Carry out interventions as prescribed by developmental specialist, physical therapist, occupational therapist, or speech therapist (repeated exposure to the activities or exercises is needed to make developmental progress)
   - Provide support to parents of infants with developmental concerns, as developmental progress can be slow, and it is difficult for families to stay motivated and maintain hope.

6. **Nursing diagnosis:** Caregiver role stain, risk for (risk factors such as first baby, knowledge deficit about newborn care, lack of prior exposure, fatigue if premature, ill, or developmentally delayed infant).
   Outcome identification and evaluation: Parent will experience competence in role; will demonstrate appropriate caretaking behaviors and verbalize comfort in new role.
   Interventions: Preventing caregiver role stain.
   - Assess parent's knowledge of newborn/infant care and the issues that arise as a part of normal development to determine parent's needs
   - Provide education on normal newborn/infant care, so that parents have the knowledge they need to expect next and how to intervene
   - Encourage respite for parents (even a few hours away from the demands of an infant's care can rejuvenate the parents).

7. **Nursing diagnosis:** Injury, risk for (risk factors such as developmental age, infant curiosity, rapidly progressing motor abilities).
   Outcome identification and evaluation: Infant safety will be maintained; infant will remain free from injury.
   Interventions: Preventing injury.
   - Encourage car seat safety to decrease risk of injury related to motor vehicles
   - Child proof home—as infant becomes more mobile, he/she will want to explore everything, increasing risk of injury
   - Never leave an infant unattended in the sink, bathtub, or swimming pool to prevent drowning
   - Tech parents first aid measures and infant CPR to minimize consequences of injury should it occur
   - Parents should always watch the infant (no amount of childproofing can replace the watchful eye of a caring parent).

PRACTICE QUESTIONS

1. Write nursing care plan for a 4-month-old child by applying nursing process.
2. Write nursing care plan for a 9-month-old child by applying nursing process.

CHAPTER 5

Nursing Care for a Toddler

LEARNING OBJECTIVES

- To understand the age specific needs of the toddler.
- To establish nursing diagnosis based on the needs of the toddler.
- To plan the nursing interventions for a toddler.
- To evaluate the nursing interventions.

NURSING PROCESS FOR THE TODDLER

1. **Nursing diagnosis:** Risk for injury related to curiosity, increased mobility, and development immaturity.
   Outcome identification and evaluation: Toddler safety will be maintained; toddler will remain free from injury.
   Interventions: Preventing injury.
   - Teach and encourage appropriate use of forward-facing car seat to decrease risk of toddler injury related to motor vehicles
   - Teach toddlers to stay away from the street and to cross the street only when holding the hand of an adult, to prevent pedestrian injury
   - Require use of bicycle helmet for any wheeled toy to prevent head injury and form habit of helmet use
   - Child proof the home to provide a developmentally safe environment for the curious and increasingly mobile toddler
   - Postpoison control center phone number in case of accidental ingestion
   - Never leave a toddler unattended in a tub or pool or near any water body to prevent drowning
   - Teach parents first-aid measures and child cardiopulmonary resuscitation (CPR) to minimize consequences of injury which it occur
   - Provide close observation and keep side rails up on crib/bed in hospital because toddlers are at particularly high risk for falling or becoming entangled in tubing as they attempt mobility.

2. **Nursing diagnosis:** Imbalanced nutrition less than body requirements, related to inappropriate nutritional intake to sustain growth needs (excess juice or milk intake, inadequate food variety intake) as evidenced by failure to attain adequate increases in height and weight over time.
   Outcome identification and evaluation: Toddler will consume adequate nutrients while using an appropriate feeding pattern; toddler will demonstrate weight gain and increases in height.
   Interventions: Promoting appropriate nutrition.
   - Assess current feeding schedule and usual intake, as well as methods used to feed, to determine area of adequacy versus inadequacy

Nursing Care for a Toddler

- Determine toddler's ability to drink from cup, finger feed, swallow and consume textures to determine if additional exposure is needed or if further interventions such as speech or occupation therapy are required
- Weigh toddler daily on same scale if hospitalized, weekly on same scale if at home and plot growth patterns weekly or monthly as appropriate on standardized growth charts to determine if growth is improving
- Wean from bottle by 15 months of age to discourage excess milk or juice intake in toddler, who can carry bottle around
- Limit juice intake 60 to 110 mL per day and milk 110 mL per day, thereby increasing appetite for solid foods
- Provide three nutrient-dense meals and at least two healthy snacks per day to encourage adequate nutrient consumption
- Feed toddler on a similar schedule daily, without distractions and with the family. Toddlers respond well to routine and structure; and may eat better in the social context of meals, and they become distracted easily (television should be off).

3. **Nursing diagnosis:** Delayed growth and development related to motor, cognitive, language, of psychosocial concerns as evidenced by delay in meeting expected milestones.
   Outcome identification and evaluation: Development will be enhanced; toddler will make continued progress toward realization of expected developmental milestones.
   Interventions: Enhancing growth and development.
   - Screen for developmental capability to determine toddler's current level of functioning
   - Offer age-appropriate toy, play, activities (including gross motor) to encourage further developmental delay (process in achieving developmental milestones can be slow and ongoing motivation)
   - Reinforce positive attributes in the toddler to maintain motivation
   - Model age-appropriate communication skills to illustrate suitable means for parenting the toddler.

4. **Nursing diagnosis:** Risk for disproportionate growth related to excess milk or juice intake, late bottle weaning and consumption of inappropriate foods or in excess amounts.
   Outcome identification and evaluation: Toddler will grow appropriately and not become overweight or obese; toddler will achieve weight and height within the 5th to 85th percentiles on standardized growth charts.
   Interventions: Promoting proportionate growth.
   - Wean from bottle and discourage use of no spill sippy cups by 15 months of age (will keep mobile toddler from carrying around and continually drinking from cup or bottle)
   - Provide juice (4-6 ounces/day) and milk (16-24 ounces/day) from a cup drinking and limit intake of nutrient-poor, high-calorie fluids
   - Provide only nutrient-rich foods without high sugar content for meals and snacks; even if the toddler will not eat, it is inappropriate to provide high-calorie junk food just, so the toddler eats something. Ensure adequate physical activity to stimulate development of motor skills and provide appropriate caloric expenditure. This also set the stage for forming life-long habits of appropriate physical activity.

5. **Nursing diagnosis:** Interrupted family processes related to issues with toddler development, hospitalization or situational crisis as evidenced by decreased parental visitation in

hospital, parental verbalization of difficulty with current situation, possible. Crisis related to the health of family member other than the toddler.

Outcome identification and evaluation: Family will demonstrate adequate functioning; family will display coping and psychosocial adjustment.

Interventions: Enhancing family functioning.
- Assess the family's level of stress and ability to cope to determine family's ability to cope with multiple stressors
- Engage in family-centered care to provide a holistic approach to care of the toddler and family
- Encourage the family to verbalize feelings (verbalization is one method of decreasing anxiety level) and acknowledge feelings and emotions
- Encourage family visitation and provide for sleeping arrangements for a parent or caregiver to stay in the hospital with the toddler (contributes to family's sense of control of situation)
- Involve family members in toddler's care, giving them a felling of control and connectedness.

6. **Nursing diagnosis:** Readiness for enhanced parenting related to parental desire for increased skills and success with toddler as evidenced by current healthy relationships and verbalization of desire for improved skills.

Outcome identification and evaluation: Parent will provide safe and nurturing environment for the toddler.

Interventions: Increasing parenting skill set.
- Use family-centered care to provide holistic approach
- Educate parent about normal toddler development to provide basis for understanding the parenting skills needed in this time period
- Acknowledge and encourage parent's behavior to validate the normalcy of the parent's feeling
- Encourage positive parenting with respect to toddler and their development (helps parents develop approaches to toddler that can be used in place of anger and frustration)
- Acknowledge and admire positive parenting skills already present to confidence in their abilities to parent
- Role model appropriate parenting behaviors related to communicating with and disciplining the toddler (role modeling actually shows rather than just telling the parent what to do).

PRACTICE QUESTIONS

1. Write nursing care plan of a 2-year-old child by applying nursing process.
2. Write nursing care plan of a 3-year-old child by applying nursing process.

CHAPTER 6

Nursing Care for a Preschool Child

LEARNING OBJECTIVES
- To understand the age specific needs of the preschool child.
- To establish nursing diagnosis based on the needs of the preschool child.
- To plan the nursing interventions for a preschool child.
- To evaluate the nursing interventions.

NURSING PROCESS FOR A PRESCHOOL CHILD

1. **Nursing diagnosis:** Risk for injury related to developmental age, environment, and motor vehicle travel.
   Interventions: Preventing injury.
   - Teach preschoolers to stay away from street and to cross the street only when holding the hand of an adult, to prevent pedestrian injury
   - Require use of bicycle helmet, use while riding any wheeled toy to prevent head injury and form habit of helmet use
   - Teach the preschooler appropriate safety rules in the home (avoiding electric outlets, etc.); the preschooler is able to follow simple directions and carry out directives; limits help him/her to organize the environment
   - Never leave a preschool child unattended in a tub or pool or near any water body to prevent drowning
   - Provide swimming lessons of children aged 4–5 to encourage water safety, but not as a replacement for adult supervision
   - Teach parents first-aid measures and child CPR to minimize consequence of injury which it occur
   - Provide close observation and keep side rails up on bed in hospital because the preschool child continues to be at risk for falling or injuring self on equipment of tubing (because of curiosity).

   Outcome identification and evaluation: Child's safety will be maintained; child will remain free from injury.

2. **Nursing diagnosis:** Imbalanced nutrition less than body requirements, related to inappropriate nutritional intake to sustain growth needs (excess juice or milk intake, inadequate food variety intake) as evidenced by failure to attain adequate increases in height and weight over time.
   Interventions: Promoting appropriate nutrition.
   - Assess current feeding schedule and usual intake as well as methods used to feed, to determine areas of adequacy versus inadequacy
   - Determine if the preschooler is unable to drink from a cup or does not finger feed or use utensils properly, or if the child has difficulty swallowing or tolerating certain textures

of foods to determine, if further interventions such as speech or occupational therapy are required
- Weigh child daily on same scale if hospitalized, weekly on same scale if at home and plot growth patterns weekly or monthly as appropriate on standardized growth charts to determine if growth is improving
- Limit juice to 4-6 ounces per day, milk to 16-24 ounces/day, to discourage sense of fullness achieved with excess milk or juice intake, thereby increasing appetite for appropriate solid foods
- Provide three nutrient-dense meals and at least two healthy snacks per day to encourage adequate nutrient consumption
- Feed the child on a similar schedule daily, without distractions and with the family; preschool children continue to respond well to routine and structure. They are more interested in the social context of meals and are still apt to become distracted easily, so the television should be off at mealtimes.

Outcome identification and evaluation: Child will consume adequate nutrients; child will demonstrate weight gain and increases in height.

3. **Nursing diagnosis:** Delayed growth and development related to motor, cognitive, language or psychosocial concerns as evidenced by delay in meeting expected milestones.
   Interventions: Enhancing growth and development
   - Screen for developmental capabilities to determine child's current level of functioning
   - Offer age-appropriate toys, play and activities (including grass motor) to encourage further development
   - Perform interventions as prescribed by physical, occupational or speech therapist; participation in those activities helps to promote function and accomplish acquisition of developmental skills
   - Provide support to families of preschoolers with developmental delay (progress in achieving developmental milestones can be slow and ongoing motivation is needed)
   - Reinforce positive attributes in the child to maintain motivation
   - Model age-appropriate communication skills to illustrate suitable means for parenting the preschooler.

   Outcome identification and evaluation: Development will be enhanced; child will make continued progress toward realization of expected developmental milestones.

4. **Nursing diagnosis:** Risk for disproportionate growth related to excess milk or juice intake, consumption of inappropriate foods or in excess amounts.
   Interventions:
   - Discourage use of no-spill sippy cups (they contribute to dental caries and allow unlimited access to fluids, possibly decreasing appetite for appropriate solid foods)
   - Limit the juice to 60-110 mL per day and milk 110 mL per day. Encourage appropriate cup drinking and limit intake of nutrient-poor, high-calorie fluids
   - Provide only nutrient-rich foods without high sugar content for meals and snacks; even if the preschooler is a picky eater, it is inappropriate to provide high-calorie junk food, just so the child eats something
   - Teach parents to role model appropriate eating (nutrient-rich, varied diet) to encourage child to try/accept new foods as well as become familiar with a variety of food

- Severely limit the intake of fast foods and foods with high sugar and fat content to decrease intake of nutrient-poor, high calorie foods.
- Ensure adequate physical activity to stimulate development of motor skills and provide appropriate caloric expenditure; this also sets the stage for forming life-long habit of appropriate physical activity
- Teach parents to limit television viewing to 1–2 hours per day to encourage participation in physical activities.

Outcome identification and evaluation: Child will grow appropriately and not become overweight or obese; child will achieve weight and height within the 5th–85th percentiles on standardized growth charts.

5. **Nursing diagnosis:** Interrupted family processes related to issues with preschool child's development, hospitalization or situational crisis as evidenced by decreased parental visitation in hospital, parental verbalization of difficulty with current situation, possible crisis related to health of family members other than the preschool child.
   Interventions: Enhancing family functioning.
   - Assess the family's level of stress and ability to cope to determine family's ability to cope with multiple stressors
   - Engage in family-centered care to provide a holistic approach to care of the preschooler and family
   - Encourage the family to verbalize feelings (verbalization is one method of decreasing anxiety levels and acknowledge feelings and emotions
   - Use puppets or dramatic play with the child to elicit the preschooler's feelings about the current situation
   - Encourage family visitation and provide for sleeping arrangements for a parent or caregiver to stay in the hospital with the preschooler; this contributes to family's sense of control in situation
   - Involve family members in preschooler's care, giving them a feeling of control and connectedness.

   Outcome identification and evaluation: Family will demonstrate adequate functioning; family will display coping and psychosocial adjustment.

6. **Nursing diagnosis:** Readiness for enhanced parenting related to parental desire for increased skill level and success with preschool child as evidenced by current healthy relationships and verbalization of desire for improved skills.
   Interventions: Increasing parenting skill set.
   - Use family-centered care to provide holistic approach
   - Educate parent about normal preschool development to provide basis of understanding for parenting skills needed in this time period
   - Acknowledge and encourage parents' verbalization of feelings related to chronic illness of child of difficulty with normal preschool behavior; this validates the normalcy of parents' feelings
   - Encourage positive parenting and respect for preschooler and his/her normal development (helps parents develop approaches to preschoolers that can be used in place of anger and frustration)
   - Acknowledge and admire positive parenting skills already present to contribute to parents' confidence in their abilities to parent

- Role model appropriate parenting behaviors related to communicating with and disciplining the child (role modeling actually demonstrates rather than just verbalizes what the parent should strive for).

Outcome identification and evaluation: Parent will provide safe and nurturing environment for the preschool child; parents will verbalize new skills they will employ in the family.

PRACTICE QUESTIONS

1. Write nursing care plan for a 4-year-child by applying nursing process.
2. Write nursing care plan for a 5-year-child by applying nursing process.

CHAPTER 7

Nursing Care for School-Age Child

LEARNING OBJECTIVES
- To understand the age specific needs of the school-age child.
- To establish nursing diagnosis based on the needs of the school-age child.
- To plan the nursing interventions for a school-age child.
- To evaluate the nursing interventions

NURSING PROCESS FOR THE SCHOOL-AGE CHILD

1. **Nursing diagnosis:** Risk for disproportionate growth factors; caregiver knowledge deficit, frequent illnesses.
   Interventions: Promoting proportionate growth.
   - Assess parent's knowledge of nutritional needs of school-age children to determine need for further education
   - Educate mother about appropriate serving sizes and foods, so that mother is aware of what to expect for school-age children
   - Determine need for additional caloric intake if necessary (if very active in sports, if have a chronic illness)
   - Platout height, weight and body mass index (BMI) to detect possible pattern.

   Outcome identification and evaluation: School-age child will demonstrate adequate growth, appropriate weight gain for age and gender.

2. **Nursing diagnosis:** Imbalanced nutrition, more than body requirements related to lack of exercise, increased caloric intake, poor food choices.
   Interventions: Promoting nutrition.
   - Assess knowledge of parents and child about nutritional needs of school-age children to determine deficits in knowledge
   - Keep diary for child have food and exercise for 1 week to determine current patterns of eating and exercises
   - Interview parents in relationship to their eating habits and exercise habits to determine where adjustments might need to be made
   - Analyze preceding date and base recommendations for changes on these data
   - Discuss ways to decrease temptation to overeat and to make good meal choices, have child assist in meal planning and grocery shopping to allow child some sense of control in process
   - Incorporate increase in daily exercise, which will stress sense of self-improvement to increase caloric expenditure and self-esteem
   - Decrease TV/computer time to increase caloric expenditure
   - Develop reward system to increase self-esteem

- Investigate joining weight-loss program for school-age children, to increase self-esteem and to increase awareness that other children have the same problem.

  Outcome identification and evaluation: School-age child will lose weight at an appropriate rate; increase amount of exercise, make appropriate eating choices, decrease caloric intake to appropriate amount for age and gender.

3. **Nursing diagnosis:** Growth and development, delayed related to speech, motor, psychosocial or cognitive concerns as evidenced by delay in meeting expected school performances.

   Interventions: Promoting growth and development.
   - Perform scheduled evaluation of the school-age child by school and healthcare provider to determine current functioning
   - Develop realistic multidisciplinary plan to ensure maximizing resources
   - Carry out interventions as prescribed by developmental specialist, physical therapist, occupational therapist, or speech therapist at home and at school to maximize benefit of interventions
   - Have scheduled evaluation meetings to be able to adapt interventions as soon as possible.

   Outcome identification and evaluation: Development will be maximized; school-age child will make continued progress toward attainment of expected school performances.

4. **Nursing diagnosis:** Caregiver role strain, risk for (risk factors, new sibling in household, knowledge deficit about school-age issues, lack of prior exposure, fatigue, ill or developmentally delayed child).

   Interventions: Preventing caregiver role strain.
   - Assess parent's knowledge of school-age children and the issues that arise as a part of normal development to determine parent's needs
   - Provide education on normal issues of school-age children, so that parents are armed with the knowledge they need appropriately to care for their school-age child
   - Provide anticipatory guidance related to upcoming expected issues related to school-age development to prepare parents for, what to expect next and how to intervene.

   Outcome identification and evaluation: Parent will experience competence in role will demonstrate appropriate caretaking behaviors and verbalize comfort in caring for a school-age child.

5. **Nursing diagnosis:** Injury, risk for (risk factors; curiosity, increasing cognitive skills and motor abilities).

   Interventions: Preventing injury.
   - Discuss safety measures needed for the following—bikes, scooters, guns, skateboards, cars, water and playground to decrease risk of injury related to those areas. Discuss and develop a fire safety plan to decrease risk of injury related to fire
   - Discuss appropriate safety equipment needed for each sport to decrease risk of injury
   - Discuss appropriate sports to participate in depending upon age, sex and maturity of child to prevent possible injury and to promote child's self-esteem
   - Teach parents and child first-aid measures and child CPR to minimize consequences of injury, which it occur.

- Discuss influence of peers on actions of school-age children to prevent possible injury due to mimicking behavior.

Outcome identification and evaluation: School-age child's safety will be maintained, will remain free from injury.

PRACTICE QUESTIONS

1. Write nursing care plan for a 7-year-old child by applying nursing process.
2. Write nursing care plan for a 9-year-old child by applying nursing process.
3. Write nursing care plan for a 10-year-old child by applying nursing process.

CHAPTER 8

Nursing Care for an Adolescent Child

LEARNING OBJECTIVES
- To understand the age specific needs of an adolescent.
- To establish nursing diagnosis based on the needs of an adolescent.
- To plan the nursing interventions for an adolescent.
- To evaluate the nursing interventions.

NURSING PROCESS FOR AN ADOLESCENT CHILD

1. **Nursing diagnosis:** Risk for disproportionate growth (risk factors; caregiver and adolescent knowledge deficit, low self-esteem, frequent illnesses).
   Interventions: Promoting appropriate physical growth.
   - Assess parents' and adolescent's knowledge of nutritional needs of adolescents to determine need for further education
   - Educate parents and adolescent about appropriate serving sizes and foods, so that they are aware of what to expect for adolescents
   - Determine need for additional caloric intake if necessary (if very active in sports, if have a chronic illness)
   - Platout height, weight and body mass index (BMI) to detect possible pattern
   - Assess for risk factors for developing eating disorder to refer to if needed and plan interventions.

   Outcome identification and evaluation: Adolescent will demonstrate adequate growth; appropriate weight gain for age and sex.

2. **Nursing diagnosis:** Nutrition more than body requirements, imbalance, related to lack of exercise, increased caloric intake, poor food choices and stresses of adolescence.
   Interventions: Promoting appropriate nutrition.
   - Assess knowledge of parents and adolescent about nutritional needs of teenagers to determine deficits in knowledge
   - Keep a detailed food and exercise diary for 1 week to determine current patterns of eating and exercise of adolescent
   - Interview family in relationship to their eating habits and exercise habits to determine where adjustments might need to be made
   - Discuss changes in a positive manner, talk about developing healthy eating habits instead of dieting to promote compliance
   - Analyze preceding data and base recommendations for changes in these data to promote compliance and to prioritize recommendations
   - Discuss ways to decrease temptation to overeat, for example, eat slowly, put down the fork between bites, serve food in smaller plates, and count mouthfuls to allow time to realize that you are full

- Create meal plans and grocery shop to allow him or her some sense of control and decision making
- Incorporate increase in daily exercise, which will stress sense of self-improvement to increase caloric expenditure and self-esteem
- Decrease TV/computer time to increase caloric expenditure
- Encourage peer exercise activities to increase peer interactions and to realize that others are like him/her
- Develop reward system to increase self-esteem
- Investigate joining weight loss program for adolescents to increase self-esteem and to increase awareness that other adolescents have the same problem.

Outcome identification and evaluation: Adolescent will lose weight at an appropriate rate; increase amount of exercise, make appropriate eating choices, decrease caloric intake to appropriate amount for age and sex.

3. **Nursing diagnosis:** Growth and development, delayed, related to speech, motor, psychosocial or cognitive concerns as evidenced by delay in meeting expected school performances.

   Interventions: Promoting growth and development.
   - Perform scheduled evaluation of the adolescent by school and healthcare provider to determine current functioning
   - Develop realistic multidisciplinary plan to ensure maximizing resources
   - Carry out interventions as prescribed by developmental specialist, physical therapist, occupational therapist or speech therapist of home and at school to maximize benefit of interventions
   - Have scheduled evaluation meetings to be able to adapt interventions as soon as possible.

   Outcome identification and evaluation: Development will be maximized; adolescent will make continued progress toward attainment of expected school performance.

4. **Nursing diagnosis:** Caregiver role strain, risk factors—knowledge deficit about adolescent issues, lack of prior exposure, fatigue, ill or developmentally delayed child.

   Interventions: Preventing caregiver role strain.
   - Assess parent's knowledge of adolescents and the issues that arise as a part of normal development to determine parent's needs
   - Provide education on normal issues of adolescence, so that parents are armed with the knowledge they need to appropriately care for their adolescents
   - Provide anticipatory guidance related to upcoming expected issues related to adolescent development to prepare parents for what to expect next and how to intervene in an appropriate manner.

   Outcome identification and evaluation: Parent will experience competence in role; will demonstrate appropriate caretaking behaviors and verbalize comfort in caring for an adolescent.

5. **Nursing diagnosis:** Injury, risk factors—increased motor and cognitive skills and feeling of invincibility.

   Interventions: Preventing injury.
   - Discuss safety measures needed for the following: Bikes, scooters, guns, skateboards, cars and water to decrease risk of injury related to those areas

- Discuss and develop a fire safety plan to decrease risk of injury related to fire
- Discuss appropriate safety equipment needed for each sport to decrease risk of injury
- Discuss appropriate sports to participate in depending upon age, gender, sex and maturity of adolescent to prevent possible injury
- Teach parents and adolescent first-aid measures and CPR to minimize consequences of injury that it occur
- Discuss influence of peers upon actions of adolescents to prevent possible injury due to mimicking behavior.

Outcome identification and evaluation: Adolescent's safety will be maintained; will remain free from injury.

6. **Nursing diagnosis:** Coping, ineffective, for coping with normal stress of adolescence (risk factors: low self-esteem, poor relationship with parents and peers, participating in risk-taking behaviors).

    Interventions: Promoting effective coping. Assess adolescent's knowledge of normal stress facing teenagers to determine current knowledge
    - Assess adolescent's present coping skills to determine areas for improvement/support
    - Encourage parents to accept teenager as a unique individual
    - Discuss with parents and adolescent normal developmental issues facing teens to give them knowledge needed to cope
    - Provide different situations the teen might be faced with and different solutions
    - Develop with adolescent different solutions to problems
    - Allow for increasing independence and opportunities to solve own problems
    - Encourage development of friends with same values
    - Parents provide unconditional love
    - Assess for any evidence of any risk-taking behaviors (drugs, smoking and suicide).

    Outcome identification and evaluation: Adolescent will demonstrate adequate coping abilities as evident by management of stress of adolescence and no evidence of participating in risk-taking behaviors.

PRACTICE QUESTIONS

1. Write nursing care plan for a 13-years-adolescent boy by applying nursing process.
2. Write nursing care plan for a 15-years-adolescent girl by applying nursing process.

CHAPTER 9

Nursing Process for a Hospitalized Child

LEARNING OBJECTIVES
- To increase the ability to perform self-care activities.
- To relieve anxiety.
- To increase sense of family power, family in making decisions.
- To prevent injuries.
- To develop social, emotional and behavioral skills of children by applying therapeutic play.

INTRODUCTION

Hospitalization of the ill child, whether it involves repeated hospitalizations for a chronic illness or a life-threatening illness or episode, creates a crisis for the child, parents, and family members. Responses to hospitalization are related to the age of the child but generally include fear of separation, loss of control, injury, and pain. The ease of transition from home to the hospital depends on how well the child has been prepared for it and how the child's physical and emotional needs have been met **(Flowchart 9.1)**. Supporting the parents and family, providing them with information, and encouraging their participation in the child's care contributes to the adjustment and well-being of all concerned.

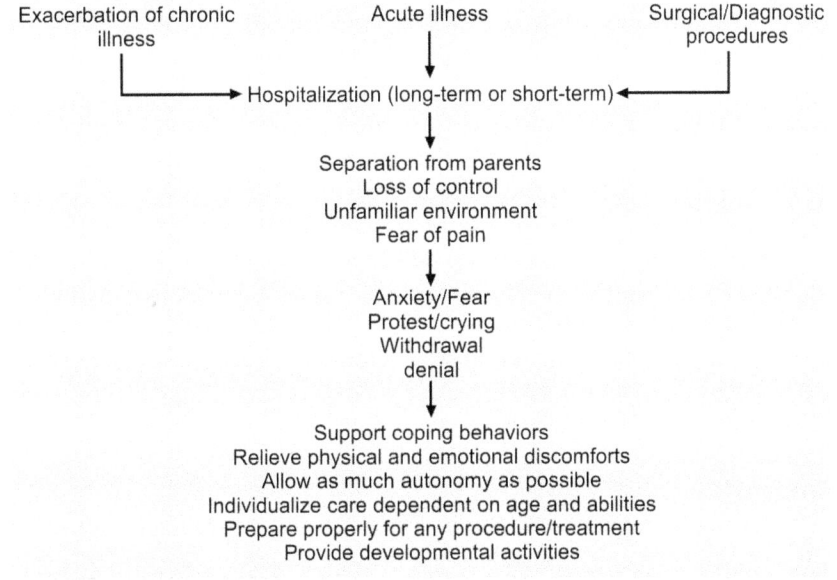

Flowchart 9.1: Consequences of hospitalization and their early preparation.

NURSING PROCESS FOR A HOSPITALIZED CHILD

1. **Nursing diagnosis:** Anxiety related to hospital situation, fear of injury or bodily mutilation, separation from family or friends, changes in routine, painful procedures and treatments, and unfamiliar events and surroundings as evidenced by crying, fussing, withdrawal or resistance.
   Goal: Minimizing anxiety.
   Interventions:
   - Orient child and family to the unit, and the child's room to familiarize them with the facility
   - Place the child in a room with another child of a similar age, developmental level and condition severity to promote sharing
   - Explain all events, treatments, procedures and activities to the parents and child (at level the child understands) in a calm, relaxed manner to help them prepare for, what is to come and decrease fear of the unknown; a calm, relaxed manner helps to establish rapport and instill trust
   - Encourage parents to room in if possible to provide the child support if parents cannot stay, encourage them to call to reduce child's fear of being alone
   - Urge parents to inform the child when they will be leaving and when they are expected to return to help child cope with their absence and promote trust
   - Assess child's usual routine at home and attempt to incorporate aspects of usual routine into hospital routine to ease the transition to the hospital and promote child participation in routine
   - Offer comfort measures such as holding, stroking and rocking to relieve distress
   - Provide a traumatic care to minimize exposure to distress, which would increase anxiety
   - Encourage the child's participation in play (unstructured and therapeutic play as necessary) to allow for expression of feelings and fears, and promote energy expenditure
   - Suggest that parents bring in a special toy or object from home to promote feelings of security
   - Provide positive reinforcement for participation in care activities to foster self-esteem
   - Assess for regression behaviors and inform parents that such behaviors are common to help alleviate their concerns about this behavior
   - Provide consistency with care measures to facilitate trust and acceptance.

   Outcome identification and evaluation: Child and family will exhibit a decrease in anxiety levels evidenced by positive coping strategies, verbalization or playing out of feelings, appropriate behaviors, positive interactions with staff, child and parent cooperation and participation, and absence of signs and symptoms of increasing anxiety and fear.

2. **Nursing diagnosis:** Risk for powerlessness related to lack of control over procedures, treatments and care, and changes in usual routine.
   Goal: Promoting control.
   Interventions:
   - Encourage child and parents to identify areas of concern to help in determining priority needs
   - Encourage parent and child to participate in care activities to promote feelings of control

- Incorporate aspects of child's routine at home and use terms similar to those used at home to foster a sense of normalcy
- Offer child choices as much as possible, such as options for foods, drinks, hygiene, activities, or clothing (if appropriate) to promote feelings of individuality and control
- Allow child opportunities for being out of bed or room within limitations as appropriate to foster independence
- Work with child, as age and development allow, and family to set up a schedule to promote structure and routine.

Outcome identification and evaluation: Child and family will demonstrate an increase in control over the situation as evidenced by participation in care activities, identification of needs and choices and incorporation of appropriate aspects of child's usual routine with that of the hospital.

3. **Nursing diagnosis:** Deficient diversional activity related to confinement in bed or healthcare facility, limited mobility, activity restrictions or equipment as evidenced by verbalization of boredom, lack of participation in play, readings or schoolwork.
   Goal: Promoting adequate diversional activities.
   Interventions:
   - Question child and family about favorite types of activities to establish a baseline for developing appropriate choices during hospitalization
   - Assist with planning activities within the limits of the child's condition to maintain muscle tone and strength without overexerting the child
   - Spend time with the child to provide stimulation and foster trust
   - Enlist the aid of a child life specialist to provide suggestions for appropriate activities
   - Encourage interaction with other children to promote sharing and avoid loneliness
   - Provide developmentally appropriate opportunities for unstructured and therapeutic play to facilitate expression of feelings
   - Encourage short trips to the playroom or activity room to provide a change of scenery and sensory stimulation.
   - Integrate play activities with nursing care to achieve therapeutic effect.

   Outcome identification and evaluation: Child will participate in diversional activities as evidenced by engagement in unstructured and therapeutic play that is developmentally appropriate, and interaction with family, staff, and other children.

4. **Nursing diagnosis:** Interrupted family processes related to separation from child due to hospitalization, increased demands of caring for an ill child, changes in role function and effect of hospitalization on other family members such as siblings as evidenced by parental verbalization of issues, parental presence in hospital or child's hospitalization requiring parent to miss work.
   Goal: Maximizing family functioning.
   Interventions:
   - Encourage parents and family members to verbalize concerns related to child's illness, diagnosis and prognosis to promote family-centered care and identify areas where intervention may be needed

- Explain therapies, procedures, child's behaviors and plan of care to parents to promote understanding of the child's status and plan of care, which helps to decrease anxiety
- Encourage parental involvement in care to promote feelings of the parents being needed and valued, providing them with a sense of control over their child's health
- Identity support system for family and child to help identify resources available for coping
- Educate family and child on additional resources available to promote a wider base of support to deal with the situation
- Suggest ways that parents can divide time between child and other siblings to prevent feelings of guilt
- Provide support and positive reinforcement to promote family coping and foster family strength
- Encourage frequent visits by family members including siblings as appropriate, to promote ongoing family functioning
- Stress the need for adequate rest, sleep, exercise, and nutrition for family members to promote family health and minimize stress of hospitalization on family
- Assist with referrals for resources and help from additional family members and friends as necessary to allow for respite or relief of care responsibilities
- Encourage family to maintain usual routine as much as possible to minimize the effects of hospitalization on family functioning.

Outcome identification and evaluation: Family will demonstrate positive coping strategies as evidenced by visiting frequently and staying with the child as necessary, sharing of family responsibilities, obtaining assistance for relief or respite, and visiting by other members of the child's family and friends.

5. **Nursing diagnosis:** Self-care deficit related to immobility, activity restrictions, regression, use of equipment, devices or prescribed treatments as evidenced by inability to feed, bath or dress self or accomplish other activities of daily living.
   Goal: Promoting self-care.
   Interventions:
   - Assess child's usual routine for self-care and self-care abilities to provide a baseline for individualizing interventions
   - Provide child-sized equipment and devices to promote child's ability to complete the self-care task
   - Encourage parents and child to do as much self-care as possible, within limitations of the child's condition and developmental level, to promote feelings of independence and foster growth and development
   - Offer praise and encouragement for activities performed to foster self-esteem, confidence and competence
   - Ensure adequate rest periods to minimize energy expenditure associated with self-care activities.

   Outcome identification and evaluation: Child will participate in self-care within limitations of condition as evidenced by assisting with bathing and hygiene, feeding, toileting and dressing and grooming.

6. **Nursing diagnosis:** Risk for delayed growth and development related to stressors associated with hospitalization, current condition or illness, separation from family and sensory overload or sensory deprivation.
   Goal: Promoting growth and development.
   Interventions:
   - Assess child's developmental stage to establish a baseline and determine appropriate strategies
   - Use unstructured and therapeutic play and adaptive toys to promote developmental functioning
   - Provide stimulating environment when possible to maximize potential for growth and development
   - Praise accomplishments and emphasize child's abilities to foster self-esteem and encourage feelings of confidence and competence
   - Include parents in techniques to foster growth and development to promote feelings of control in their child's care.

   Outcome identification and evaluation: Child will demonstrate developmentally appropriate milestones as evidenced by age-appropriate behaviors and activities.

7. **Nursing diagnosis:** Deficient knowledge related to hospitalization, surgery, treatments, procedures, required care and follow-up as evidenced by questioning and verbalization lack of prior exposure.
   Goal: Enhancing knowledge.
   Interventions:
   - Assess child's and family's willingness to learn to ensure effective teaching
   - Providing family with time to adjust to diagnosis to facilitate their ability to learn and participate in the child's care
   - Repeat information to promote multiple opportunities for child and family to learn
   - Teach in short sessions to prevent overloading the child and parents with information
   - Gear teaching to a level of understanding for the child and the family (depends on age of child, physical condition, memory) to promote learning
   - Provide reinforcement and rewards to help facilitate the teaching/learning process
   - Use multiple modes of learning such as written information, verbal instruction, demonstrations and media, when possible to facilitate learning and retention of information
   - Provide the child and family with written step-by-step instructions for procedures or care to allow for reference at a later date
   - Have child and family provide return demonstrations of care procedures to ensure effectiveness of teaching
   - Arrange for trial home care during hospitalization and after discharge as appropriate to ensure understanding and provide opportunities for additional teaching and learning.

   Outcome identification and evaluation: Child and family will demonstrate understanding of all aspects of child's current situation as evidenced by identification of child's and family's needs, verbal statements of understanding and/or need for additional information, return demonstration of procedures and treatments, and verbalization of instructions for follow-up and continued care.

Nursing Management
Specific Nursing Diagnoses and Nursing Process
Nursing diagnosis

Anxiety of child, parent(s) and family related to change in health status, change in environment, threat to self-concept, situational crisis **(Table 9.1)**.

Assessment: Increased apprehension; fear; helplessness; uncertainty; distress over hospitalization; restlessness; expressed concern over procedures, pain, loss of control, pain, separation from significant others; crying; clinging; refusal to interact with staff; changes in vital signs.

Evaluation
- Expression of reduction in anxiety by child, parent(s), and family
- Expresses feelings and fears about hospitalization
- Modifies hospital environment to include home routines
- Prepares child and family for procedures and treatments
- Verbalizes pre and postoperative procedures and expectations
- Participates in decision making, planning, and implementing care
- Minimizes fear of bodily injury, pain, separation anxiety, loss control and independence
- Visits or stays with child
- Interacts with staff and develops trust and rapport
- Exhibits understanding of instructions and information given.

Nursing diagnosis

Self-care deficit, bathing/hygiene, dressing/grooming, feeding, toileting related to impaired ability to perform ADL, intolerance to activity pain and discomfort **(Table 9.2)**.

Assessment: Inability to wash body, take off or put on clothing, feed self, positioning or mechanical restrictions, weakness, fatigue, imposed bed rest, inability to carry out toileting with use of bedpan or go to bathroom.

Evaluation
- Anticipates child's needs
- Helps child to remain as independent as possible in ADL
- Provides aids and devices to assist child in performance of ADL and self-care
- Promotes rest periods before and after activity
- Promotes independence in self-care activities.

Nursing diagnosis

Diversional activity deficit related to environmental lack of diversional activity, long-term hospitalization **(Table 9.3)**.

Assessment: Boredom, desire for something to do because usual hobbies and activities cannot be undertaken in hospital.

Evaluation
- Schedules play and diversional activities in care plan
- Provides diversional activities for child according to abilities and age

Table 9.1: Nursing interventions for anxiety of child, parent(s), and family.

Interventions	Rationales
Assess child's parental and family level of anxiety, developmental level, understanding of illness and reason for hospitalization, responses to this and previous hospitalizations	Provides information about sources and level of anxiety related to illness and hospitalization; sources of anxiety and responses vary with age of child and include separation, pain and bodily injury, loss of control, enforced dependence, fear of unknown, fear of equipment, unfamiliar environment and routines, guilt, fear and concern for child's recovery, feelings of powerlessness
Assess social and emotional history of child, parent(s), and family for strengths and successful coping ability	Provides information about strengths and weaknesses to draw upon to cope with hospitalization
Allow expression of feelings and concerns about illness and procedures and listen individually to child, parent(s), and family members	Provides opportunity to vent feelings and fears to reduce anxiety and promote adaptation to hospitalization
Provide a calm, accepting environment and avoid rushing through interactions and care	Assists child and family in establishing trust and obtaining emotional stability
Provide orientation to hospital environment and room, routines, meal and play time, introduction to staff members, forms to sign, and hospital policies	Familiarizes child and family with environment, promotes secure feeling, and reduces fear of unknown
Have same personnel following written care plan, care for child; schedule personal contact with child within workday	Promotes continuity and consistency of care to support trusting relationship
Encourage involvement of child and parent(s) in planning and interventions of care; allow parents to remain with child or have open visitations; allow to hold and cuddle the child	Promotes participation in and adaptation to hospitalization, reduces anxiety; allows demonstration of love and affection for child
Allow child and parent(s) to incorporate home routines as much as possible; bring toys, tapes, photographs and favorite foods from home as appropriate	Promotes security and reduces anxiety associated with new experiences
Maintain a quiet environment, control visitors and interactions as needed	Decreases stimuli that increase anxiety
Allow child to play out feelings, accept feelings and responses expressed by the child	Permits child to express feelings without fear of punishment
Approach child in a positive way; use child's proper name; avoid communicating, either verbally or nonverbally, any rejection, judgments, or negativism	Promotes rapport and trust and maintains identity
Identify and recognize regressive behavior as a part of the illness and assist child in dealing with dependency associated with the hospitalization	Allows for behaviors common to hospitalization and loss of control
Provide support to child during any procedures or distressing features associated with care, including intrusive procedures, exposure of body parts, need for personal privacy and privacy of others	Reduces anxiety and fear caused by possible body injury

Nursing Process for a Hospitalized Child

Table 9.2: Nursing interventions for self-care deficit, bathing/hygiene, dressing/grooming, feeding, toileting.

Interventions	Rationales
Assess physical tolerance and abilities to perform ADL, and play activities and restrictions imposed by the illness and medical protocol	Provides information about amount of energy and effect of illness on activity level
Anticipate child's personal needs for toileting, feeding, brushing teeth, bathing and other care if unable to manage on own; allow child to do as much as possible	Prevents embarrassing experiences with toileting and maintain comfort with personal cleanliness and appearance
Provide personal care for infant and small child; assist child and encourage parent(s) to assist child that needs help with ADL, and adjust times and methods to fit home routines	Provides needed assistance using patterns and articles that child is accustomed to using and doing
Praise child for participation in own care according to age, developmental level, and energy	Promotes self-esteem and independence
Provide assistive aids or devices to perform ADL; allow choices when possible	Assists child in performing self-care for ADL
Balance activities with rest as needed; place needed articles and call light within reach	Prevents fatigue by conserving energy and promoting rest

(ADL: activities of daily living)

Table 9.3: Nursing interventions for diversional activity deficit.

Interventions	Rationales
Assess type of activities allowed and desired and amount of motor activity needed; check medical protocol for bed rest or limitations imposed by illness	Provides information about type of activities and play to suggest
Show playroom to child and introduce child and family to other children and families with similar illness	Provides a familiar environment for child
Place child in a room with another child of same age if possible	Promotes interaction and diversion while hospitalized
Schedule care and treatments to allow for play activities	Provides opportunity for play and diversion
Provide age-appropriate play activities according to amount of energy of child and activity allowed, including quiet play with games, television, reading, soft toys, favorite toy	Prevents fatigue resulting from over activity while ill and in need of rest and quiet
Encourage family to play with child or interact with child	Promotes diversion for child
Provide play activities that include educational needs for school age child; bring schoolwork from home if appropriate	Promotes therapy that includes educational needs
Provide a play therapist for assistance in planning activities and assessing child's play needs	Promotes age-appropriate diversional activities

- Engages in activities appropriate for age, desires and limitations imposed by illness
- Provides play therapist or other workers to plan and assist with diversional activities.

Nursing Process for a Hospitalized Child

Table 9.4: Nursing interventions for powerlessness of child and parent(s).

Interventions	Rationales
Encourage parent(s) and child to verbalize feelings in an accepting environment	Allows for venting of feelings about loss of control and frustrations over loss of ability to perform activities
Allow for input from child and parent(s) in care goals, care plan, and scheduling of activities, and integrate this input into routines as much as possible	Allows for as much control as possible for child and family
Encourage parent(s) to participate in child's care as much as desired; and to visit or remain with child continuously	Promotes support of child and allows family some control over the situation
Provide encouragement and praise to child and parent(s) for their participation; encourage and defend expression of their true feelings	Promotes positive feedback and reduces fear of rejection by staff because of their behavior
Allow child to perform simple tasks in hospital unit and for own care, such as pouring own water and marking amounts on record at bed side	Promotes independence and control of the environment

Nursing diagnosis

Powerlessness of child and parent(s) related to healthcare environment, illness-related regimen **(Table 9.4)**.

Assessment: Expression of loss of control over situation, expression or behavior indicating dissatisfaction with inability to perform activities and dependence on others, reluctance to express true feelings, fear of alienation from others in the hospital environment.

Evaluation
- Visits or remains with child as able
- Participates in goal development, care, and scheduling of treatments
- Incorporates suggestions of child and parent(s) in care
- Verbalizes increase in control over situation and decreased feelings of powerlessness and helplessness
- Accepts responsibility for actions, behaviors that contribute to adaptation to hospitalization
- Complies with medical protocol while hospitalized.

Play/Therapeutic Play

Play provides the child with fun and stimulation. It also helps the child develop satisfying relationships with people and learn how to function in the environment. As the child grows and matures, play develops intelligence, sensorimotor function, awareness of self and others, morality, and creativity. Toys provide the medium for play by helping the child learn about activities and roles in life that are difficult to understand. Toys should proceed from simple to complex in content as the child grows and develops. Play that is directed to serve as a release from stress, to teach child to express emotions in a socially accepted manner, to test situations that have produced fear, and to help child communicate needs is therapeutic play **(Flowchart 9.2)**.

Nursing Process for a Hospitalized Child

Flowchart 9.2: Pathophysiology of play/therapeutic play.

```
Play activity                                    Therapeutic play
     ↓                                                  ↓
Selected by child purely              Selected to stimulate growth
    for enjoyment                          and development,
     ↓                                    Express emotions,
Exploration, pleasure,               Releases tension/stress,
imitation, socialization            Communication of fears/needs
    group games                                     ↓
   ↓         ↓                         Sensorimotor development
Passive    Active                      Intellectual development
   ↓         ↓                              Self-awareness
Television  Motor activity        ──── Moral development ────
Radio        ↓                       ↓            ↓             ↓
Board games  Riding tricycle      Teaching    Diversional    Expressive
Cards        Swimming             activities  activities     activities
Music        Climbing                ↓            ↓             ↓
Puzzles      Skating              Hospital     Toys        Creative drawing
Crafts toys  Sports               equipment,   Games        and painting
                                  anatomically Books       Making cards or
                                  correct dolls, Radio,TV, Tapes  gifts
                                  play telephone, Weaving    Dramatic play
                                  drawings,   Crayons and    Puppets
                                  models.     coloring books dolls
                                                             Clay modeling
```

Nursing Management

Specific Nursing Diagnoses and Nursing Process

Nursing diagnosis

High-risk for trauma related to internal factors of lack of safety precautions or education. External factors of playing with unsafe toys, injury from contact games **(Table 9.5)**.

Assessment: Request for guidelines for toys selection and provision for safe environment for play.

Table 9.5: Nursing interventions for high-risk for trauma.

Interventions	Rationales
Assess age of child and reason for particular selection of type and article of play, and intended purpose of play (enjoyment, development, therapy)	Provides information needed to select appropriate toy or activity for play based on age; infants grasp and hold articles and stuffed toys; young child plays with replicas of adult tools and other toys, plays pretend, and later moves from toys to games, hobbies, sports; older child continues with games and sports and begins to daydream. Play provides fun, diversion, and learning about procedures for the child who is hospitalized
Select safe toys appropriate for age and amount of activity allowed (active or passive play) and that suit the skills and interest of the child	Provides guidelines for quiet play or play that involves motor activity

Contd...

Contd...

Interventions	Rationales
Encourage play and allow parent(s) to bring favorite toy, game, or other play materials from home	Promotes learning and skill development, and facilitates expression of feelings
In a quiet environment, use play kit to prepare child for a procedure, to observe child's behavior, or to allow child to reveal fears and concerns with or without someone in attendance	Promotes therapeutic play with a selection of toys and articles that include dolls or puppets (nurse, doctor, child, family members); hospital supplies (syringe, dressings, tape, tubes); paper, crayons, and paints; stuffed toys, toy telephone
Remove all unsafe, sharp, broken toys, toys with small parts that can be swallowed, toys inappropriate for age	Prevents trauma or injury to the child
Allow child to communicate type of toy desired and to assist in the selection of toys and play activities	Promotes independence and control over play situation

Evaluation
- Provides environment for safe play
- Selects play materials related to age and individual needs
- Verbalizes criteria for safe toys and play activities
- Absence of trauma or injury resulting from play.

PRACTICE QUESTIONS

1. Write the nursing process for a 5-year-old child admitted in pediatric ward.
2. Write the nursing process for a 3-year-old child applying therapeutic play.

CHAPTER 10

Nursing Process for the Child with Genetic Disorder

LEARNING OBJECTIVES

- Obtain a detailed family history and construct a pedigree.
- Assess and analyze hereditary and nonhereditary disease risk factors.
- Identify potential genetic conditions or genetic predisposition to disease.
- Provide genetic information and psychosocial support to individuals and families.
- Provide nursing care for patients and families at risk for or affected by diseases with a genetic component.
- Provide genetic counseling.
- Facilitate genetic testing and interpret genetic test results and laboratory reports.

NURSING PROCESS FOR THE CHILD WITH GENETIC DISORDER

1. **Nursing diagnosis:** Deficient knowledge related to lack of information regarding complex, technical medical condition, prognosis and medical needs as evidenced by verbalization, questions, or actions demonstrating lack of understanding about child's condition or care.
   Outcome identification and evaluation: Child and family will verbalize accurate information and understanding about condition, prognosis, and medical needs. Child and family demonstrate knowledge of condition, prognosis and medical needs including possible causes, contributing factors, and treatment measures.
   Intervention: Providing patient and family teaching.
   - **Assess child's and family's willingness to learn:** Child and family must be willing to learn for teaching to be effective.
   - **Provide family with time to adjust to diagnosis:** Will facilitate adjustment and ability to learn and participate in child's care.
   - **Repeat information:** Allows time to family and child to learn and understand.
   - **Teaching short sessions:** Many short sessions are more helpful than one long session. Gear teaching to the child and family's level of understanding (depends on age of child, physical condition, memory) to ensure understanding.
   - **Provide reinforcement and rewards:** Facilitates the teaching/learning process.
   - **Use multiple modes of learning involving many senses (written, verbal, demonstration and videos) when possible:** Child and family are more likely to retain information when presented in different ways using many senses.
   - **Refer child and family to a genetics specialist:** Genetic information is highly technical; the field is advancing at a rapid pace and information needs to be the most current and accurate. A genetic specialist can provide this along with expertise, support, and resources.
2. **Nursing diagnosis:** Decisional conflict related to treatment options, conflicting values and ethical, legal, and social issues surrounding genetic testing as evidenced by verbalization of

uncertainty about choices, verbalization of undesired consequences of alternative actions being considered, delayed decision-making, physical signs of stress.
Outcome identification and evaluation: Family will state they are able to make an informed decision: Family will state advantages and disadvantages of choices and share fears and concerns regarding choices.
Intervention: Providing decision-making support.
- Give family time and encourage them to express their feelings associated with decision making. The decision-making process becomes more difficult if feelings are not expressed.
- Encourage family to list advantages and disadvantages of each alternative.
- **Initiate health teaching and referral to genetic specialist when needed:** Genetic testing information is often technical and complex. Families need accurate and up-to-date information to aid in decision making.
- **Maintain a nondirective manner:** This is a difficult decision that the family must make for themselves; the nurse should provide all the necessary information while maintaining an unobtrusive role.
- **Validate the family's feelings regarding the decisional conflict:** Validation is a therapeutic communication technique that promotes the nurse-patient relationship.
3. **Nursing diagnosis:** Risk for delayed growth and development related to physical disability, activity restrictions secondary to genetic disorder.
Outcome identification and evaluation: Child's growth and development will be enhanced: Child will demonstrate adequate growth patterns within parameters of disease, child will make continued progress toward attainment of developmental milestones and will not suffer regression in abilities. Child will demonstrate developmental milestones within age parameters and limits of disease. Child will make steady gains in growth patterns (e.g., height and weight) within disease parameters. Child expresses interest in the environment and people around him/her. Interacts with environment appropriately for developmental level.
Intervention: Promoting growth and development.
- Screen for developmental capabilities to determine child's current level of functioning
- Offer age-appropriate toys, play and activities (including gross motor) to encourage further development
- Perform exercises or interventions as prescribed by physical or occupational therapist: These activities promote functional and developmental skills
- Provide support to families: Due to immobility and extremity deficits, the child's progress toward developmental milestones may be slow
- Use therapeutic play and adaptive toys to facilitate developmental functioning
- Provide stimulating environment when possible to maximize potential for growth and development
- Praise accomplishments and emphasize child's abilities to improve self-esteem and encourage feeling of confidence and competence
- Monitor height and weight and plot on growth chart to identify growth patterns and deviations in these patterns.
4. **Nursing diagnosis:** Fear related to outcome of genetic testing as evidenced by reports of apprehension and increased tension.

Outcome identification and evaluation: Family will state they can cope with the results of the genetic testing or demonstrate reduced fear. Family accurately discusses chances of offspring having genetic disease, demonstrates positive coping, and asks questions about genetic testing and meaning of results.

Intervention: Managing fear.
- Empathize with the family and avoid false reassurances; be truthful. Allows family to recognize that fear is a reasonable response. Giving false information or reassurance will actually increase fear
- Explore coping skills used previously by the family to cope with fear. Reinforce these skills and explore other outlets such as relaxation breathing and physical activity. Encourage use of coping mechanisms that help control fear
- Encourage verbalization of feelings and concerns about genetic testing. Allow time for questions. Provide a safe outlet to express feelings and encourage open communication between the family members
- Explain all procedures and review results as available: Knowledge deficit contributes to fear
- Refer to appropriate support groups and genetic counseling. Talking with families who have gone through similar situations can help decrease fear and provide methods of coping. Genetic counseling provides information along with support and additional resources.

5. **Nursing diagnosis:** Family process interrupted, related to child's hospitalization, diagnosis of genetic illness as evidenced by inadequate family coping.
   Outcome identification and evaluation: Family will maintain functional system of support, demonstrate adequate coping, adaptation of rates and functions and decreased anxiety. Parents are involved in child's care, ask appropriate questions, express fears and concerns, and can discuss child's care and condition calmly.
   Intervention: Promoting family coping.
   - Encourage family verbalize concerns about child's illness, diagnosis and prognosis. Allow the nurse to identify concerns and areas where further education may be needed and demonstrate family-centered care
   - Explain therapies, procedures, child's behaviors and plan of care to parents. Understanding the child's current states and plan of care helps decrease anxiety
   - Encourage parental involvement in care, which allows parents to feel needed and valued and gives them a sense of control over their child's health
   - Identify support system for family and child, which helps nurse identify needs and resources available for coping
   - Educate family about resources available to help them develop a wide base of support.

PRACTICE QUESTIONS

1. Baby Roshini 7-year-old admitted in pediatric medical ward diagnosed with thalassemia. Explain the nursing management of baby Roshini by applying of nursing process.
2. Baby Lakshmi 1-month-old admitted in surgical ward with cleft lip and palate. Discuss the pre- and postoperative management of baby Lakshmi with cleft lip and palate by applying nursing process.

CHAPTER 11

Nursing Process for the Child with Respiratory Disorder

LEARNING OBJECTIVES
- To identify the signs and symptoms of a child with respiratory disorder.
- To frame nursing diagnosis based on the needs of the child.
- To plan nursing interventions and outcome identification.

INTRODUCTION

The respiratory tract is a common site of major and minor disorders in infants and children, and any alteration in respiratory structure or function has a profound effect on the ability to supply the body with oxygen and remove carbon dioxide. A constant supply of oxygen is necessary to sustain organ function and survival, and any decrease in or cessation oxygen intake will threaten the life of an infant or child. Smaller, narrower airways are predisposed to obstruction and infection, which compromise airway patency and pattern. This in turn changes the respiratory rate and efficiency. This tendency gradually decreases after the age of 5.

Each stage of life and its associated changes resulting from growth and developmental patterns establish different pulmonary parameters and susceptibility to diseases. Although the system generally functions the same as in an adult, anatomic changes that occur with growth influence chronic illnesses related to this system.

NURSING PROCESS FOR THE CHILD WITH RESPIRATORY DISORDER (IN GENERAL)

1. **Nursing diagnosis:** Ineffective airway clearance related to inflammation, increased secretions, mechanical obstruction or pain as evidenced by presence of secretions, productive cough, tachypnea and increased work of breathing.
   Goal: Child will be able to maintain patent airway.
   Interventions: Maintaining a patent airway.
   - Position with airway open (sniffing position if supine), open airway allows adequate ventilation
   - Humidify oxygen or room air and ensure adequate fluid intake (intravenous or oral) to help liquefy secretions for ease in clearance
   - Suction with bulb syringe or via nasopharyngeal catheter as needed, particularly prior to bottle-feeding to promote clearance of secretions
   - If tachypneic, maintain nil per orals (NPO) status to avoid risk of aspiration
   - In older child, encourage expectoration of sputum with coughing to promote airway clearance
   - Perform chest physiotherapy if ordered to mobilize secretions
   - Ensure emergency equipment is readily available to avoid delay should airway become unmaintainable.

Evaluation: Free from secretions or obstruction, easy work of breathing, respiratory rate within parameters forage.

2. **Nursing diagnosis:** Ineffective breathing pattern related to inflammatory or infectious process as evidenced by tachypnea, increased work of breathing, nasal flaring, retractions, diminished breath sounds.
   Goal: Child will be able to exhibit adequate ventilation.
   Interventions: Promoting effective breathing patterns.
   - Assess respiratory rate, breath sounds and work of breathing frequently to ensure progress with treatment and, so that deterioration can be noted early
   - Use pulse oximetry to monitor oxygen saturation in the least invasive manner to note adequacy of oxygenation and ensure early detection of hypoxemia
   - Position for comfort with open airway and room for lung expansion and use pillows or padding if necessary to maintain position, to ensure optimal ventilation via maximum lung expansion
   - Administer supplemental oxygen and/or humidity as ordered to improve oxygenations
   - Allow for adequate sleep and rest periods to conserve energy
   - Administer antibiotics as ordered, may be indicated in the case of bacterial respiratory infection
   - Encourage incentive spirometry and coughing with deep breathing (can be accomplished through play) to maximize ventilation (play enhances the child's participation).

   Evaluation: Respiratory rate within parameters for age, easy work of breathing (absence of retractions, accessory muscle use, grunting), clear breath sounds with adequate aeration, oxygen saturation more than 94% or within prescribed parameters.

3. **Nursing diagnosis:** Gas exchange, impaired, related to airway plugging, hyperinflation, atelectasis as evidenced by cyanosis, decreased oxygen saturation and alterations in arterial blood gases.
   Goal: Child will be able to maintain adequate gaseous exchange.
   Interventions: Promoting adequate gas exchange.
   - Administer oxygen as ordered to improve oxygenation
   - Monitor oxygen saturation via pulse oximetry to detect alterations in oxygenation
   - Encourage clearance of secretions via coughing, expectoration, chest physiotherapy and suctioning; mobilization of secretions may improve gas exchange
   - Administer bronchodilators if ordered (albuterol, levalbuterol and racemic epinephrine) to treat bronchospasm and improve gas exchange
   - Provide frequent contact and support to the child and family to decrease anxiety, which increases the child's oxygen demands
   - Assess and monitor mental status (confusion, lethargy, restlessness, combativeness); hypoxemia can lead to changes in mental status.

   Evaluation: Pulse oximetry reading on room air is within normal parameters for age, blood gases within normal limits, absence of cyanosis.

4. **Nursing diagnosis:** Risk for infection related to presence of infectious organisms as evidenced by fever or presence of virus or bacteria on laboratory screening.
   Goal: Child will be able to exhibit no signs of secondary infection and will not spread infection to others.

Interventions: Preventing infection.
- Maintain aseptic technique, practice good hand washing and use disposable suction catheters to prevent introduction of further infectious agents
- Limit number of visitors and screen them for prevent further infection
- Administer antibiotics if prescribed to prevent or treat bacterial infection
- Encourage nutritious diet according to child's preferences and ability to feed orally to assist body's natural infection-fighting mechanisms
- Isolate the child as required to prevent nosocomial spread of infection
- Teach child and family preventive measures such as good hand washing, covering mouth and nose when coughing or sneezing, adequate disposal of used tissues to prevent nosocomial or community spread of infection.

Evaluation: Symptoms of infection decreased over time and others remain free from infection.

5. **Nursing diagnosis:** Risk for fluid volume deficit related to decreased oral intake, insensible losses via fever, tachypnea or diaphoresis.
   Goal: Child will be able to maintain hydration status.
   Interventions: Maintaining adequate fluid volume.
   - Administer intravenous fluids if ordered to maintain adequate hydration in NPO state
   - When allowed oral intake, encourage oral fluids; popsicles, favorite fluids and games can be used to promote intake
   - Assess for signs of adequate hydration (elastic skin turgor, moist mucosa, adequate urine output)
   - Strict intake and output monitoring can help identify fluid imbalance
   - Urine specific gravity, urine and serum electrolytes, blood urea nitrogen, creatinine and osmolality are reliable indicators of fluid status.

   Evaluation: Oral mucosa moist and pink, skin turgor elastic, urine output adequate and reached to 1–2 mL/kg/h.

6. **Nursing diagnosis:** Nutrition altered; less than body requirements related to difficulty feeding as evidenced by poor oral intake, tiring with feeding.
   Goal: Child will be able to maintain adequate nutritional intake.
   Interventions: Promoting adequate nutritional intake.
   - Weigh on same scale at same time daily; weight gain or maintenance can indicate adequate nutritional intake
   - Calorie counts over a 3-day period are helpful in determining if caloric intake is sufficient
   - Assist family and child to choose higher-calorie, protein-rich foods to optimize growth potential
   - Coax young children to eat better by playing games and offering favorite foods resulting in improved intake.

   Evaluation: Weight gained. Child consumed adequate diet for age.

7. **Nursing diagnosis:** Activity intolerance related to high respiratory demand as evidenced by increased work of breathing and requirement for frequent rest when playing.
   Goal: Child will be able to resume normal activity level.
   Interventions: Increasing activity tolerance.

- Provide rest periods balanced with periods of activity; group nursing activities and visits to allow for sufficient rest; activity increases myocardial oxygen demand so must be balanced with rest
- Provide small, frequent meals to prevent overtiring (energy is expended while eating)
- Encourage quiet activities that do not require exertion to prevent boredom
- Allow gradual increase in activity as tolerated, keeping pulse oximetry reading within normal parameters, to minimize risk for further respiratory compromise.

Evaluation: Activity is tolerated without difficulty breathing. Pulse oximetry readings and vital signs within parameters for age and activity level.

8. **Nursing diagnosis:** Fear related to difficulty breathing, unfamiliar personnel, procedures and environment (hospital) as evidenced by clinging, crying, fussing, verbalization or lack of cooperation.
   Goal: Fear/anxiety will be reduced.
   Interventions: Relieving fear.
   - Establish trusting relationship with child and family to decrease anxiety and fear
   - Explain procedures to child at developmentally appropriate level to decrease fear of unknown
   - Provide favorite blanket or bear to patient, as well as comfort measures preferred by client such as rocking or music for added security
   - Involve parents in care to give child reassurance and decrease fear.

   Evaluation: Decreased episodes of crying or fussing, happy and playful at times.

9. **Nursing diagnosis:** Family processes, altered, related to child's illness or hospitalization as evidence by family's presence in hospital, missed work, demonstration of inadequate coping.
   Goal: Parents demonstrate adequate coping and decreased anxiety.
   Interventions: Promoting adequate family processes.
   - Encourage parents' verbalization of concerns related to child's illness; allows for identification of concerns and demonstrates to the family that the nurse also cares about them, not just the child
   - Explain therapy, procedures, and child's behavior to parents; developing an understanding of the child's current status helps decrease anxiety
   - Encourage parental involvement in care so that parents may continue to feel needed and valued.

   Evaluation: Parents are involved in child's care, ask appropriate questions and are able to discuss child's care and condition calmly.

NURSING PROCESS FOR RESPIRATORY DISORDERS (SPECIFIC CONDITIONS)

Asthma

Asthma in children is a reversible airway-reactive disease characterized by bronchospasm, increased mucus production, and edema of the mucosa of the bronchioles. The result is obstruction, air trapping, respiratory distress, and changes in ventilation. Asthma is the leading chronic disorder in children. Most children experience their first attacks between two and seven years of age with the onset of the most severe cases occurring after the age of 7 years. The onset of an attack may be gradual or immediate; continuous, with wheezing present at all times; or spasmodic, with intermittent attacks separated by intervals without symptoms.

As an attack progresses, alveoli that are hyperinflated and poorly ventilated may lead to impaired gas exchange, hypoxemia, hypercapnia, and eventual respiratory acidosis and failure. The two types of asthma are extrinsic (immune mechanisms) and intrinsic (imbalance in the autonomic nervous system), both of which affect the bronchial tissue and mast cell function that produces the characteristic symptoms of the disease.

Status asthmaticus is an acute condition characterized by an asthma attack that fails to respond to treatment and continues and increases in severity. It requires hospitalization of the child **(Fig. 11.1)**.

Symptoms of Asthma in Children

Common childhood asthma signs and symptoms include:
- Frequent, intermittent coughing
- A whistling or wheezing sound when exhaling
- Shortness of breath
- Chest congestion or tightness
- Chest pain, particularly in younger children
- Trouble sleeping caused by shortness of breath, coughing or wheezing

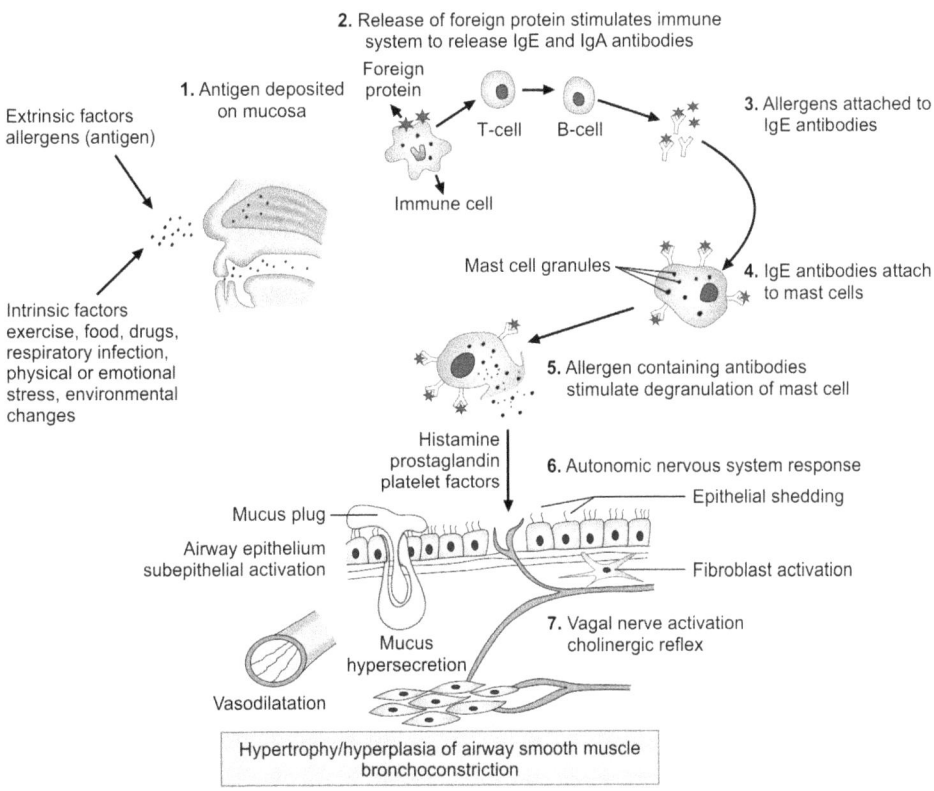

Fig. 11.1: Pathophysiology of asthma.

- Bouts of coughing or wheezing that get worse with a respiratory infection, such as a cold or the flu
- Delayed recovery or bronchitis after a respiratory infection
- Trouble breathing that may limit play or exercise
- Fatigue, which can be caused by poor sleep.

Complications

Asthma may cause a number of complications, including:
- Severe asthma attacks that require emergency treatment or hospital care
- Permanent narrowing of the airways (bronchial tubes)
- Missed school days or getting behind in school
- Poor sleep and fatigue
- Symptoms that interfere with play, sports or other activities.

Nursing Management

A. Essential Nursing Diagnoses and Nursing Process Associated with this Condition

Nursing diagnosis

Ineffective airway clearance related to tracheobronchial infection, obstruction secretion (Table 11.1).

Table 11.1: Nursing interventions for ineffective airway clearance.

Interventions	Rationales
Assess respirations for rate (count for one full minute), depth and ease, presence of tachypnea (50–80/min), dyspnea and if it occurs during sleep or quiet time; note panting, nasal flaring, grunting, slowing, deep (hyperpnea) or shallow (hypopnea) breathing, stridor on inspiration, head bobbing during sleep	Reveals rate and type of respirations (baselines or deviations that are related to age and size of the infant/child and presence of anxiety in the child, changes that indicate obstruction and consolidation of airways and lungs resulting in a decrease in lung surface are for gas diffusion, extreme changes in depth are abnormal, head bobbing indicates dyspnea in the infant and fatigue causing neck flexion, grunting indicates chest pain or impending respiratory failure
Assess breath sounds by auscultation, consolidation by percussion and fremitus	Provides indication of patent airways by auscultation, revealing crackles heard in the presence of secretions (fine and coarse) rhonchi (audible and palpable) in larger airway obstruction and wheezes in small bronchiolar narrowing (inspiration and expiration), diminished breath sounds in presence of decreased air flow and lung consolidation indication of consolidation by presence of dullness on percussion and increased fremitus, decreased functional lung area by presence of tympany on percussion

Contd...

Contd...

Interventions	Rationales
Assess skin color changes, distribution and duration of cyanosis (nail beds, skin, mucous membranes, circumoral) or pallor	Reveals presence and degree of cyanosis, indicating an uneven distribution of gas and blood in the lungs, and alveolar hypoventilation resulting from airway obstruction, the weakness of muscles used in respiration or respiratory center depression
Assess cough (moist, dry, hacking, paroxysmal, brassy, or croupy), onset, duration, frequency, if occurs at night, during day, or during activity; mucus production, when produced, amount, color (clear, yellow, green), consistency (thick, tenacious, frothy); ability to expectorate or if swallowing secretions, stuffy nose or nasal drainage	Reveals characteristics of cough as an indication of a respiratory condition that may be produced by infection or inflammation; small and narrow airways of an infant/child and the difficulty to cough up secretions cause obstruction from the stasis of secretions, which lead to infection and change in respiratory status
Elevate head of be bed child and hold infant and young child in lap or in an upright position with head on shoulder; older child may sit up and rest head on a pillow on over bed table	Facilitates chest expansion and respiration efficiency by reducing pressure of abdominal organs on diaphragm
Reposition on sides q2h	Prevents accumulation and pooling of secretions
Provide cool steam vaporizer at bed side or mist tent	Promotes environmental air humidification that soothes dried mucous membranes and aids in liquefaction of secretions for easier removal as inspiration of dry air reduces ciliary action and causes the retention of secretions
Provide fluids at frequent intervals over 24 hours time periods; encourage clear liquids, and avoid milk as much as possible	Maintains hydration status, and clear liquids liquefy and mobilize secretions; milk tends to thicken secretions
Provide for periods of rest by organizing procedures and care and disturbing infant/child as little as possible in acute stages of illness	Prevents unnecessary energy expenditure resulting in fatigue
Perform postural drainage between meals using gravity, percussion, and vibration unless contraindicated; hold infant on lap; support child with pillows	Promotes removal of secretions and sputum from airways; percussion and vibration loosen and dislodge secretions, and gravity drains the airways and lung segments through positioning
Assist to perform deep breathing and coughing exercises in child when in a relaxed position for postural drainage unless procedures are contraindicated; use incentive spirometer in older child, blowing up balloon or blowing bubbles in younger child	Promotes deeper breathing by enlarging tracheobronchial tree and initiating cough reflex to remove secretions

Contd...

Contd...

Interventions	Rationales
Suction nasal and/or pharyngeal, if needed and appropriate, using correct catheter and method, amount of negative pressure, and time limits; orotracheal with the administration of oxygen before and after suctioning if needed; use bulb syringe to suction mucus from infant's nose	Removes secretions when cough is nonproductive (older child) if unable to regulate cough or breathe through mouth if nose obstructed by mucus (infant or young child), type of suctioning dependent on amount, ability to drain or cough up, breath sounds in upper airways; catheter size is age dependent, maximum negative pressure of 60–90 cm H_2O with time limit of 5–10 seconds for infant, and 90–110 cm H_2O with 10–15 seconds for child; prolonged suctioning causes vagal stimulation and bradycardia, and the use of high pressure damages the mucous membrane lining of airways
Provide mouth care QID and after suctioning	Prevents drying of oral mucous membranes
Provide toys, games for quiet play, and a quiet environment	Prevents excessive energy expenditure and need for additional oxygen consumption, which changes respiratory status while still providing moderate activity and diversion of play
Place airway maintenance equipment and supplies at bedside (resuscitation bag, oxygen and suction equipment, endotracheal tube, tracheotomy tube, and supplies)	Provides immediate access to emergency equipment for interventions to treat airway obstruction if needed
Administer medications (mucolytics, bronchodilators, antibiotics, expectorants, decongestants, and/or antihistamines) orally, parenterally, via aerosol therapy with hand-held measured dose inhaler, small volume nebulizer, intermittent positive pressure breathing (IPPB) according to physician order	Treats conditions affecting secretions, infection by liquefying secretions and enhancing outflow and removal of secretions (mucolytics, expectorants), relieving bronchospasms (bronchodilators), destroying infectious agents by interfering with cell way synthesis (antibiotics), reducing allergic responses and discomfort of nose stuffiness (decongestants, antihistamines), and by suppressing cough (cough suppressants) unless cough is desired to bring up secretions

Assessment: Dyspnea; tachypnea; cough with or without sputum; uncontrollable cough, that is hacking and paroxysmal, becomes ratting, and produces a clear, frothy sputum; abnormal breath sounds (wheezing on expiration and inspiration, fine and coarse crackles); nail bed cyanosis; fever; assuming orthopneic position.

Evaluation
- Takes respirations for rate, depth, and ease and notes deviations from baseline parameters
- Maintains thin, clear secretions that can be coughed up or removed from airways by suctioning
- Performs deep breathing and coughing exercises, postural drainage, and vibration/percussion if appropriate
- Maintains proper care and disposal of supplies and prevention of transmission of infectious agents to child

- Complies with daily medication regimen via correct route and method, using correct dosage and form of drug(s)
- Maintains hydration status with increases in intake when needed.

Nursing diagnosis

Ineffective breathing pattern related to inflammatory process, tracheobronchial obstruction, anxiety.

Assessment: Dyspnea, tachypnea, cough, nasal flaring, prolonged expiratory phase, intercostal and suprasternal retractions in infant, hyperresonance on percussion, shallow and irregular respirations, barrel chest configuration, abnormal arterial blood gases (ABGs), cyanosis, anxiety, restlessness, apprehension, speaks in short, broken phrases or unable to speak.

(Refer Table 14.2 from chapter 14)

Nursing diagnosis

Impaired gas exchange related to ventilation perfusion imbalance **(Table 11.2)**.

Assessment: Restlessness, irritability, hypoxemia, hypercapnia, confusion, somnolence.

Table 11.2: Nursing interventions for impaired gas exchange.

Interventions	Rationales
Assess respiratory status for rate, depth, and ease, (count for one minute), presence of dyspnea, tachypnea, chest movement, periods of apnea	Reveals respiratory effort, rate and depth, (baselines or deviations), symmetry of movements, and use of accessory muscles, which affect the amount of air that reaches the alveoli for ventilation process and diffusion of oxygen (external respiration)
Assess for presence of cyanosis (skin, nail beds, circumoral, and mucous membranes), ABGs for decreased pH and PO_2 and increased PCO_2 levels, transcutaneous monitoring for $tcPO_2$ and $tcPCO_2$, pulse oximeter sensor for O_2 saturation level	Reveals status of hypoxemia and hypercapnia and potential for respiratory failure: cyanosis in children results hypoventilation or an uneven distribution of gas and circulation through the lungs, usually caused by disease and breathing abnormalities; gas levels provide the basic for oxygen administration adjustment, need for position change; continuous monitoring by oximetry or transcutaneous electrode reduces need for arterial punctures to determine hypoxemia and hypercapnia
Assess changes in consciousness and activity, presence of irritability and restlessness	Reveals hypoxic state as oxygen level in blood reduces causing decrease of oxygen to brain
Place child in semi- or high-Fowler's position, orthopneic position for older child unless contraindicated	Promotes chest expansion and ease of breathing, gas distribution, and pulmonary blood flow, all of which enhance gas exchange
Administer oxygen via hood (infant), tent (young child), cannula, or face mask (older child) at rate prescribed, and adjust according to blood gas levels	Ensures adequate oxygen intake to maintain desired level, a PO_2 of less than 60 mm Hg and PCO_2 of >50–55 mm Hg may indicate need for repositioning, stimulation, suctioning, or ventilator support

Contd...

Contd...

Interventions	Rationales
Provide sedation for restlessness, irritability as ordered unless respirations are depressed	Promotes rest and ease of respiratory effort to support ventilation, especially if anxiety present
Determine effect of disease process on gas exchange	Reveals any condition that may interfere with ventilation and the diffusion process will affect gas exchange
Note early stages of hypoxemia and effects on nervous system (mood changes, anxiety, confusion), circulatory system (tachycardia, hypertension), respiratory system (altered depth and pattern, dyspnea, retractions, grunting, prolonged expiration), gastrointestinal system (anorexia)	Promotes careful evaluation of early signs and symptoms of insufficient alveolar ventilation and prevention of respiratory failure or arrest

Evaluation
- Takes respiratory rate, depth, and ease, and notes deviations from baseline parameters
- Maintains position of comfort and optimal chest expansion and ventilation
- Complies with safe oxygen administration via correct method, device, and amount as needed whether continuous or intermittent
- Reports signs and symptoms of respiratory changes, skin color changes, mentation changes
- Monitors infant during sleep for apneic periods by correct use of apnea monitor
- Calls upon assistance from respiratory therapist available from durable medical equipment resource for oxygen administration
- Maintains proper cleansing and care of equipment and supplies and disposal of contaminated articles used in oxygen administration.

Nursing diagnosis
High-risk for fluid volume deficit related to loss of fluid through normal routes, altered intake.

Assessment: Difficulty in drinking, tachypnea, and dyspnea; thirst; dry skin and mucous membranes; diaphoresis; insensible loss.

(Refer Table 14.11 from chapter 14)

Nursing diagnosis
Sleep pattern disturbance related to internal factors of chronic illness.

Assessment: Interrupted sleep form dyspnea, tachypnea, irritability, restlessness, inability to remain in prone or supine positions.

(Refer Table 14.10 from chapter 14)

Nursing diagnosis
Altered nutrition: Less than body requirements related to inability to ingest food because of biological factors.

Assessment: Anorexia, nausea, vomiting, weight loss, dyspnea and tachypnea preventing intake of food.

(Refer Table 14.3 from chapter 14)

Nursing Process for the Child with Respiratory Disorder

Table 11.3: Nursing interventions for anxiety of parent(s) and child.

Interventions	Rationales
Assess level of parental and child anxiety before, during, and after attack	Provides information about anxiety level of child and parent(s) as respirations become more difficult and fear of suffocation is present, and about fear of subsequent attacks
Provide calm, supportive, and nonjudgmental environment, especially during an attack	Reduces anxiety and calming effect slows and eases respirations for improved ventilation
Allow parent(s) and child to express fears and concerns and to ask questions about disease and what to expect	Provides opportunity to vent feelings and secure information to reduce anxiety, especially if they know how to prevent or reduce frequency of attacks
Prepare parent(s) and child before all procedures and treatments	Relieves anxiety caused by fear of unknown
Stay with child during acute attack	Provides comfort and support to the child
Encourage quiet play and avoid any disciplinary actions	Provides distractions from changes in breath emotional upsets, which increase respiratory difficulty or may initiate an acute attack
If hospitalized, allow open visitation, and telephoning; encourage parent(s) to stay with child if possible, to bring toy or blanket from home, and to maintain home schedules for sleep, feeding, play as appropriate	Relieves anxiety for parent(s) and child when familiar people and routines are available

B. Specific Nursing Diagnoses and Nursing Process

Nursing diagnosis

Anxiety of parent(s) and child related to threat of or change in health status **(Table 11.3)**.

Assessment: Increased apprehension, fear with asthma attack, change in respiratory status, exposure to known or unknown allergens, tension and uncertainty about possible hospitalization for acute attack.

Evaluation
- Expresses reduction in anxiety about possible attack
- Resolves misconceptions about the disease by verbalizing what causes the disease, what to expect, and how to prevent attack
- Supports and comforts child during an attack with calmness and understanding
- Participates in anxiety controlling measure like breathing exercises quiet play.

Nursing diagnosis

High-risk for activity intolerance related to respiratory problem, fatigue **(Table 11.4)**.

Assessment: Prolonged dyspnea form asthma attack; lethargy; exhausted appearance, inability to eat, speak, play.

Evaluation
- Controls activities that cause fatigue or precipitate attack
- Provides rest and activity periods scheduled daily
- Fatigue minimized or absent.

Nursing Process for the Child with Respiratory Disorder

Table 11.4: Nursing interventions for high-risk for activity intolerance.

Interventions	Rationales
Assess presence of weakness and fatigue caused by respiratory changes	Provides information about energy reserves as dyspnea and work of breathing over period of time exhausts these reserves
Schedule and provide rest periods in a quiet environment	Promotes adequate rest and reduces stimuli
Disturb only when necessary, perform all care at one time instead of spreading over a long period of time, avoid performing any care or procedures during an attack	Conserves energy and prevents interruption in rest
Provide for quiet play, reading, TV, games while at rest	Prevents alteration in respiratory status and energy depletion caused by excessive activity

Nursing diagnosis

Health-seeking behaviors (prevention of asthma attack and secondary infections of respiratory tract) related to lack of understanding of preventative measures and need for behavior changes **(Table 11.5)**.

Assessment: Expressed desire for increased control of health practices and effect of current environmental conditions and behaviors on health status, increased frequency of attacks.

Evaluation
- Demonstrates age-related measures to take to prevent transmission of infectious agents
- Avoids exposure to known allergens
- Complies with medication regimen and correctly administers medications via tablet, liquid, metered dose, or small volume nebulizer inhaler, subcutaneous injections as prescribed
- Verbalization of understanding of disease and importance of control of precipitating factors and symptoms of an attack

Table 11.5: Nursing interventions for health seeking behaviors (prevention of asthma attack and secondary infections of respiratory tract).

Interventions	Rationales
Assess for knowledge of factors related to attacks, past history of respiratory infections and measures taken to maintain health of child	Provides basis for information needed for health maintenance, as respiratory changes or infection can trigger an asthma attack
Assess for use of over-the-counter medications, type used and effects	Identifies whether products available for treatment of respiratory diseases should or should not be used, as they may interact with prescribed medications, causing attack to become more severe
Assess health history of allergies in family members, what does or does not precipitate attack, and what behaviors result from the attack	Identifies familial tendency to airway reactive disease or history of allergic rhinitis, eczema, urticaria
Assess for knowledge of long-term effects of disease, which may eventually lead to obstructive disease of the lungs	Provides information related to prognosis, which depends on severity and frequency of attacks, and possible relationship to future health

- Verbalized understanding of daily requirements to prevent attack
- Maintains infection-free health status
- Maintains school schedule within limitations imposed by disease, with notification of condition to school nurse, teacher, coach and other appropriate staff.

Bronchiolitis

Bronchiolitis is an acute viral inflammation of the lower respiratory tract involving the bronchioles and alveoli. Accumulated thick mucus, exudate, and cellular debris and the mucosal edema from the inflammatory process obstruct the smaller airways (bronchioles). This causes a reduction in expiration, air trapping, an hyperinflation of the alveoli. The obstruction interferes with gas exchange, in severe cases causing hypoxemia and hypercapnia, which could lead to respiratory acidosis. Children in a debilitated state experiencing this disorder with other or serious diseases are hospitalized (**Fig. 11.2**).

Symptoms of Bronchiolitis

Bronchiolitis usually develops following one to three days of common cold symptoms, including the following:
- Nasal congestion and discharge
- A mild cough
- Fever (temperature higher than 100.4°F or 38°C).
- Decreased appetite.

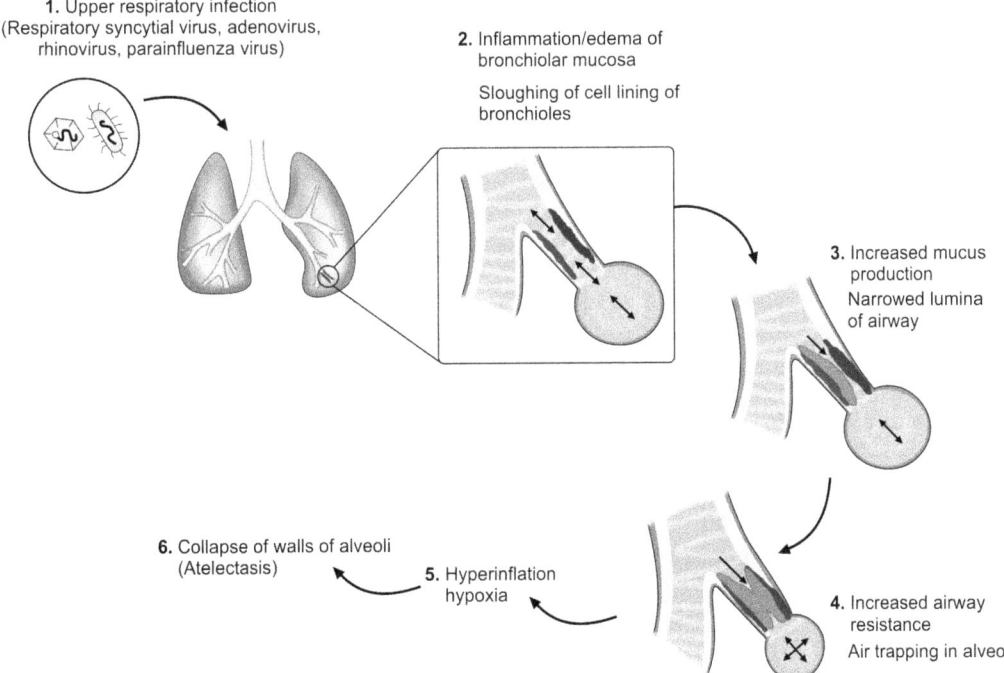

Fig. 11.2: Pathophysiology of bronchiolitis.

As the infection progresses and the lower airways are affected, other symptoms may develop, including the following:
- Breathing rapidly (60 to 80 times per minute) or with mild to severe difficulty
- Wheezing, which usually lasts about seven days
- Persistent coughing, which may last for 14 or more days
- Apnea (a pause in breathing for more than 15 or 20 seconds)
- Retractions (sucking in of the skin around the ribs and the base of the throat)
- Nasal flaring (when the nostrils enlarge during breathing)
- Grunting
- Hypoxia
- Cyanosis

Complications

Complications of severe bronchiolitis may include:
- Cyanosis
- Apnea
- Dehydration
- Fatigue and respiratory failure.

Nursing Management

A. Essential Nursing Diagnoses and Nursing Process Associated with this Condition

Nursing diagnosis

Ineffective airway clearance related to tracheobronchial infection, obstruction, secretion.

Assessment: Abnormal breath sounds (diminished or absent, crackles, wheezes); audible and palpable rhonchi; hyper-resonance; change in rate and depth of respirations; tachypnea (50–80 minutes); paroxysmal, non-productive, and harsh hacking cough; dyspnea and shallow respiratory excursion; fever; increased mucus and nasal discharge.

(Refer Table 11.1)

Nursing diagnosis

Ineffective breathing pattern related to inflammatory process, tracheobronchial obstruction.

Assessment: Dyspnea, tachypnea, cough, nasal flaring, shallow respiratory excursion, suprasternal and subcostal retractions, abnormal ABGs.

(Refer Table 14.2 from chapter 14)

Nursing diagnosis

Impaired gas exchange related to ventilation perfusion imbalance.

Assessment: Hypoxia, hypercapnia, irritability, restlessness, fatigue, inability to move secretions.
(Refer Table 11.3)

Nursing diagnosis

Altered nutrition: Less than body requirements related to inability to ingest food because of biological factors.

Nursing Process for the Child with Respiratory Disorder

Assessment: Dyspnea, fatigue, and weakness, causing difficulty in feeding, anorexia.

(Refer Table 14.3 from chapter 14)

Nursing diagnosis

High-risk for fluid volume deficit related to excessive losses through normal routes, altered fluid intake.

Assessment: Tachypnea, fatigue, increased temperature, dry skin and mucous membranes, increased pulse rate, weight loss.

(Refer Table 14.11 from chapter 14)

Nursing diagnosis

Hyperthermia related to illness of lower respiratory infection.

Assessment: Low-grade, moderate fever; malaise.

(Refer Table 14.18 from chapter 14)

B. Specific Nursing Diagnoses and Nursing Process

Nursing diagnosis

Anxiety of parent(s) and child related to change in health status of infant or small child, threat of or actual hospitalization of infant/small child **(Table 11.6)**.

Assessment: Increased apprehension that condition might worsen; expressed concern and worry about impending hospitalization, need for treatment such as mist tent, IV therapy while hospitalized.

Table 11.6: Nursing interventions for anxiety of parent(s) and child.

Interventions	Rationales
Assess source and level of anxiety, how anxiety is manifested, and need for information that will relieve anxiety	Provides information about anxiety level and the need for interventions to relieve it; sources of anxiety may include fear and uncertainty about treatment and recovery, guilt for presence of illness, possible loss of parental role, and loss of responsibility if hospitalized
Allow expression of concerns and opportunity to ask questions about condition and recovery of ill infant/small child	Provides opportunity to vent feelings, and to secure information needed to reduce anxiety
Communicate with parent(s) and answer questions calmly and honestly	Promotes calm and supportive environment
Encourage parent(s) to remain calm and involved in care and decision-making regarding infant/small child noting any improvement that results	Promotes constant monitoring of infant/small child for improvement or worsening of symptoms
Allow parent(s) to stay with infant/small child or allow open visitation and telephoning, have parents assist in care (holding, feeding, diapering) and suggest routines and methods of treatment	Allows parent(s) to care for and support infant/small child; absence and wondering about condition of infant/small child may increase anxiety

Table 11.7: Nursing interventions for fatigue.

Interventions	Rationales
Assess for extreme weakness and fatigue; ability to rest, and sleep, movement in bed	Provides information to determine effects of dyspnea and work of breathing over period of time, which becomes exhaustive and depletes infant/small child energy reserves and ability to rest, eat, drink
Disturb infant/small child only when necessary, perform all care at one time instead of spreading over a long period of time	Conserves energy and prevents interruptions in rest
Schedule and provide rest periods in a quiet, comfortable environment (temperature and humidity)	Promotes adequate rest and reduces stimuli in order to decrease risk for fatigue
Allow quiet play with familiar toy while maintaining bed rest	Rest decreases fatigue and respiratory distress; quiet play prevents excessive activity, which depletes energy and increases respirations

Evaluation
- Expresses reduction in anxiety about disease process. Therapy and prognosis
- Participates in care and decision-making regarding infant/small child
- Verbalized positive effect of caring for and supporting ill infant/small child
- Visits and/or telephones the hospital if unable to stay.

Nursing diagnosis

Fatigue related to states of respiratory discomfort and effort **(Table 11.7)**.

Assessment: Lethargy or listlessness, emotional lability or irritability, exhausted appearance, inability to eat, limpness.

Evaluation
- Decreased respiratory rate and excursion
- Provides rest and sleep periods imposed by illness
- Reduces and/or minimizes fatigue
- Participates in activities that do not compromise energy and breathing pattern
- Maintains ability to eat, drink, and play within limits imposed by illness.

Nursing diagnosis

Knowledge deficit related to lack of information on how to prevent transmission of respiratory syncytial virus **(Table 11.8)**.

Assessment: Direct or indirect contact with the virus, cross-infection of family members, parent(s) request for information about preventive measures.

Evaluation
- Protects self, family members, and child from exposure to the virus
- Verbalized methods of preventing small child from touching face and other areas with hands and hand washing procedure for child
- Verbalized how virus is transmitted and precautions necessary to take to prevent spread of disease and/or secondary infection.

Table 11.8: Nursing interventions for knowledge deficit.

Interventions	Rationales
Assess existing knowledge of disease prevention and transmission	Provides baseline for type of information needed to prevent infection transmission to child
Inform that the virus is transmitted by direct and indirect contact via the nose and eyes, and that hands should be kept away from these areas	Explains that kissing and cuddling infant/small child, and fomites that are on hard, smooth surfaces are sources of contact with the virus
Instruction in hand washing technique for child, family members and staff	Prevents transmission by the hands, which are the main sources of contamination and carriers of organisms to the face area
Advise that plastic goggles may be worn when caring for infant/small child	Prevents risk of contact with virus via the eyes
Inform of potential for spread of virus to other family members and need for segregation of infant/small child from others	Explains that virus is easily transmitted, with an incidence as high as half of family members acquiring viral infections
If hospitalized, isolate and use gloves, gown precautions; confine care assignments to patients with respiratory conditions	Protects from exposure to secretions and transmission of virus to other patients

Epiglottitis

Epiglottitis is the acute inflammation of the epiglottis and surrounding laryngeal area with the associated edema that constitutes an emergency situation as the supraglottic area becomes obstructed. It results in respiratory distress that must be relieved by endotracheal intubation or tracheotomy in severe cases. Onset is rapid (over 4–12 hours) and breathing pattern usually re-established within 72 hours following intubation and antimicrobial therapy. Children most commonly affected are between 3 and 7 years of age **(Fig. 11.3)**.

Symptoms of Epiglottis
- A sever sore throat
- Difficulty and pain when swallowing
- Difficulty breathing, which may improve when leaning forwards
- Breathing that sounds abnormal and high pitched (stridor)
- A high temperature (fever) of 38°C (100.4°F) or above
- Irritability and restlessness
- Muffled or hoarse voice
- Drooling.

Complications
- Respiratory failure
- Spreading infection—pneumonia, meningitis or a blood infection (sepsis).

Nursing Process for the Child with Respiratory Disorder

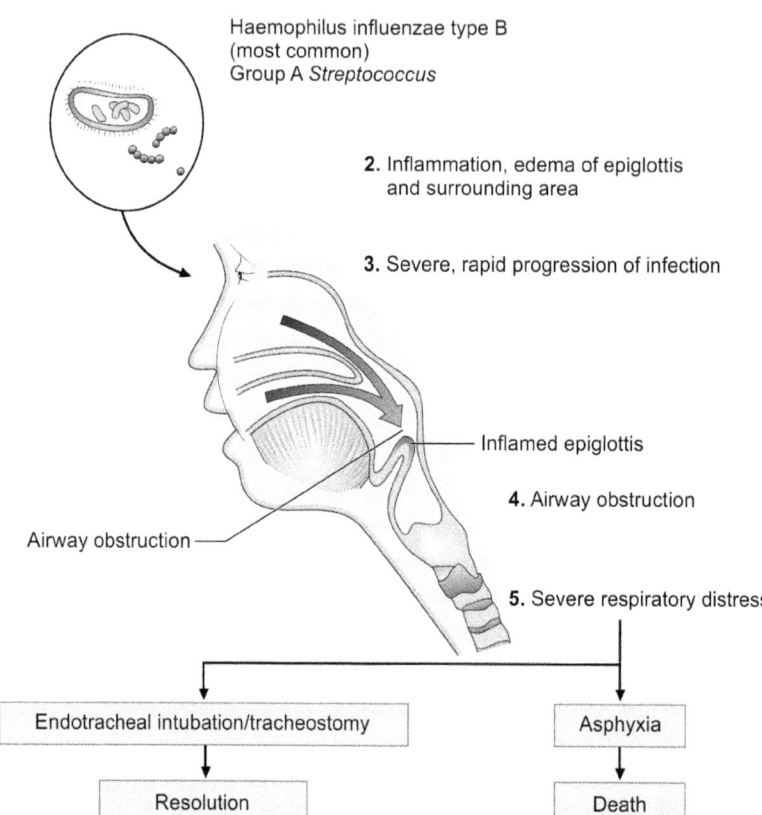

Fig. 11.3: Pathophysiology of epiglottitis.

Nursing Management

A. Essential Nursing Diagnoses and Nursing Process Associated with this Condition

Nursing diagnosis

Ineffective airway clearance related to epiglottis infection, obstruction, secretion.

Assessment: Sudden increase in temperature, dyspnea, tachypnea, drooling, difficulty in swallowing, bright red epiglottis with edema, decreased breath sounds, muffled voice, sore throat, presence of tracheotomy or endotracheal tube.

(Refer Table 11.1)

Nursing diagnosis

Ineffective breathing pattern related to inflammatory process, obstruction.

Assessment: Air hunger, dyspnea, tachypnea, use of accessory muscles (intercostal, sub or suprasternal retractions), cough, assumption of three-point position, sitting up with mouth open and chin forward, stridor or croaking sound on inspiration.

(Refer Table 14.2 from chapter 14)

Nursing diagnosis

High-risk for fluid volume deficit related to loss of fluid through normal routes (respirations and temperature), altered intake.

Assessment: Increased body temperature, dry skin and mucous membranes, decreased skin turgor, increased pulse and respirations, sore throat and difficulty in swallowing, refusal to drink fluids.

(Refer Table 14.11 from chapter 14)

Nursing diagnosis

Hyperthermia related to illness of inflammation/infection of epiglottal area.

Assessment: Sudden increase in body temperature above normal range, as high as 101°F, warm to touch, increased pulse and respirations, positive culture.

(Refer Table 14.18 from chapter 14)

B. Specific Nursing Diagnoses and Nursing Process

Nursing diagnosis

Anxiety (parent[s] and child) related to change in health status of child change in environment (hospitalization) change in role functioning (parenting) **(Table 11.9)**.

Assessment: Verbalization of extreme fear and apprehension by parent(s); agitation, crying, irritability, air hunger and extreme expression of fear (child).

Evaluation
- Expresses a reduction in anxiety as acute stage of disease is relieved
- Parent(s) stays and supports child while hospitalized
- Child's fear and air hunger relieved and progressive calmness of child is established.

Table 11.9: Nursing interventions for anxiety of parent(s) and child.

Interventions	Rationales
Assess severity of fear and anxiety of patent(s) and child	Provides information about presence of extreme anxiety present as symptoms of disease become more acute and breathing more difficult
Provide calm and supportive environment and inform parent(s) that best care is being given to child	Provides reassurance and reduces anxiety of parent(s)
Allow child to assume position of comfort, provide familiar object (toy, blanket)	Promotes comfort and security for child
Remain with child at all times during acute stages	Provides constant assessment for emergency interventions and reassurance for parent(s)
Allow parent(s) to stay with child, provide a place for rest	Promotes security needs for child and assists in reducing parental anxiety
Inform of all procedures, care, and changes in the child's condition	Reduces anxiety caused by fear of the unknown
Avoid any care or procedures that are not necessary during acute stage	Prevents increase of anxiety which increases respiratory distress
Allow for expression of fears and feelings of parent(s) and child and for behaviors caused by severe anxiety	Reduces anxiety and embarrassment

Table 11.10: Nursing interventions for high-risk for suffocation.

Interventions	Rationales
Assess for changes in skin color from pallor to cyanosis, severe dyspnea and sternal and intercostal retractions, lethargy, increased pulse	Provides information about increasing airway obstruction
Allow to sit up and avoid forcing child to lie down	Lying down may cause epiglottis to fall backward, causing airway obstruction
Avoid inspecting throat with tongue blade or obtaining throat culture unless immediate emergency equipment and personnel at hand	Leads to airway spasms and obstruction
Administer O_2 and monitor via pulse oximeter	Promotes oxygenation of tissues and prevents hypoxemia
Have emergency intubation equipment at hand and assist with end tracheal intubation or tracheostomy if necessary, or prepare for procedure in surgery	Establishes airway if obstruction present and respiratory failure and asphyxia imminent

Nursing diagnosis

High-risk for suffocation related to disease process **(Table 11.10)**.

Assessment: Supraglottic edema; obstruction; dysphasia; hypoxia; cyanosis; extreme anxiety, with struggle to breathe.

Evaluation
- Prevents airway obstruction and maintains airway potency
- Prevents suffocation as a result of endotracheal intubation or tracheotomy procedure
- Respiratory/ventilatory status within normal parameters established.

Laryngotracheobronchitis

Laryngotracheobronchitis is the most common form of croup. It is characterized by an acute viral infection of the larynx, trachea, and bronchi which causes obstruction below the level of the vocal cords. Spasmodic croup is croup of sudden onset, occurring mainly at night and characterized by laryngeal obstruction at the level of the vocal cords caused by viral infections or allergens, both occur as a result of upper respiratory infection, edema, and spasms that cause respiratory distress in varying degrees depending on the amount of obstruction. The disease most commonly affects infants and small children between 3 months and 3 years of age and occurs in the winter months. Hospitalization is reserved for those with severe symptoms and compromised respiratory function caused by the obstruction **(Fig. 11.4)**.

Symptoms of Laryngotracheobronchitis

Clinical findings:
- Hoarseness of voice
- Brassy cough
- Inspiratory or even an expiratory stridor
- Fever
- Rhinorrhea

Nursing Process for the Child with Respiratory Disorder

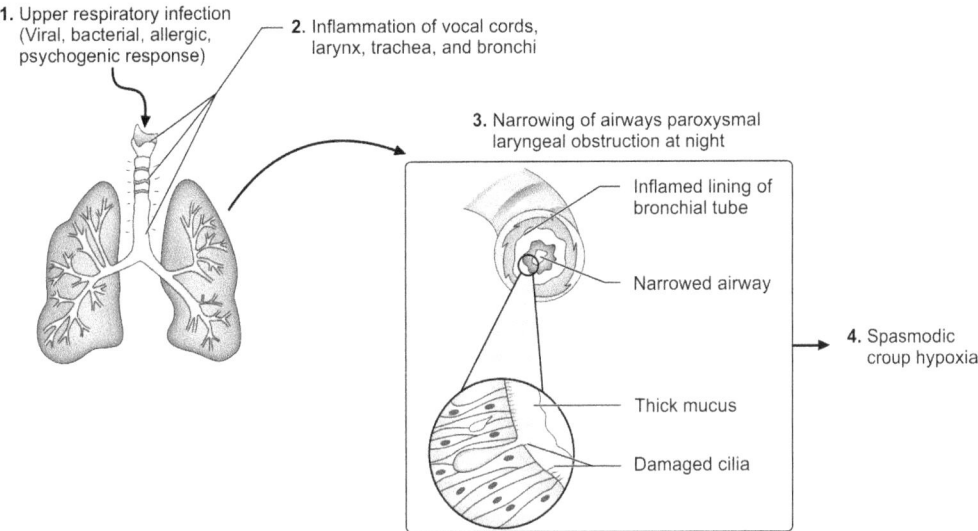

Fig. 11.4: Pathophysiology of laryngotracheobronchitis.

- Sore throat
- Cough
- Pulmonary examination may reveal rhonchi, crepitations, or wheezing.

Nursing Management

A. Essential Nursing Diagnoses and Nursing Process Associated with this Condition

Nursing diagnosis

Infective airway clearance related to tracheobronchial obstruction, secretions.

Assessment: Dyspnea; thick secretions; tachypnea; hoarseness; persistent barking cough; diminished breath sounds, with scattered crackles and rhonchi; cyanosis; restlessness; tachycardia; hypoxemia; hypercapnia.

(Refer Table 11.1)

Nursing diagnosis

Ineffective breathing pattern related to inflammatory process, larygotracheobronchial constriction and obstruction.

Assessment: Dyspnea, tachypnea, abnormal ABGs, barking, metallic sounding cough, nasal flaring, inspiratory stridor, subclavicular and substernal retractions, cyanosis or pallor, restlessness, irritability.

(Refer Table 14.2 from chapter 14)

Nursing diagnosis

High-risk for fluid volume deficit related to loss of fluid through normal routes (respirations and temperature), altered intake.

Assessment: Low grade temperature, dry skin and mucous membranes, increased pulse and respirations, difficult swallowing, poor skin turgor, sunken fontanels, and absence of tears.

(Refer Table 14.11 from chapter 14)

Nursing diagnosis

Sleep pattern disturbance related to internal factor of illness (difficulty breathing).

Assessment: Interrupted sleep caused by cough, restlessness, irritability.

(Refer Table 14.10 from chapter 14)

B. Specific Nursing Diagnoses and Nursing Process

Nursing diagnosis

Anxiety (parent[s] and child) related to change in health status of infant/small child threat to or change in environment (hospitalization) **(Table 11.11)**.

Assessment: Increased apprehension that condition might worsen and hospitalization might be necessary (parental); crying and clinging behaviors, refusal to eat or play (infant or small child); persistent cough and breathing difficulty (infant/small child).

Evaluation
- Expresses a reduction in anxiety with explanations of disease and therapy
- Verbalizes the positive effect of caring for and supporting their sick infant/small child
- Visits, calls hospital when unable to stay with child.

Nursing diagnosis

Fatigue related to states of discomfort (dyspnea) **(Table 11.12)**.

Assessment: Lethargy or listlessness, emotional lability or irritability, exhausted appearance, inability to eat.

Table 11.11: Nursing interventions for anxiety (parent[s] and child).

Interventions	Rationales
Assess level and sources of anxiety of parent(s) and child and identify behaviors caused by anxiety	Provides information about need for interventions to relieve anxiety and concern
Allow parents to express concern and to ask questions about course of disease and what to expect	Provides opportunity to vent feelings, secure information needed to reduce anxiety
Encourage parent(s) and child to remain calm and provide a quiet environment	Anxiety affects respirations and calm environment reduces anxiety
Inform parent(s) and child of all procedures, especially use of croup tent, care and any changes in condition	Relieves anxiety resulting from fear of the unknown
Allow parent(s) to stay with infant/small child if hospitalized, bring toy, blanket from home; allow visits from siblings	Allows parent(s) to care for and support child and provide familiar objects and people to reduce child's anxiety
If hospitalized, carry out home routines for feeding, sleep	Prevents anxiety associated with changes in daily rituals

Table 11.12: Nursing interventions for fatigue.

Interventions	Rationales
Assess for extreme weakness and fatigue, ability to rest and sleep	Dyspnea and work of breathing over period of time exhausts the infant/child's energy reserves affecting ability to rest, eat, drink
Disturb only when necessary, perform all care at one time instead of spreading over a long period of time	Conserves energy and prevents interruptions in rest
Schedule and provide rest periods in a quiet, comfortable environment (temperature and humidity)	Promotes adequate rest and reduces stimuli to decrease fatigue
Allow quiet play while maintaining bed rest	Rest decreases fatigue and respiratory distress; quiet play prevents excessive activity, which depletes energy and increases respirations

Evaluation
- Minimized fatigue with rest and sleep periods provided
- Infant/small child eats and drinks within limits and methods imposed by illness
- Participates in activates that do not compromise energy and breathing pattern
- Maintains respiratory status at baseline parameters.

Pneumonia

Pneumonia is a lower respiratory condition characterized by the inflammation or infection of the pulmonary parenchyma. It is caused by bacteria, viruses, or fungi, or by the aspiration of a foreign substance. It may occur as a primary infection or secondary to another illness or infection.

Pneumonia is most common in infants and small children, but it can occur throughout childhood. Signs and symptoms of the disease depend on the age, causative agent, extent of the disease, the degree of obstruction it causes and the systemic reaction to the infection. The treatment and care is similar for all types of pneumonia **(Figs. 11.5A and B)**.

Signs and Symptoms of Pneumonia
- High fever
- Chills
- Shortness of breath
- Increased breathing rate
- A worsening cough that may produce discolored or bloody sputum (phlegm)
- Sharp chest pains—caused by inflammation of the membrane that lines the lungs
- Lethargic
- Have difficulty with feeding.

Complications
- Bacteria in the blood stream (bacteremia)
- Lung abscess

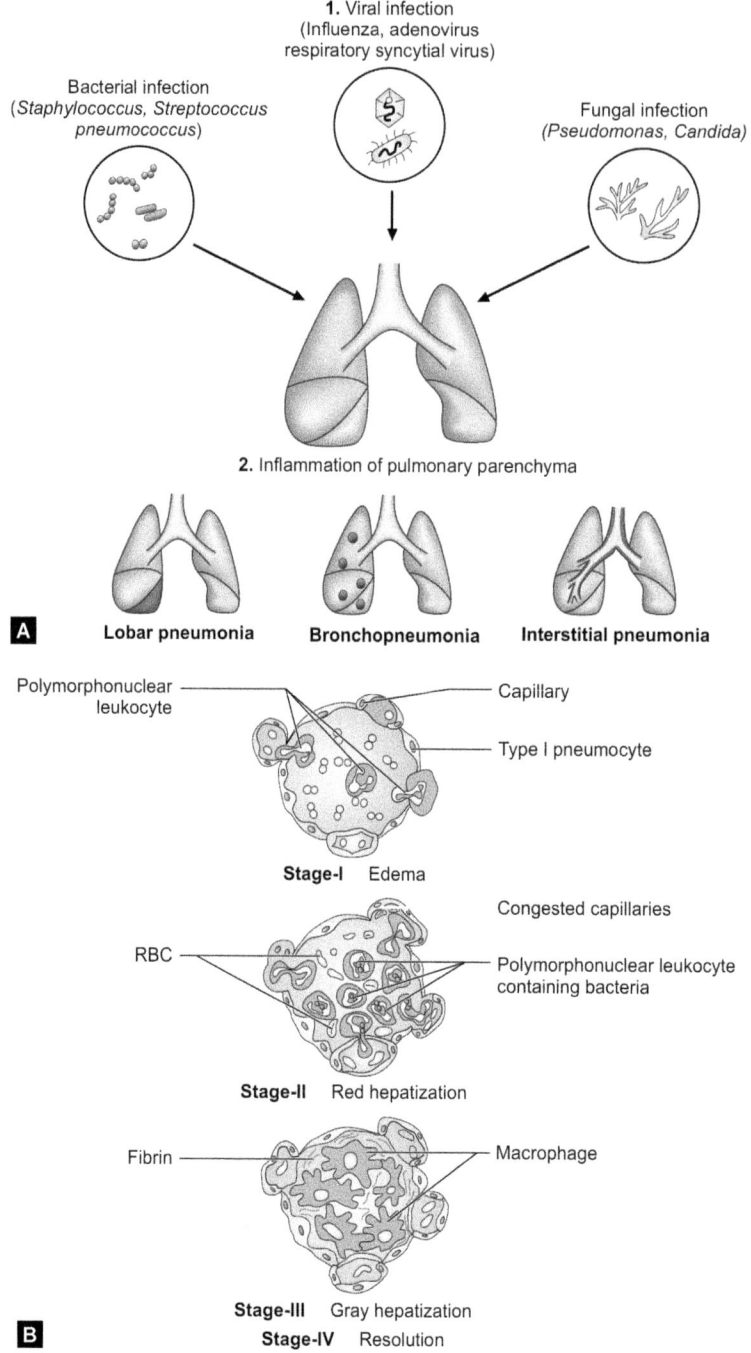

Figs. 11.5A and B: (A) Pathophysiology of pneumonia; (B) Pathophysiology of lobar pneumonia.

- Fluid accumulation around lungs (pleural effusion)
- Difficulty breathing.

Nursing Management

A. Essential Nursing Diagnoses and Nursing Process Associated with this Condition

Nursing diagnosis

Infective breathing pattern related to inflammatory process.

Assessment: Dyspnea, tachypnea, nasal flaring, decreased dull breath sounds, crackles, productive cough in older child, use of accessory muscles with retractions, circumoral cyanosis, shallow respirations, increased fremitus.

(Refer Table 14.2 from chapter 14)

Nursing diagnosis

High-risk for fluid volume deficit related to excessive losses through normal routes; altered fluid intake.

Assessment: Increased temperature and pulse rate, tachypnea, vomiting and diarrhea in young child, reduced fluids in proportion to output.

(Refer Table 14.11 from chapter 14)

Nursing diagnosis

Altered nutrition: Less than body requirements related to inability to ingest food or digest food because of biological factors.

Assessment: Lack of interest in food, anorexia, cough, abdominal pain, vomiting and diarrhea in younger child.

(Refer Table 14.3 from chapter 14)

Nursing diagnosis

Hyperthermia related to illness of lower respiratory tract infection.

Assessment: Abrupt onset of high body temperature (102–105°F in infants and 104–105°F in older child), tachycardia, tachypnea, chills, myalgia, warm to touch, flushed cheeks, convulsions in infant/young child.

(Refer Table 14.18 from chapter 14)

B. Specific Nursing Diagnoses and Nursing Process

Nursing diagnosis

Anxiety of parent(s) and child related to threat to or change in health status; threat to or change in environment (hospitalization) **(Table 11.13)**.

Assessment: Increased apprehension that condition of child might worsen, expressed concern and worry about actual or impending hospitalization of child.

Nursing Process for the Child with Respiratory Disorder

Table 11.13: Nursing interventions for anxiety of parent(s) and child.

Interventions	Rationales
Assess sources and level of anxiety, how anxiety is manifested, and need for information and support	Provides information about the need for interventions to relieve anxiety and concern
Allow to express concerns and ask questions regarding condition of ill child	Provides opportunity to vent feelings, secure information needed to reduce anxiety
Encourage to remain calm and involved in care and decision making regarding child's needs and to note any improvements that result	Promotes constant, monitoring of child's condition for improvement or worsening of symptoms
Allow parent to stay with child or visit when able and to call when concerned if hospitalized; assist in care (hold, feed, bathe, clothe, and diaper) and provide information about child's daily routines	Allows parent to care for and support child instead of increasing anxiety, if not with child

Evaluation
- Reduces parental and child anxiety with understanding of disease and what can be expected until illness is resolved.
- Participates in care of child, visits and/or calls hospital, if unable to stay.

Nursing diagnosis

High-risk for injury related to internal factor of pulmonary complications in infant/child (Table 11.14).

Assessment: Fluid accumulation in the pleural cavity, dyspnea, pneumothorax, empyema, decreased breath sounds with crackles, seizure activity with high temperature, staphylococcal-type pneumonia in infant, pneumococcal-type pneumonia in child.

Evaluation
- Respirations within baseline parameters according to age for rate, depth and ease, absence of crackles, dyspnea
- Temperature within normal range for 24–48 hours.

Table 11.14: Nursing interventions for high-risk for injury.

Interventions	Rationales
Assess vital signs and breath sounds, cough and ability to cough up secretions	Changes revealed in early stages of complications and reveals airway patency and dyspnea caused by fluid accumulation in pleural cavity and secretion accumulation in airways
Prepare infant/child for procedure and assist with thoracentesis; use therapeutic play to prepare child	Performed to drain fluid to be cultured or to instill antibiotics, if infection present
Monitor temperature for sudden rise	Reveals a sudden, rapid rise in temperature which may trigger a febrile seizure
Report detection of possible respiratory complications early (chest pain, dyspnea, cyanosis, abdominal distention)	Allows for immediate preventative measures to be taken during course of disease

Table 11.15: Nursing interventions for knowledge deficit of parent(s) and caretaker.

Interventions	Rationales
Assess knowledge of disease and methods to control and resolve disease; willingness and interest of parent(s) to implement care	Promotes plan of instruction that is realistic to ensure compliance of medical regimen; prevents repetition of information
Provide information and explanations in clear, under stable language; use pictures, pamphlets, video tapes, model in teaching about disease	Ensures understanding based on readiness and ability to learn; visual aids reinforce learning
Instruct in administration of medications including action of drugs, dosages, times, frequency, side effects, expected results, methods to give medications; provide written instructions and schedule to follow and inform to administer full course of antibiotic to child	Provides information about drug therapy, which is the most important treatment for the cure of pneumonia, and about prevention of lung complications resulting from the disease; bacterial pneumonia is treated with antibiotic therapy
Instruct and assist to plan feedings and/or develop menus for appropriate inclusion of nourishing fluids, daily caloric and basic four requirements for age group	Promotes proper diet, which enhances health status, and adequate fluid intake, which prevents dehydration
Inform of importance of activity or activity restrictions and of adequate rest during illness and convalescence	Promotes more rest and possible restriction of activity needed during more acute stages of disease
Instruct in care of used tissues and to cover mouth and nose when coughing or blowing nose, proper handwashing technique for parent and child	Prevents transmission of microorganism by droplets dispersed into the air or by hands

- Absence of signs and symptoms of pulmonary complication
- Culture of chest fluid negative for infectious organisms.

Nursing diagnosis

Knowledge deficit of parent(s), caretaker related to unfamiliarity with disease and complications, measures to control and prevent transmission of respiratory disease **(Table 11.15)**.

Assessment: Verbalization of need for information about medications, activity and rest, nutritional and fluid requirements and medical asepsis techniques to prevent spread of infection.

Evaluation
- Statements of knowledge of diseases, medications, dietary and exercise requirements of child
- Adaptation and compliance of parent(s) with medical regimen
- Precautions taken to prevent spread of infection or contraction of other upper respiratory infections
- Secures pneumonia vaccination, if underlying chronic conditions exist and risk for recurrences is high for child over 2 years of age
- Verbalized signs and symptoms of disease progression or recurrence.

Tuberculosis

Tuberculosis in children is usually contracted from an infected adult by droplets expelled from the respiratory tract and dispersed into the air. Although its incidence and death rate are greater most cases are managed at home with drug therapy. Only patients with more serious forms of the disease or who need special diagnostic tests are hospitalized (**Fig. 11.6**).

Symptoms of Tuberculosis

Common symptoms include:
- Coughing that lasts longer than 2 weeks with green, yellow, or bloody sputum
- Weight loss
- Fatigue

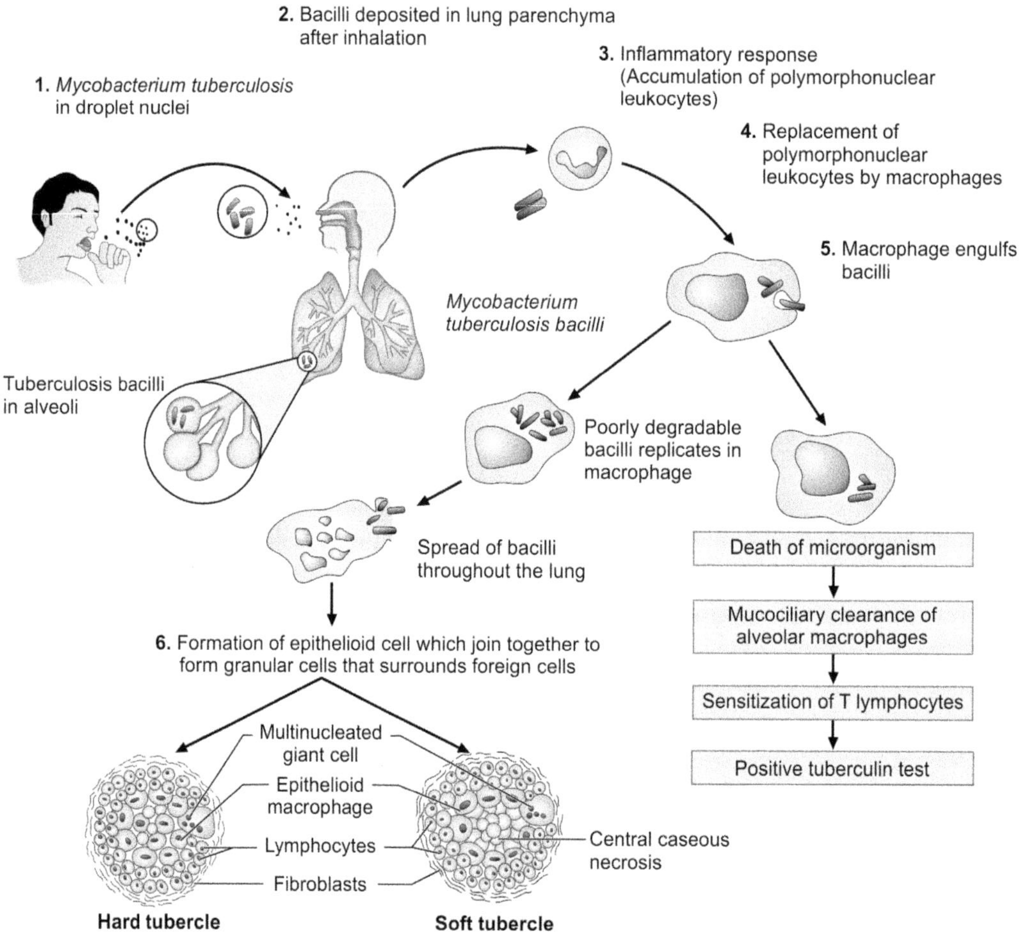

Fig. 11.6: Pathophysiology of pulmonary tuberculosis.

- Fever
- Night sweats
- Chills
- Chest pain
- Shortness of breath
- Loss of appetite.

The occurrence of additional symptoms depends on where the disease has spread beyond the chest and lungs.

Nursing Management

A. Essential Nursing Diagnosis and Nursing Process Associated with this Condition

Nursing diagnosis

Altered nutrition: Less than body requirements related to inability to ingest food because of biological, economic factors.

Assessment: Inadequate food intake, lack of food, pyridoxine deficiency as result of drug therapy.

(Refer Table 14.3 from chapter 14)

B. Specific Nursing Diagnosis and Nursing Process

Nursing diagnosis

Knowledge deficit of parent(s), caretaker related to unfamiliarity with disease and treatment (Table 11.16).

Assessment: Verbalization of need for information about medications, activity and rest, nutritional requirements, and infection transmission prevention.

Evaluation
- Verbalizes knowledge of disease, medications, dietary and exercise requirements
- Adaptation and compliance of parent(s) with medication regimen of daily or twice weekly administration of drugs
- Appropriate growth and development advances for age group
- Maintains follow-up schedule for physician visits, laboratory testing for culture
- Precautions taken to prevent spread of infection or contracting other upper respiratory infections
- Continues with activities (play, school) or limits activities such as contact sports or strenuous games.

Table 11.16: Nursing interventions for knowledge deficit of parent(s) and caretaker.

Interventions	Rationales
Assess knowledge of disease and methods to control and resolve disease; willingness and interest of parent(s) to implement care	Promotes plan of instruction that is realistic to ensure compliance of medical regimen; prevents repetition of information

Contd...

Nursing Process for the Child with Respiratory Disorder

Contd...

Interventions	Rationales
Provide information and explanations in clear, understandable language; use pictures, pamphlets, video tapes, model in teaching about disease	Ensures understanding based on readiness and ability to learn; visual aids reinforce learning
Instruct in administration of medications, including action of drugs, dosages, times, frequency, side effects, expected results, methods to give medications; provide written instructions and schedule to follow	Provides information about drug therapy which is the most important treatment for the cure of tuberculosis and is administered for at least 9 months during the course of the disease and for 6 months after negative cultures secured; isoniazid alone or in combination with other antituberculosis drugs administered for active tuberculosis and conversion from negative to positive skin testing
Instruct and assist in planning feedings and/or developing menus for appropriate inclusion of meat and milk and daily caloric and basic four requirements for age group	Ensures proper diet that enhances health status, and adequate amounts of meat and milk supply pyridoxine in those receiving isoniazid to prevent peripheral neuritis
Inform of importance of activity or activity restrictions and adequate rest during convalescence	More rest and possible restrictions of activity needed during active stage of disease, but school or nursery school attendance is encourage if asymptomatic
Instruct in care of used handkerchiefs and to cover mouth and nose when coughing or blowing nose, proper hand washing technique	Prevents transmission of microorganism by droplets dispersed into the air
Inform of importance of testing of family members and follow-up skin tests for exposed contacts	Provides early detection of disease and possible source of disease, and prevents potential spread of disease
Inform parent(s) of importance of maintaining the treatment regimen over long period of time; offer information and support for continued care	Recovery required extended period of time and support helps to ensure compliance with regimen

PRACTICE QUESTIONS

1. Baby Malar 3-years-old child admitted with epistaxis. Write nursing management of child by applying nursing process.
2. Master Raghu 7-years-old admitted with the condition of asthma. Write a care plan by using nursing process.

CHAPTER 12

Nursing Process for the Child with Neurological Disorder

> **LEARNING OBJECTIVES**
> - To identify the signs and symptoms of a child with neurological disorder.
> - To frame nursing diagnosis based on the needs of the child.
> - To plan nursing interventions and outcome identification.

INTRODUCTION

The neurologic system includes the central nervous system (CNS), consisting of the cerebrum, cerebellum, brain stem, and spinal cord; the peripheral nervous system, consisting of the motor (efferent) and sensory (afferent) nerves; and the autonomic nervous system (ANS), consisting of the sympathetic and parasympathetic systems, which provide the control of vital body functions. Any alteration in the system affects the process of receiving, integrating, and responding to stimuli that enter the system. This results in disturbances of which signs and symptoms are dependent on the type and site of the impairment and the normal functioning of the system. The disturbances may be manifested by alterations in consciousness or muscle function. Changes in the system also occur as the child develops neurologically and completes the growth and development requirements for adulthood. The neurologic system is one of the last body systems to finish development after birth.

NURSING PROCESS FOR THE CHILD WITH NEUROLOGICAL DISORDER (IN GENERAL)

1. **Nursing diagnosis:** Decreased intracranial adaptive capacity related to compression of brain tissue due to increased CSF or cerebral edema secondary to increased ICP resulting from brain injury. Congenital structural defects, brain tumor, decreased reabsorption of CSF or shunt malfunction as evidenced by vomiting. Headache, complaints of visual disturbances, decreased pulse and consciousness, increased head circumference or bulging fontanel.
   Goal: Child will be free from signs and symptoms of increased intracranial pressure.
   Interventions: Promoting adequate intracranial adaptive capacity.
   - *Assess neurologic status closely, monitor for signs and symptoms of increased ICP:* Changes in level of consciousness, signs of irritability or lethargy, changes in papillary reaction can indicate changes in ICP
   - *Monitor vital signs:* Decreased pulse and respiratory rate and increased blood pressure or pulse pressure can indicate increased ICP
   - Measure head circumference in children less than 3 years of age: Increases in head circumference outside parameters for age can indicate increased ICP
   - Elevate head of bed 15°–30° to facilitate venous return and can help to reduce ICP

- Minimize environmental stimuli and noise, avoid pain-producing procedures if possible, which can increase ICP
- *Have emergency equipment ready and available:* Increased ICP can result in respiratory or cardiac failure
- *Notify physician immediately if changes in assessment are noted:* Early intervention is critical to prevent neurologic damage and death.

Evaluation: Signs and symptoms of increased intracranial pressure reduced as evidenced by remaining free of headache, vomiting, vision disturbances, vital signs within parameters for age, no signs of altered levels of consciousness, free of excessive irritability or lethargy, head circumference is within parameters for age.

2. **Nursing diagnosis:** Risk for ineffective (cerebral) tissue perfusion related to increase ICP, alteration in blood flow secondary to hemorrhage, vessel malformation, cerebral edema.
   Goal: Child will be able to exhibit adequate cerebral tissue perfusion.
   Interventions: Promoting adequate tissue perfusion.
   - *Assess neurologic status closely, monitor for signs and symptoms of increased ICP:* Changes in level of consciousness, signs of irritability or lethargy, changes in papillary reaction can indicate decreased cerebral tissue perfusion
   - *Monitor vital signs:* Decreased pulse and respiratory rate and increased blood pressure of pulse pressure can indicate ICP, which can lead to decreased cerebral perfusion
   - *Measure specific gravity of urine:* Can detect an over secretion or under secretion of anti-diuretic hormone
   - *Have emergency equipment ready and available:* Decreased cerebral perfusion can result in respiratory or cardiac failure
   - *Notify physician immediately if changes in assessment are noted:* Early intervention is critical to prevent neurologic damage and death.

   Evaluation: Child remains alert and oriented with no signs of altered level of consciousness; vital signs within parameters for age; motor, sensory and cognitive function within parameters for age; head circumference within parameters for age.

3. **Nursing diagnosis:** Risk for injury related to altered level of consciousness, weakness, dizziness, ataxia, loss of muscle coordination secondary to seizure activity.
   Goal: Child will be free from injury.
   Interventions: Preventing injury.
   - Ensure child has patent airway and adequate oxygenation (have suction, oxygen available at bedside) and place child in side-lying position if possible; a child with altered level of consciousness may not be able to manage the secretions and is at risk for aspiration and ineffective airway clearance, providing suction and oxygenation can help ensure an open airway and the side-lying position can help secretions drain and prevent obstruction of airway or aspiration
   - Protect child from hurting self during seizure or changes in level of consciousness by removing environment obstacles, easing child to lying position, and padding side rails; helps to keep environment safe
   - Institute seizure precautions for any child at risk for seizure activity; to help prevent injury that can result from acute seizure activity
   - With seizure activity do not insert a tongue blade or restrain child: can lead to injury to caregiver and child

- *Administer anticonvulsant medications as ordered:* Will help to promote cessation and prevention of seizure activity
- *Assist child with ambulation:* Help prevent injury in child with weakness, dizziness and ataxia
- *Allow for periods of rest:* To prevent fatigue and decrease risk of injury.

Evaluation: Child is free of injury as evidenced by no signs of aspiration or traumatic injury.

4. **Nursing diagnosis:** Disturbed sensory perception related to presence of neurologic lesion or pressure on sensory or motor nerves secondary to increased ICP, presence of tumor, swelling postoperatively as evidenced by visual disturbances (i.e. reports of double vision), pupillary changes, nystagmus, ataxia, balance disturbances or loss of response to stimuli.
   Goal: Child will be free of changes in sensory perception.
   Interventions: Managing disturbed sensory perception.
   - *Assess for changes in sensory perception:* Provides baseline data and allows nurse to recognize change in sensory perception early
   - *Monitor child for risk of injury secondary to changes in sensory perception:* Visual changes, disturbances of gait or balance increase child's risk for injury
   - *Notify physician of changes in sensory perception:* Can indicate increased ICP and medical emergency
   - Assist child to learn to use adaptive methods to live with permanent changes in sensory perception (i.e., use of eyeglasses) and maximize the use of intact senses; adaptive devices can enhance sensory input and intact senses can often compensate for impaired senses
   - *Provide familiar sounds (voices, music):* Can help relieve anxiety related to changes in sensory perception, especially visual changes.

   Evaluation: No complaints of double vision, no disturbances of gait or balance noted, and no increased in loss of responses to stimuli.

5. **Nursing diagnosis:** Risk for infection related to surgical interventions, presence of foreign body (i.e. shunt), trauma to skull, nutritional deficiencies, stasis of pulmonary secretions and urine. Presence of infectious organisms as evidenced by fever, poor feeding, decreased responsiveness and presence of virus or bacteria on laboratory screening.
   Goal: Child will be free from signs or symptoms of local or systemic infection.
   Interventions: Preventing infection.
   - *Monitor vital signs:* Elevation in temperature can indicate presence of infection
   - *Monitor incision sites for signs of local infection:* Redness, warmth, drainage, swelling, pain at incision site can indicate presence of infection
   - *Maintain aseptic technique:* Practice good hand washing, use proper technique when managing postoperative incisions and external shunts to prevent introduction of further infectious agents
   - *Administer antibiotics as prescribed:* To prevent or treat bacterial infection
   - *Encourages nutritious diet and proper hydration according to child's preferences and ability to feed orally:* To assist body's natural defenses against infection
   - *Isolation of child as required:* To prevent nosocomial spread of infection
   - Teach child and family preventive measures such as good hand washing, covering mouth and nose upon cough or sneeze, adequate disposal of used tissues: to prevent nosocomial or community spread of infection.

Evaluation: Child exhibited no signs or symptoms of local or systemic infection and did not spread infection to others, symptoms of infection decreased over time and others remained free of infection.

6. **Nursing diagnosis:** Self-care deficit related to neuromuscular impairments; cognitive deficits as evidenced by an inability to perform hygiene care and transfer self independently.
   Goal: Child will be able to care for self within age parameters.
   Interventions: Maximizing self-care.
   - *Introduce child and family to self-help methods as soon as possible:* Promotes independence from the beginning
   - *Encourage family and staff to allow child to do as much as possible:* Allows child to gain confidence and independence
   - *Teach specific measures for bowel and urinary elimination as needed:* Promotes independence, increases self-care abilities and self-esteem
   - Collaborate with physical therapy, occupational therapy, and speech therapy departments to provide child and family with appropriate tools to modify environment and methods *to promote transferring and self-care:* Allows for maximum functioning
   - *Praise accomplishments and emphasize child's abilities:* Helps improve self-esteem and encourages feeling of confidence and competence
   - *Balance activity with periods to rest:* To reduce fatigue and increase energy for self-care.

   Evaluation: Child is able to feed, dress, manage elimination within limits of disease and age.

7. **Nursing diagnosis:** Impaired physical mobility related to muscle weakness, hypertonicity, impaired coordination, loss of muscle function or control as evidenced by an inability to move extremities, to ambulate without assistance, to move without limitations.
   Goal: Child will be able to engage in activities within age parameters.
   Interventions: Maximizing physical mobility.
   - *Encourage gross and fine motor activities:* Facilitates motor development
   - *Collaborate with physical therapy, occupational therapy, and speech therapy departments to strengthen muscles and promote optimal mobility:* Facilities motor development
   - *Utilize passive and active range of motion (ROM) and teach child and family how to perform:* Prevent contractures, facilitate joint mobility and muscle development (active ROM) to help increase mobility
   - *Praise accomplishments and emphasize child's abilities:* Helps improve self-esteem and encourages feeling of confidence and competence.

   Evaluation: Child is able to move extremities, move about environment and participate in exercise programs within limits of age and disease.

8. **Nursing diagnosis:** Risk for delayed development related to physical disability, cognitive deficits, activity restrictions.
   Goal: Child will be able to demonstrate developmental milestones within age parameters.
   Interventions: Maximizing development.
   - *Use therapeutic play and adaptive toys:* Helps facilitate developmental functioning
   - *Provide stimulating environment when possible:* To maximize potential for growth and development
   - *Praise accomplishments and emphasize child's abilities:* Helps improve self-esteem and encourages feeling of confidence and competence.

Evaluation: Child expressed interest in the environment and people around him or her, and interacts with environment age appropriately.

9. **Nursing diagnosis:** Nutrition, imbalanced; less than body requirements related to vomiting and difficulty feeding secondary to increased ICP; difficulty sucking, swallowing, or chewing; surgical incision pain or difficulty assuming normal feeding position; inability to feed self as evidenced by decreased oral intake, impaired swallowing, weight loss.
   Goal: Child will be able to exhibit signs of adequate nutrition.
   Interventions: Promoting adequate nutrition.
   - Monitor height and weight; insufficient intake will lead to impaired growth and weight gain
   - *Monitor hydration status (moist mucous membranes, elastic skin turgor and adequate urine output):* Insufficient intake can lead to dehydration
   - *Use techniques to promote caloric and nutritional intake and teach family (i.e., positioning, modified utensils, soft or blended foods, allow extra time):* These techniques can facilitate intake
   - *Assess respiratory system frequently:* To assess for aspiration
   - *Monitor for nausea and vomiting and medicate if ordered:* To help reduce vomiting and increase intake
   - *Monitor for pain and medicate if ordered:* To help reduce pain related to surgical incisions and trauma, and increase intake
   - *Assist family to assume as normal a feeding position as possible:* To help increase oral intake.

   Evaluation: Weight remained within parameters for age, skin turgor good, vomiting ceased or decreased.

10. **Nursing diagnosis:** Fluid volume deficit, risk for, related to vomiting, altered level of consciousness, poor feeding or intake, insensible loss due to fever, failure of regulatory mechanisms (as in diabetes insipidus) as evidenced by dry oral mucosa, decreased skin turgor, sudden weight loss, hypotension and tachycardia.
    Goal: Fluid volume will be maintained and balanced.
    Interventions: Promoting adequate fluid balance.
    - *Administer IV fluids if ordered:* To maintain adequate hydration in children who are nil per orals (NPO) or unable to tolerate oral intake
    - *When oral intake is allowed and tolerated, encourage per orals (PO) fluids:* To promote intake and maintain hydration
    - *Strict intake and output monitoring:* Can help identify fluid imbalance and also detect signs of abnormal pituitary secretions resulting in conditions like syndrome of inappropriate anti-diuretic hormone secretion (SIADH) and diabetes insipidus (DI).
    - *Maintain minimum hydration and avoid over hydration in clients, where cerebral edema is a concern:* Fluid overload can contribute to cerebral edema
    - *Urine specific gravity, urine and serum electrolytes (especially serum sodium), blood urea nitrogen, creatinine and osmolality, and daily weights:* Are reliable indicators of fluid status and can also detect signs of abnormal pituitary secretions resulting in conditions like SIADH and DI.

Evaluation: Oral mucosa moist and pink, skin turgor elastic, urine output reached to 1–2 cc/kg/h.

11. **Nursing diagnosis:** Knowledge deficit related to lack of information regarding complex medical condition, prognosis, and medical needs as evidenced by verbalization, questions, or actions demonstrating lack of understanding regarding child's condition or care.
    Goal: Child and family will be able to verbalize accurate information and understanding about condition, prognosis and medical needs.
    Interventions: Providing client and family teaching.
    - *Assess child's and family's willingness to learn:* Child and family must be willing to learn for teaching to be effective
    - *Provide family with time to adjust to diagnosis:* Will help facilitate adjustment and ability to learn and participate in child's care
    - *Repeat information:* Allows family and child time to learn and understand
    - *Teach in short session:* Many short sessions are found to be more helpful than one long session
    - *Give teaching to a level of understanding of the child and also the family (depends on age of child, physical condition and memory):* To ensure understanding
    - *Provide reinforcement and rewards:* Help facilitate the teaching-learning process
    - *Use multiple modes of learning involving many senses (provide written, verbal, demonstration and videos) when possible:* Child and family more likely to retain information when presented in different ways using many senses.
    Evaluation: Child and family verbalized regarding knowledge of condition and prognosis and medical needs including possible causes, contributing factors and treatment measures.

12. **Nursing diagnosis:** Family processes, interrupted related to child's illness, hospitalization, diagnosis of chronic illness in child and potential long-term effects of illness as evidenced by family's presence in hospital, missed work, demonstration of inadequate coping.
    Goal: Family will be able to maintain adequate coping, adaptation of roles and function, and decreased anxiety.
    Interventions: Promoting adequate family processes.
    - *Encourage parents and family members to verbalize concerns related to child's illness, diagnosis and prognosis:* Allows the nurse to identify concerns and areas where further education may be needed. Demonstrates family-centered care
    - Explain therapies, procedures, child's behaviors and plan of care to parents; understanding the child's current status and plan of care helps decrease anxiety
    - *Encourage parental involvement in care:* Allow parents to feel needed and valued with a sense of control over their child's health
    - *Identify support system for family and child:* Helps nurse identify needs and resources available for coping
    - *Educate family and child on additional resources available:* To help them develop a wide base of support.
    Evaluation: Parents are involved in child's care, ask appropriate questions, express fears and concerns, and are able to discuss child's care and condition calmly.

NURSING PROCESS FOR SPECIFIC NEUROLOGICAL DISORDERS

Hydrocephalus

Hydrocephalus is the enlargement of the intracranial cavity caused by the accumulation of cerebrospinal fluid in the ventricular system. This results from an imbalance in the production and absorption of the fluid, causing an increase in intracranial pressure as the fluid builds up. Fluid may accumulate as a result of blockage of the flow (non-communicating hydrocephalus) or impaired absorption (communicating hydrocephalus). In the infant, as the head enlarges to an abnormal size, he experiences lethargy, changes in level of consciousness, and lower extremity spasticity and opisthotonos. If the hydrocephalus is allowed to progress, the infant experiences difficulty in sucking and feeding, as well as emesis, seizures sunset eyes, and cardiopulmonary complications, as lower brainstem and cortical function are disrupted or destroyed. In the child, increased intracranial pressure (ICP) focal manifestations that are experienced related to space-occupying focal lesions include headaches, emesis, ataxia, irritability, lethargy, and confusion. Treatment may include surgery to provide shunting for drainage of the excess fluid from the ventricles to an extra-cranial space such as the peritoneum or right atrium (in older children). ICP, if progression of the disease is slow or surgery is contraindicated, ICP may be reduced or managed with medications **(Fig. 12.1)**.

Symptoms of Hydrocephalus

The signs and symptoms of hydrocephalus vary generally by age of onset:

Infants

Common signs and symptoms of hydrocephalus in infants include:
- An unusually large head
- A rapid increase in the size of the head
- A bulging or tense soft spot (fontanel) on the top of the head
- Vomiting
- Sleepiness
- Irritability
- Poor feeding
- Seizures
- Eyes fixed downward (sun setting of the eyes)
- Deficits in muscle tone and strength, responsiveness to touch, and expected growth.

Toddlers and Older Children

Among toddlers and older children, signs and symptoms may include:
- Abnormal enlargement of a toddler's head
- Headache
- Nausea or vomiting
- Fever
- Delays in walking or talking
- Problems with previously acquired skills, such as walking or talking

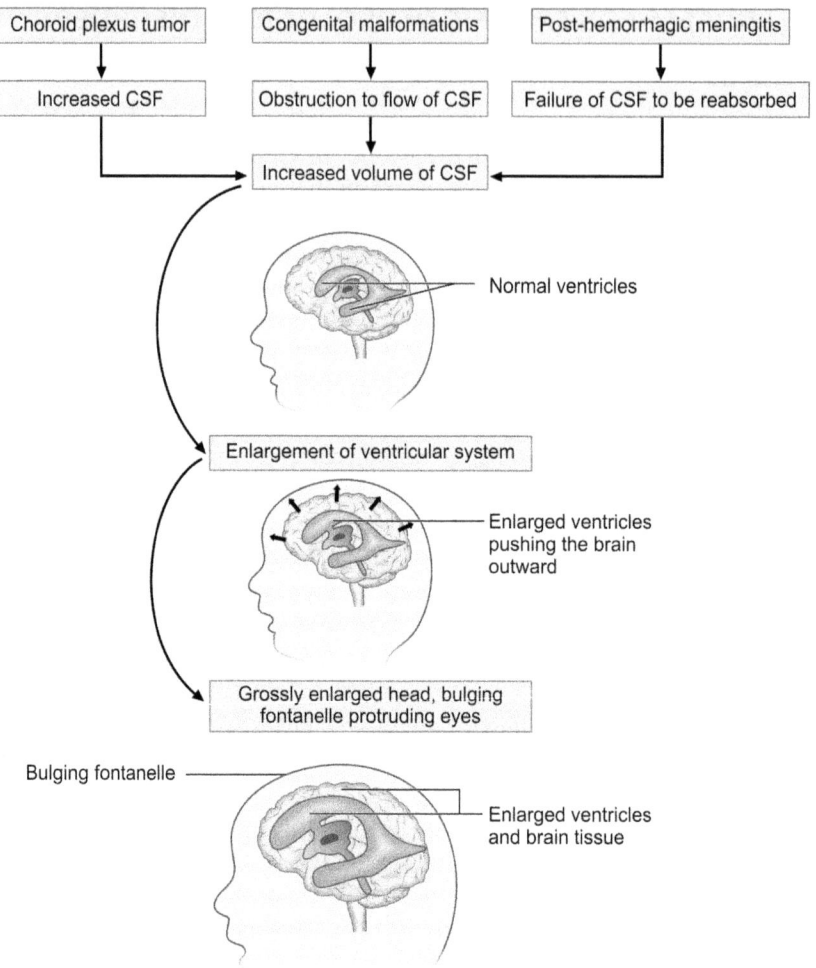

Fig. 12.1: Pathophysiology of hydrocephalus.

- Blurred or double vision
- Unstable balance
- Poor coordination
- Irritability
- Change in personality
- Problems with attention
- Decline in school performance
- Poor appetite
- Seizures
- Sleepiness
- Difficulty remaining awake or waking up.

Young and Middle-aged Adults

Common signs and symptoms in this age group include:
- Headache
- Difficulty in remaining awake or waking up
- Loss of coordination or balance
- Loss of bladder control or a frequent urge to urinate
- Impaired vision
- Decline in memory, concentration and other thinking skills that may affect job performance.

Nursing Management

A. Essential Nursing Diagnoses and Nursing Process Associated with this Condition

Nursing diagnosis

Fluid volume excess related to compromised regulatory mechanism shunt placement—ventriculoatrial **(Table 12.1)**.
Assessment: Decreased cardiac output, change in respiratory pattern, tachycardia, tachypnea, dyspnea, weight gain, chest pain, cardiac arrhythmias, pulmonary congestion.
(Refer Table 14.9 from chapter 14)

Nursing diagnosis

High-risk for fluid volume deficit related to excessive losses through normal routes.
Assessment: Postoperative vomiting or diarrhea, use of diuretics, altered intake, thirst, dry skin and mucous membranes.
(Refer Table 14.11 from chapter 14)

Nursing diagnosis

Altered nutrition: Less than body requirements related to inability to ingest food/feedings.
Assessment: Advanced stage of hydrocephalus, postoperative vomiting, NPO status.
(Refer Table 14.3 from chapter 14)

Nursing diagnosis

High-risk for impaired skin integrity related to physical immobilization and external factor of pressure **(Table 12.1)**.
Assessment: Decreased movement of head, disruption of skin surface by surgical procedure (shunt insertion) or diagnostic procedure.

Evaluation
- Absence of skin impairment with intactness maintained
- Skin and mucous membranes free of inflammation, irritation, infection
- Skin breakdown or wound healing in progress
- Prevents or reduces pressure on skin
- Maintains appliances, devices, prosthesis, cast within parameters to safeguard skin integrity
- Provides nutritional, fluid requirements for skin healing and integrity
- Maintains skin, hair, nail cleanliness
- Provides protective measures, devices and topical applications to ensure skin and mucous membrane integrity

Table 12.1: Nursing interventions for high-risk for impaired skin integrity.

Interventions	Rationales
Assess skin and mucous membranes for color changes, warmth, dryness, firmness, swelling or edema, lesions or breaks, and infection or inflammation of the oral cavity, nose, eyes, ears and scalp	Provides information about potential for disruption of skin integrity in any part of the body to ensure identification and intervention before impairment becomes too severe or extensive
Assess mobility status, ability to move in bed, use of restraints and length of time restraint used, enforced bed rest as part of medical regimen, presence of any immobilization device	Reveals ability for movement, external factors that produce pressure leading to skin breakdown as circulation of oxygen and nutrients is reduced
Assess for any skin rashes, dermatitis, pruritus and scratching	Reveals skin conditions that lead to impairment
Assess for open wounds and type of drainage (serosanguineous or purulent), peristomal skin, diarrhea and effect on perianal area, diaper rash from prolonged exposure to ammonia from urine decomposition	Reveals presence of secretions and excretions that lead to skin impairment especially in infants and young children who have thinner, more sensitive skin
Assess skin under cast edges, tightness of cast, color and sensation in toes or fingers, redness and discomfort under any immobilization or assistive (prosthetic) device caused by improper fit	Reveals skin impairment causes and neurocirculatory effects of cast, splint, brace application
Assess nutritional and hydration status including dehydration or fluid imbalances and obesity or emaciation with muscle wasting and weakness	Reveals information regarding ability to maintain healthy skin and mucous membranes with proper nutrition and circulation to tissues and the preservation of muscle mass and strength needed to pad bony prominences and allow movement and position change
Assess effect of radiation therapy, presence and extent of burns, chemotherapy on skin and mucous membranes and areas of vulnerability	Provides rationale for preventive measures to treat risk for burns, stomatitis, impairment, and infection caused by immunosuppression
Assess skin cleanliness and examine bony prominences for changes, condition of hair and nails, use of cleansing products, and skin response; include assessment of effect of contact allergens that cause skin changes	Provides information about removal of dirt, irritants, bacteria, sweat, urine, feces to promote skin integrity and offers an assessment opportunity
Provide bathing in bed, tub, or shower; use warm water and mild soap and rinse well, with a soft towel pat dry and (avoid rubbing) including all folds, crevices, and creases	Promotes health and cleanliness of skin, reduces accumulation of body secretions and excretions, and reduces bacteria in skin folds where bacterial growth is enhanced
Provide careful cleansing of eyes with either warm, sterile water or saline and soft cloth from inner to outer aspect of eye; nasal mucosa with warm water and application of a protective lubricant; oral mucosa with a peroxide solution mouthwash	Promotes intact mucous membranes from irritation and breakdown caused by pressure or inflammation from tubes or by sanctioning, chemotherapy, or NPO status: rapidly dividing epithelial tissue of oral and nasal mucosa leads to breakdown when receiving chemotherapeutic agents

Contd...

Contd...

Interventions	Rationales
Provide hair shampooing, nail trimming as needed; cut nails straight across with round-tipped scissors; dry hair well with hair dryer, rubbing gently with soft towel	Promotes cleanliness and prevents skin irritation or break caused by scratching with long nails
Apply emollients, lotions to skin, bony prominences with gentle massage using fingers and/or hands	Protects and softens skin and promotes circulation to vulnerable parts
Apply skin adhesive barrier to peristomal area including tracheotomy, urinary or bowel diversion and over bony prominences, if immobilized or too weak or ill to move in bed	Protects skin that is exposed to secretions and excretion or pressure
Provide position change q12h as indicated with prone, supine, side or elevated position utilized; if child is able, encourage to change positions on own	Prevents prolonged pressure on any one area leading to skin and tissue breakdown
Maintain body alignment and encourage to maintain correct posture when sitting, lying, and walking	Promotes even pressure on body parts
Pad bony prominences and susceptible parts with sheepskin, foam rubber, pillows, alternating pads and mattress, special apparatus such as stryker frame	Protects vulnerable parts from pressure and redistributes weight and improves circulation
Maintain tight, wrinkle free linens and bed free of crumbs, sharp toys, and dampness from urine or feces	Prevents irritation and excoriation of skin
Correct tight dressings by loosening tape, correct dry and sticking dressings with saline solution before removing, secure tubing away from skin contact, correct fit of any prosthesis or immobilization device, petal edges of cast with soft adhesive material	Reduces external sources of pressure that decrease circulation or irritate skin
Apply topical skin medications (ointments, solutions) as ordered; bathe or soak area or extremity	Promotes healing and prevents infection
Provide bath with oatmeal or other emollients, mitts on hands, temporary soft restraints as needed	Soothes pruritus and prevents scratching
Provide nutritional diet that is high in protein and calories and includes vitamins A and C	Promotes tissue healing with synthesis of protein to meet metabolic needs and information of collagen and connective tissue by vitamins A and C
If wound present, provide dressing change, irrigations, debridement, wet or dry dressing, opsite as indicated specific to wound	Promotes healing and prevents infection and further skin breakdown

- Maintains body alignment and body posture conducive to preventing skin breakdown
- Provides effective wound care and dressing change without contamination of site
- Complies with medical regimen to treat any skin eruption or destruction to tissues.

Nursing diagnosis

Hyperthermia related to illness (infection).
Assessment: Increase in body temperature above normal range.
(Refer Table 14.18 from chapter 14)

Nursing diagnosis

Altered growth and development related to effects of disorder or disability.
Assessment: Altered physical growth; mental retardation; delay or difficulty in performing motor, social skills typical of age; dependence.
(Refer Table 14.4 from chapter 14)

B. Specific Nursing Diagnoses and Nursing Process

Nursing diagnosis

Anxiety of parent(s) and child related to threat to or change in health status, threat to or change in environment (hospitalization) **(Table 12.2)**.

Table 12.2: Nursing interventions for anxiety of parent(s) and child.

Interventions	Rationales
Assess source and level of anxiety and need for information and support about condition and impending surgery	Provides information about severity of anxiety and need for interventions and support; allows for identification of fear and uncertainty about condition and/or surgery, treatments, and recovery; guilt about condition, possible loss of infant/child or of parental role and responsibility; children with this condition are often disable with intellectual deficits
Allow expressions of concerns and opportunity to ask questions about condition and recovery of ill infant/child	Provides opportunity to vent feelings, secure information needed to reduce anxiety
Communicate with parent(s) and answer questions calmly and honestly	Promotes calm and supportive environment
Encourage parent(s) to remain calm and involved in care and decision making regarding infant/child, noting any improvement that results	Promotes constant monitoring of infant/child for improvement of worsening of symptoms
Allow parent(s) to stay with infant/child or visit when able if hospitalized, and to assist in care (hold, feed, diaper) and suggestions for routines and methods of treatment	Allows parent(s) to care for and support child instead of becoming increasingly anxious due to absence from child and wondering about infant/child's condition
If surgery planned, answer all questions from parent(s) and child with honesty and hope; refer to physician for answers and explanations if needed	Promotes supportive environment and reduces anxiety caused by fear of unknown

Nursing Process for the Child with Neurological Disorder

Assessment: Increased apprehension that condition of infant might worsen or condition may develop in child as a complication, expressed concern and worry about preoperative preparation and the surgical procedure, concern about possible or actual physical, neurological, and mental deficits.

Evaluation
- Expression of reduction in anxiety about condition, therapy and prognosis
- Participates in care and decision making regarding infant/child
- Verbalizes positive effect of caring for and supporting infant/child
- Visits or telephones, if unable to stay
- Verbalizes understanding of surgical procedure and preoperative care
- Participates in infant/child care following surgery
- Utilizes social services, counseling services, clergy for support.

Nursing diagnosis

High-risk for injury related to internal factors of sensory, integrative, and effector dysfunction preoperatively **(Table 12.3)**.

Table 12.3: Nursing interventions for high-risk for injury related to internal factors of sensory, integrative, and effector dysfunction preoperatively.

Interventions	Rationales
Assess for rapidly increased circumference of head, tense, bulging fontanels, widening suture lines, irritability; lethargy, "cracked pot" sound on percussion, sunset sign, opisthotonos, spasticity of lower extremities, seizures	Indicates in increasing ICP in infant/small child
Assess vomiting, papilledema, ataxia, irritability, lethargy, apathy, confusion, change in level of consciousness, headache, cranial nerve palsies, spinal cord dysfunction with upper extremity spasticity	Indicates increasing ICP in children with symptoms related to cause of hydrocephalus
Perform neurologic and vital sign assessment q4h or as needed	Provides data indicating an increasing ICP, which causes decreased respirations, increase in blood pressure and pulse
Position with head elevated to 30° and support head when handling or changing position. Monitor skin integrity with position change	Promotes drainage of and reduces accumulation of CSF; infant may not be able to lift and move head
Carry out seizure precautions, such as crib/bed padding, remove toys and objects from bed, maintain suction and oxygen at bedside, and note and report characteristics of seizure	Prevents injury to self during seizures caused by increased ICP, and facilitates treatment of apnea during seizure activity
Support an enlarged head by cradling it in an arm when holding, place infant on a pillow when moving, move head and body of infant at the same time	Protects infant's head from trauma and neck from strain

Nursing Process for the Child with Neurological Disorder

Table 12.4: Nursing interventions for high-risk for injury related to internal factor of shunt placement and potential complications of shunt functioning.

Interventions	Rationales
Assess for signs and symptoms of increased ICP, swelling along shunt tract	Provides data that indicates shunt malfunction
Pump device by compressing reservoir or antechamber of the valve mechanisms, which forces fluid into the catheter, with fluid moving out of the chamber if catheter is patent; perform only if ordered by surgeon, and notify physician if pump refilling cannot be felt with finger	Test for shunt patency; relieve pressure by flushing and pumping valve; the correct valve pressure prevents too rapid ICP reduction
Note vomiting, drowsiness, irritability, swelling at pump site; redness, exudate, and temperature of child	Indicates shunt blockage
Position on nonoperative side and maintain on complete bed rest for 1–3 days, elevate head and shoulders, if ordered	Maintains proper functioning of shunt

Assessment: Neuromuscular, neurosensory, and behavioral changes; increased ICP; CSF accumulation; vital signs changes; seizure activity.

Evaluation
- Identification of signs and symptoms of increasing ICP
- Maintains stable neurologic status
- Prevents injury resulting from seizure activity or positioning of enlarged head
- Complies with follow-up care and visits to physician and other professionals.

Nursing diagnosis

High-risk for injury related to internal factor of shunt placement and potential complications of shunt functioning **(Table 12.4)**.

Assessment: Increased ICP, kinking or plugging of shunt tubing, separation of tubing, changing of position of tubing, obstruction of shunt, displacement with growth.

Evaluation
- Absence of shunt malfunction
- Recognizes signs and symptoms of increased ICP and shunt malfunction
- Monitors pump for patency
- Maintains and supports postoperative measures to ensure success of surgery and decrease infection
- Maintains follow-up appointments with physician and diagnostic procedures to monitor condition and shunt function.

Nursing diagnosis

High-risk for infection related to invasive procedure of shunt insertion **(Table 12.5)**.

Assessment: Elevated temperature, swelling, redness at shunt tract or operative site, nausea, vomiting, lethargy, excessive drainage on dressing, poor feeding.

Nursing Process for the Child with Neurological Disorder

Table 12.5: Nursing interventions for high-risk for infection.

Interventions	Rationales
Assess site for inflammatory process, temperature for elevation, WBC for increases, characteristics of drainage on dressings	Provides data indicating presence or potential for infection, which affects shunt function
Follow principles of asepsis when performing procedures like dressing changes	Prevents transmission of microorganisms to shunt site
Monitor temperature q4h	Elevation of temperature indicates infection
Avoid positioning head on valve site for at least 2 days postoperatively	Alleviates the risk of infection

Evaluation
- Measures taken to prevent infection
- Preventive antibiotics administered for 2 days postoperatively
- Protects site and shunt from contamination and trauma
- Absence of infection leading to shunt malfunction and externalization of shunt.

Intracranial Tumor

A brain tumor is a solid tumor that may be benign, malignant, or a metastatic growth from a tumor in another part of the body. Most central nervous system tumors occur in the cerebellum or brainstem, causing increased intracranial pressure and the symptoms associated with it. Other tumors occur in the cerebrum. Brain tumors are most prevalent in children, 3–7 years of age. A malignant brain tumor is the second most common type of cancer in children. It has a poor prognosis, because the tumor is the second most common type of cancer in children. It has a poor prognosis, because the tumor usually enlarges to an advanced stage before signs and symptoms, which are easily missed, are detected. Signs and symptoms are site and size dependent. Treatment includes surgery, although total removal is not usually possible; or chemotherapy and radiation, which may decrease the size of the tumor before surgery. One or a combination of these procedures may be tried, with each resulting in possible residual neurologic deficits **(Fig. 12.2)**.

Symptoms of an Intracranial Tumor

The following are the most common symptoms of a brain tumor. However, each child may experience symptoms differently. Symptoms vary depending on size and location of tumor. Many symptoms are related to increase in pressure in or around the brain. There is no spare space in the skull for anything except the delicate tissues of the brain and its fluid. Any tumor, extra tissue, or fluid can cause pressure on the brain and result in the following symptoms:

Increased intracranial pressure (ICP)—caused by extra tissue or fluid in the brain. Pressure may increase because one or more of the ventricles that drain cerebrospinal fluid (CSF, the fluid that surrounds the brain and spinal cord) has been blocked, causing the fluid to be trapped in the brain. Increased ICP can cause the following:
- Headache
- Nausea
- Personality changes

Nursing Process for the Child with Neurological Disorder

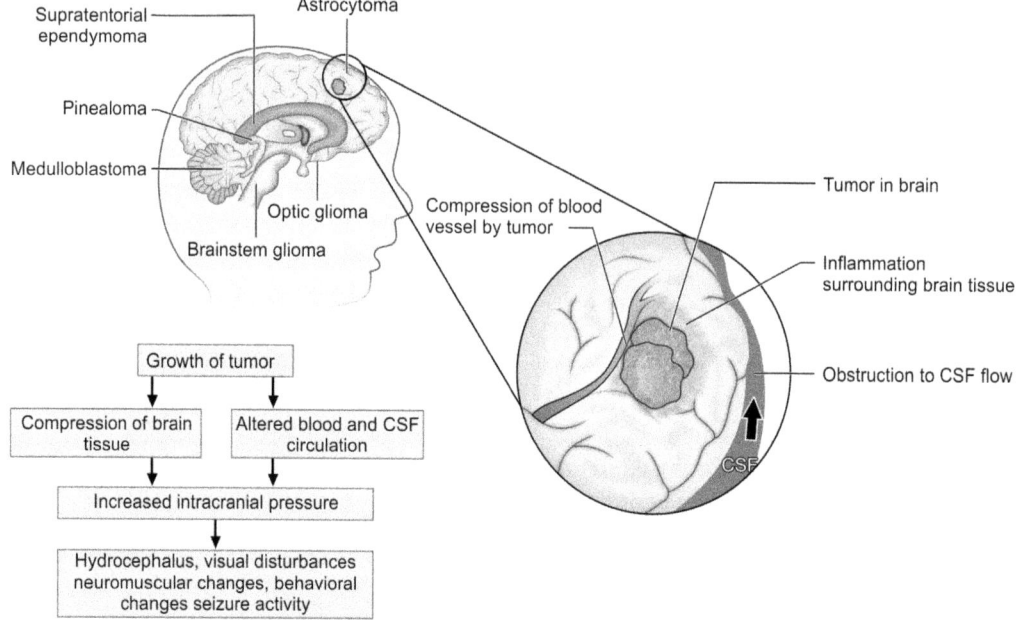

Fig. 12.2: Pathophysiology of intracranial tumors.

- Irritability
- Drowsiness
- Depression
- Decreased cardiac and respiratory function and eventually coma if not treated.

Symptoms vary depending upon which part of the brain the tumor found

Symptoms of brain tumors in the cerebrum (front of brain):
- Seizures
- Visual changes
- Slurred speech
- Paralysis or weakness on behalf of the body or face
- Increased intracranial pressure (ICP)
- Drowsiness or confusion
- Personality changes.

Symptoms of brain tumors in the brainstem (middle of brain):
- Seizures
- Endocrine problems (diabetes or hormone regulation)
- Visual changes or double vision
- Headaches
- Paralysis of nerves/muscles of the face or half of the body
- Respiratory changes
- Increased intracranial pressure (ICP).

Symptoms of brain tumors in the cerebellum (back of brain):
- Increased intracranial pressure (ICP)
- Vomiting (usually occurs in the morning without nausea)
- Headache
- Uncoordinated muscle movements
- Problems walking (ataxia).

Nursing Management

A. Essential Nursing Diagnoses and Nursing Process Associated with this Condition

Nursing diagnosis

Hyperthermia related to illness.

Assessment: Increase in body temperature above normal range, presence of infection (meningitis or upper respiratory), surgical procedure (anesthesia, brainstem, or hypothalamus area).
(Refer Table 14.18 from chapter 14)

Nursing diagnosis

Sleep pattern disturbance related to sensory alternations caused by internal factors of illness.

Assessment: Lethargy, restlessness, irritability, disorientation, coma, frequent napping.
(Refer Table 14.10 from chapter 14)

Nursing diagnosis

High-risk for fluid volume deficit related to excessive losses through normal routes.

Assessment: Vomiting, altered intake, diuresis with use of diuretic, diabetes insipidus, thirst, dry skin and mucous membranes.
(Refer Table 14.11 from chapter 14)

Nursing diagnosis

Altered nutrition: Less than body requirements related to inability to ingest food.

Assessment: Vomiting, nausea, choking and possible aspiration with facial paralysis or edema, refusal to eat or drink, gavage feedings, depressed gag reflex.
(Refer Table 14.3 from chapter 14)

Nursing diagnosis

Impaired physical mobility related to neuromuscular impairment.

Assessment: Inability to purposefully move within physical environment, impaired coordination, loss of balance, decreased muscle strength and control, spasticity, hypo or hyperreflexia, paralysis, general weakness, ataxia following surgery.
(Refer Table 14.19 from chapter 14)

Nursing diagnosis

Altered growth and development related to effects of disorder or disability following surgery/other therapy.

Nursing Process for the Child with Neurological Disorder

Table 12.6: Nursing interventions for pain.

Interventions	Rationales
Assess severity and length of headache, recurrence, progressive characteristics, and precipitating factors	Provides information regarding presence of tumor since headache is most common symptom in child
Administer analgesic to treat, or anticipate headache based on assessment	Relieves headache and promotes rest and comfort
Provide toys, games for quiet play	Provides diversional activity to detract from pain
Apply cool compress to head for low to moderate pain	Provides comfort and relief from headache

Assessment: Delay or difficulty in performing skills typical of age group (motor, social, or expressive), inability to perform self-control activities appropriate for age behavior and/or intellectual deficits, presence of somnolence syndrome.
(Refer Table 14.4 from chapter 14)

B. Specific Nursing Diagnoses and Nursing Process
Nursing diagnosis

Pain related to biologic injuring agents **(Table 12.6)**.

Assessment: Verbal descriptor of pain, headache in frontal or occipital area that is worse in the morning and becomes worse if head lowered or with straining, increased VS, restlessness, hostility, inability to relax.

Evaluation
- Pain is absent or relieved
- Complies with analgesic regimen to prevent or control headache
- Limits activities that initiate or increase headache
- Participates in quiet play.

Nursing diagnosis

High-risk for injury related to internal factors of sensory, integrative, and effector dysfunction **(Table 12.7)**.

Assessment: Neuromuscular, neurosensory, and behavioral changes; increased ICP; seizure activity; vital signs changes.

Evaluation
- Symptoms of brain tumor assessed and identifies
- Prepares for diagnostic and surgical procedures
- Maintains safe environment with absence of injury.

Nursing diagnosis

Anxiety of parent(s) and child related to change in health status and threat to self-concept **(Table 12.8)**.

Nursing Process for the Child with Neurological Disorder

Table 12.7: Nursing interventions for high-risk for injury related to internal factors of sensory, integrative and effector dysfunction.

Interventions	Rationales
Assess head circumference in the infant/small child for increases as fluid obstruction caused by tumor will increase head size	Provides data indicating an increase in ICP as tumor with a poorer prognosis, grows because tumor becomes large before diagnosis is made
Assess vital signs including increased BP; decreased pulse pressure, pulse and respirations; when monitoring pulse and respirations, take for 1 full minute	Provides changes indicating presence of brain tumor depending on type and location of tumor
Assess changes in gross and fine motor control, weakness, ataxia, spasticity, paralysis, changes in balance or coordination	Provides neuromuscular status changes indicating presence of brain tumor
Assess changes in vision (visual acuity, strabismus, diplopia, nystagmus), head tilt, papilledema	Provides changes in neurosensory status indicating presence of brain tumor
Assess for irritability, lethargy, loss of consciousness or coma, fatigue, napping	Provides behavior changes indicating presence of tumor
Assess for increased ICP including, for infant: irritability, poor feeding, vomiting, head enlargement, lethargy, high-pitched cry; and in child: vomiting, diplopia, behavioral changes, change in VS, seizure activity	Provides information about ICP changes caused by brain distortion or shifting caused by tumor
Alter environment by padding bed or crib, reduce light and stimulation	Prevents injury if seizure activity possible
Place in comfortable position with head elevated	Promotes comfort and decreases ICP by gravity

Table 12.8: Nursing interventions for anxiety of parent(s) and child.

Interventions	Rationales
Assess level of anxiety and need for information that will relieve anxiety following surgery	Provides information about degree of anxiety and need for interventions and support; allows for identification of fear and uncertainty about surgery, treatments, recovery, guilt about illness, possible loss of child, parental role and responsibility
Allow expression of concerns, and inquiries about condition of ill child, possible consequences, and prognosis	Provides opportunity to vent feelings, secures information needed to reduce anxiety
If surgery planned, answer all question from parent(s) and child with honesty	Promotes supportive environment
Allow parent(s) to stay with infant/child or open visitation; encourage participation in care of infant/child	Promotes care and support of child by parent(s)
If surgery planned, orient to special care unit, equipment, and staff	Reduces anxiety caused fear of unknown

Assessment: Increased apprehension as diagnosis is confirmed and condition worsens; expressed concern and worry about postoperative residual tumor and effects, hair removal before surgery, insomnia, social isolation.

Evaluation
- Expresses reduction in anxiety and adjustment to diagnosis and treatments
- Participates in care and supports infant/child
- Maintains child's self-concept and body image
- Asks questions, expresses concern about treatment and prognosis.

Guillain–Barré Syndrome

Guillain-Barré syndrome (infectious polyneuritis) is an acute inflammation of the spinal and cranial nerves manifested by motor dysfunction that predominates over sensory dysfunction. The disease most commonly occurs in children between 4 and 10 years of age. The actual cause is unknown, but it is associated with a previously existing viral infection or vaccine administration. Neurologic symptoms include muscle cramps and paresthesia, with weakness progressing to paralysis, the severity of the disease ranges from mild to severe, with the course of the disease dependent on the degree of paralysis present at the peak of the condition, recovery is usually complete and may take weeks or months. Treatment is symptom-dependent, with hospitalization required in the acute phase of the disease to observe and intervene for respiratory or swallowing complications **(Fig. 12.3)**.

Symptoms of Guillain–Barré Syndrome
- Decreased feeling or pain in fingers and toes
- Leg weakness or pain progressing to the arms
- Problems walking
- Irritability
- Breathing problems
- Facial weakness.

Nursing Management

A. Essential Nursing Diagnoses and Nursing Process Associated with this Condition

Nursing diagnosis

Decreased cardiac output related to effects of autonomic dysfunction on cardiac activity.

Assessment: Variations in homodynamic readings (tachycardia, bradycardia, hypotension, hypertension), decreased peripheral pulses, oliguria, cyanosis, pallor of skin and mucous membranes, ECG changes (arrhythmias), diaphoresis, dizziness, orthostatic hypotension.
(Refer Table 14.1 from chapter 14)

Nursing diagnosis

Ineffective breathing pattern related to neuromuscular impairment.
Assessment: Altered chest expansion, respiratory depth changes, cyanosis, abnormal ABG's.
(Refer Table 14.2 from chapter 14)

Nursing Process for the Child with Neurological Disorder

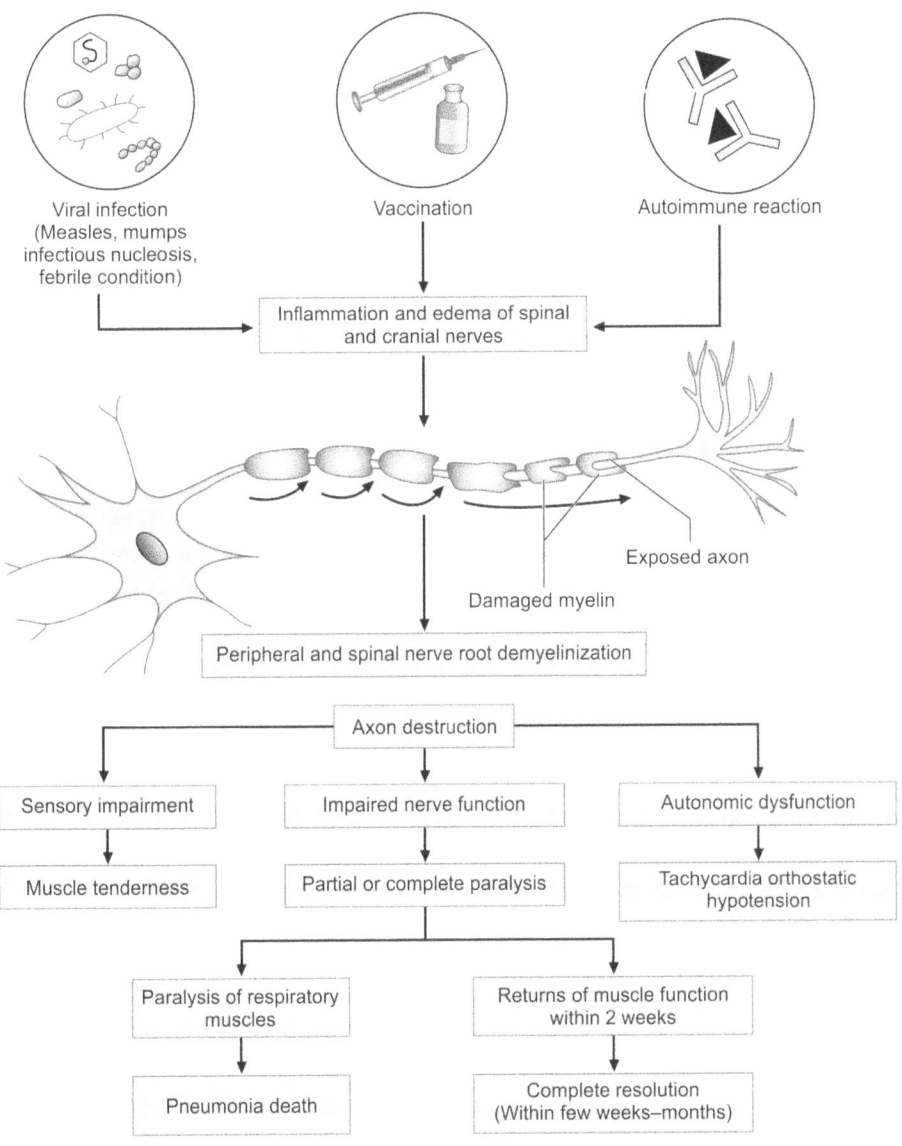

Fig. 12.3: Pathophysiology of Guillain–Barré (GB) syndrome.

Nursing diagnosis

Ineffective airway clearance related to tracheobronchial obstruction, secretions.

Assessment: Abnormal breath sounds (crackles, wheezes), changes in rate or depth of respiration, paralysis of chest muscles, tachypnea, cough, dyspnea, inability to clear secretions from airway, inability to swallow secretions, weakness in speech, gag reflex, aspiration.

(Refer Table 11.1 from chapter 11)

Nursing diagnosis

Altered nutrition: Less than body requirements related to inability to ingest food, absorb nutrients.

Assessment: Anorexia, diarrhea, weakness of chewing and swallowing muscles, dysesthesia of hands with inability to feed self, weight loss, loss of muscle tone, paralysis (ascending).
(Refer Table 14.3 from chapter 14)

Nursing diagnosis

Constipation related to neuromuscular impairment **(Table 12.9)**.
Assessment: Paralysis, hard formed stools, decreased bowel sounds.

Table 12.9: Nursing interventions for constipation.

Interventions	Rationales
Assess normal pattern of bowel elimination and characteristics of stool (frequency, amount, shape and consistency), presence of diseases or abnormalities of the bowel caused by congenital defects	Provides information that indicates baseline parameters for comparison; frequency varies among children depending on age and foods ingested but may be as few as 3–5/day in infant, as few as 6/week in child less than 3 years of age and as few as 4/week in older child; presence of constipation may be associated with disorders in children that lead to obstruction
Assess abdomen for hard mass or distention, measure abdominal girth, auscultate for bowel sounds that are diminished or absent	Indicates accumulation of stool in bowel or reduction in peristalsis
Assess for toilet training techniques, change in diet, change in environment	Provides information that may lead to reasons for constipation
Assess for intentional stool withholding, discomfort in defection, word the child uses to indicate need to defecate	Provides information about reason child might have for suppressing the urge to defecate
Assess parent(s) attitude about bowel habits and toilet training	Provides information about child's reaction to parental attitudes and may cause bowel elimination suppression
Provide privacy during bowel elimination	Promotes elimination by preserving privacy which a child considers important for a very private and intimate activity
Allow child to sit up during bowel elimination on a bedpan, if necessary or on a commode or toilet, if possible	Provides a normal position for easier bowel elimination
Encourage fluid intake and activity within limitations imposed by illness; add fiber, prune juice to diet	Provides fluid and exercise for bowel motility and prevents hard, dry stool if water is reabsorbed because of lack of fluids, bulk in stool provide by fiber in the diet promotes motility
Add sugar in formula of infant; administer stool softeners, suppositories or isotonic enema as ordered for child; explain procedure and what to expect to the child before administering	Promotes bowel evacuation when unable to control by fluids and diet; preparation by explanation encourages cooperation

Nursing Process for the Child with Neurological Disorder

Evaluation
- Absence of suppression of bowel elimination and relief of constipation
- Return of baseline bowel elimination pattern with soft formed stool
- Appropriate administration of oral or rectal relief measures
- Dietary, fluid and activity modifications for prevention of constipation or resolution of exiting constipation
- Modifies bowel elimination pattern to establish regularity and comfort.

Nursing diagnosis

Impaired physical mobility related to neuromuscular impairment.

Assessment: Paralysis, inability to purposefully move within physical environment, including bed mobility and transfer, ambulation, limited ROM, decreased muscle strength and control trauma from falls.
(Refer Table 14.19 from chapter 14)

Nursing diagnosis

Hyperthermia related to illness causing autonomic instability.

Assessment: Increase in body temperature above normal range or decrease below normal range, warm or cool to touch.
(Refer Table 14.18 from chapter 14)

B. Specific Nursing Diagnoses and Nursing Process

Nursing diagnosis

Altered urinary elimination patterns related to neuromuscular impairment **(Table 12.10)**.

Assessment: Paralysis, retention of urine.

Evaluation
- Maintains 1:0 ratio within baseline
- Promotes urinary elimination program
- Monitors presence of retention and reports to physician
- Absence of urinary retention and of signs of increased infection.

Nursing diagnosis

Pain related to biological injuring agent (inflammation of nerves) **(Table 12.11)**.

Table 12.10: Nursing interventions for altered urinary elimination pattern.

Interventions	Rationales
Assess continuing extent of paralysis and effect on urinary elimination	Provides information about effect of motor weakness, which travels upward from extremities
Assess 1:0 q4 8h and palpate bladder q2h: cloudy, foul-smelling urine	Provides monitoring for 1:0 ratio and presence of urinary retention (ITI as paralysis progress)
Provide urinary elimination rehabilitation program	Promotes urine elimination and return to normal pattern as soon as possible
Catheterize as last resort; maintain indwelling catheter if needed to maintain elimination	Relieves distention and retention

Nursing Process for the Child with Neurological Disorder

Table 12.11: Nursing interventions for pain.

Interventions	Rationales
Assess pain and ability to participate in activities	Provides information about degree of pain or presence of progressive paralysis
Reposition q2h; support extremities and maintain clean, comfortable bed with mattress and padding to bony prominences as needed	Promotes comfort and reduces risks for skin impairment
Administer analgesics based on pain assessment and respiratory status; evaluate effect	Eliminates or controls pain and promotes comfort
Apply moist heat to painful areas as ordered	Promotes circulation to area and relieves pain

Assessment: Communication of pain descriptors of discomfort in hand and feet, guarding behavior, alteration in muscle tone, autonomic responses of diaphoresis, VS changes.

Evaluation
- Absence of pain in extremities
- Control of pain sensation with proper use of analgesics
- Participates in ADL and other activities
- Distracts child from dwelling on pain.

Nursing diagnosis

Anxiety of parent(s) and child related to change in health status and threat to self-concept (Table 12.12).

Table 12.12: Nursing interventions for anxiety of parent(s) and child.

Interventions	Rationales
Assess source and level of anxiety, how anxiety is manifested, and need for information that will relieve it	Provides information about degree of anxiety and needed interventions; sources may include fear and uncertainty about treatment and recovery, guilt about presence of illness, fear of possible loss of parental role and responsibility while child hospitalized
Allow expression of concerns and opportunity to ask questions about child's condition and recovery	Provides opportunity to vent feelings, secure information needed to reduce anxiety
Communicate with parent(s) and child and answer questions calmly and honestly	Promotes supportive environment
Encourage parent(s) and child to note improvements resulting from treatments	Promotes positive attitude and optimistic look for recovery
Allow parent(s) to stay with child or open visitation and telephoning, and allow to assist in care of child	Allows for care and support of child which decreases anxiety is caused by absence and lack of knowledge about child's condition
Allow child to participate in own care depending on ability and/or paralysis; allow to make choices about ADL as soon as possible	Promotes independence and control, and preserves developmental status

Table 12.13: Nursing interventions for high-risk for altered parenting.

Interventions	Rationales
Assess for presence of permanent disability or possibility of long-term recovery and effect on parent(s)	Identifies factors associated with long recovery period
Encourage parent(s) to express feelings and unmet needs, and ability to meet and develop self-expectations	Identifies potential for social deprivation of parent(s) and development of strategies to achieve realistic expectations
Encourage touching and play activities between parent(s) and child	Enhances comfort and positive parental behaviors
Encourage and praise positive parental behaviors; support any participation in care or decision making on behalf of the child	Reduces anxiety for and enhances learning about child's needs and care

Assessment: Increased apprehension as condition worsens and paralysis spreads, expressed concern and worry about permanent effects of disease, treatments during hospitalization, expressed feeling of increased helplessness and uncertainty.

Evaluation
- Express reduction in anxiety concerning disease process, therapy, and prognosis
- Participates in care and decision making regarding child
- Visits or calls hospital if unable to stay
- Verbalizes that anxiety decreases as resolution of disease begins
- Maintains child's self-concept and developmental status
- Allows for optimal self-care by child.

Nursing diagnosis

High-risk for altered parenting related to lack of knowledge **(Table 12.13)**.

Assessment: Verbalization of decreased interactions with hospitalized child and inability to provide care, lack of control over situation, request for information about parenting skills for long recovery period or permanent residual disability.

Evaluation
- Maintains parental role as illness is resolved
- Participates in care and physical rehabilitation
- Verbalizes positive effects of treatment and participation in care
- Adapts to long-term therapy and any loss of function
- Attends parenting classes if appropriate
- Maintains decision making and control over care and child rearing practices.

Meningitis

Meningitis, the inflammation of the meninges, is the most common infection of the central nervous system (CNS). Those at greatest risk for this disease are infants between 6 and 12 months of age, with most cases occurring between 1 month and 5 years of age. Meningitis may be bacterial or viral in origin. Bacterial causes include infections such as *Haemophilus influenzae* (type B), *Streptococcus pneumoniae*, *Neisseria meningitidis*, or *Staphylococcus*

Nursing Process for the Child with Neurological Disorder

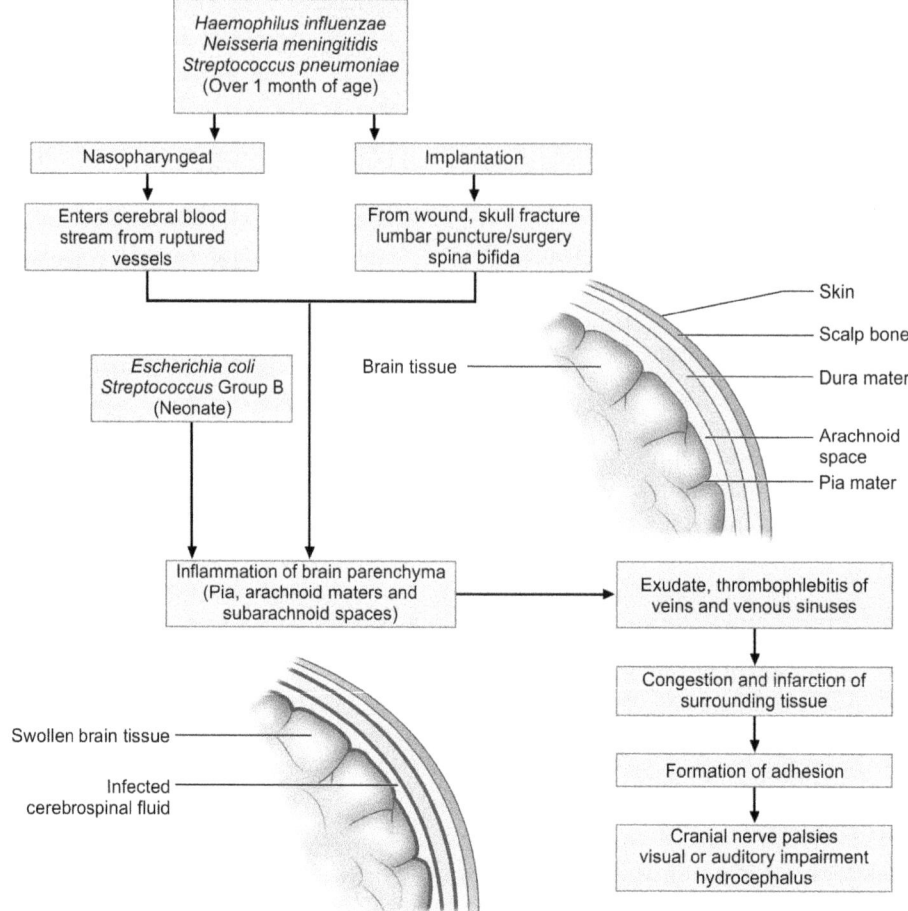

Fig. 12.4: Pathophysiology of meningitis.

aureus. The most common route of infection is vascular dissemination from an infection in the nasopharynx or sinuses. In addition, infection may be implanted as a result of skull fracture wounds, lumbar puncture or surgical procedure. Meningitis may also be caused by a variety of viral (aseptic) agents and is usually associated with measles, mumps, herpes, or enteritis. This form of meningitis is self-limiting and is treated symptomatically for 3–10 days. Treatment includes hospitalization to differentiate between the two types of meningitis, isolation, management of types of meningitis, isolation, management of symptoms, and prevention of complications **(Fig. 12.4)**.

Common Signs and Symptoms of Meningitis

- Fever
- Severe, persistent headache
- Neck stiffness and pain
- Nausea and vomiting

- Confusion and disorientation (acting "goofy")
- Drowsiness or sluggishness
- Sensitivity to bright light
- Poor appetite
- More severe symptoms include seizure and coma

In infants symptoms may include fever, irritability, poor feeding and lethargy.

Other Potential Signs and Symptoms of Meningococcal Meningitis

These are additional signs and symptoms of Meningococcal Meningitis that has entered the blood stream:
- Abnormal skin color
- Stomach cramps
- Ice-cold hands and feet
- Skin rash
- Muscle ache or joint pain
- Rapid breathing
- Chills.

Nursing Management

A. Essential Nursing Diagnoses and Nursing Process Associated with this Condition

Nursing diagnosis

Hyperthermia related to illness.

Assessment: Increase in body temperature above normal range, warm to touch, increased respiratory and pulse rate.

(Refer Table 14.18 from chapter 14)

Nursing diagnosis

High-risk for fluid volume deficit related to:
1. Excessive losses through normal routes
   Assessment: Vomiting, diarrhea.
2. Deviations affecting intake of fluids
   Assessment: Decreased intake, fluid restrictions, change in level of consciousness.
3. Failure of regulatory mechanisms
   Assessment: Secretion of antidiuretic hormone, increased specific grade and osmolality, reduced output, dehydration.

(Refer Table 14.11 from chapter 14)

Nursing diagnosis

Altered thought processes related to physiological changes **(Table 12.14)**.

Assessment: Disorientation to time, place, person, events, changes in consciousness; behavior changes.

Evaluation
- Mental and psychologic functions at optimal level
- Absence of increased intracranial pressure

Nursing Process for the Child with Neurological Disorder

Table 12.14: Nursing interventions for altered thought process.

Interventions	Rationales
Assess history for neurological conditions or infection, cognitive functioning	Provides information about reason for mentation changes
Assess for increased ICP and effects on orientation, mentation, intellectual function, motor function	Provides information about increased ICP, which results from brain edema, shift or distortion, and brain hypoxia
Perform neurological checks q2h, orientation, grip and grasp and pain response, presence of irritability, confusion, memory loss; include cranial nerve function, if indicated	Provides data about changes in thought processes that indicate serious pathology
Elevate head of bed to 30° and maintain proper head and neck alignment	Promotes blood flow to brain and prevents hypoxia
Provide toys and stimulation that are age appropriate and modified for illness	Promotes development level with in prescribed limitations to improve orientation and attention span
Limit sensory and motor expectations, if unable to maintain thought processes and independence in activities	Prevents frustration and insecure feelings

- Awareness of environment and orientation preserved
- Thought processes returned to baseline level
- Absence of residual effects (mental retardation) of brain disease.

B. Specific Nursing Diagnoses and Nursing Process

Nursing diagnosis

Anxiety of parent(s) related to threat to or change in health status of child; threat to or change in environment (hospitalization of child) **(Table 12.15)**.

Assessment: Increased apprehension that condition of child might worsen, expressed concern and worry about actual hospitalization of child and seriousness of illness.

Evaluation
- Express a reduction in anxiety with explanations of disease process and therapy
- Verbalizes the positive effect of caring for and supporting their sick infant/small child
- Participates in care and decision making regarding infant/small child
- Visits and/or telephones the hospital if unable to stay.

Nursing diagnosis

High-risk for injury related to internal factor of altered neurologic regulatory function **(Table 12.16)**.

Assessment: Increase intracranial pressure (early signs of lethargy, restlessness, increased head circumference, headache, vomiting, personality changes; or late signs of decreased level of consciousness, change in posturing, widening of pulse pressure, projectile vomiting, decreased pulse and respirations, seizures, abnormal PERL, shrill cry, bulging fontanel, changes in vision, headache).

Table 12.15: Nursing interventions for anxiety of parent(s).

Interventions	Rationales
Assess sources and level of anxiety, how anxiety is manifested and need for information and support	Provides information about the need for interventions to relieve anxiety and concern; sources may include fear and uncertainty about treatment and recovery, guilt for presence of illness, fear of possible loss of parental role and loss of responsibility when hospitalization necessary
Allow to express concerns and ask questions regarding condition of ill child	Provides opportunity to vent feelings, secure information needed to reduce anxiety
Encourage to remain calm and involved in care and decision making regarding child's needs, noting any improvements that result	Promotes constant monitoring of child's condition for improvement or worsening of symptoms
Allow parent to stay with child, or to visit when able and to call when concerned if hospitalized; allow to assist in care (hold, feed, bathe, clothe, and diaper) and provide information about child's daily routines	Allows parent to care for and support child instead of increasing anxiety by not being with child

Table 12.16: Nursing interventions for high-risk for injury related to internal factor of altered neurologic regulatory function.

Interventions	Rationales
Assess neurologic status to include vs pattern changes in consciousness, behavior patterns and papillary/ocular responses appropriate for age, measure head circumference in infant	Provides information that offers clues to possible change in intracranial pressure caused by inflammation of the brain and associated edema
Attach cardiac and respiratory monitor to assess for bradycardia and hypopnea	Increased intracranial pressure will decrease pulse and respirations, and widen the pulse pressure, with pulse becoming irregular and respirations rapid and shallow as ICP progresses and the body attempts to decrease blood flow to brain
Reposition q2h, have oxygen and suctioning equipment on hand to be administered when needed	Maintains airway potency and prevents obstruction by secretion, which increased CO_2 retention and ICP
Provide quite environment free from bright lighting, minimize handling and care of infant/child, allow for rest periods between care of procedures, restrict visiting if irritable	Promotes comfort and rest and reduces irritability
Administer antibiotics as prescribed and based on analysis of CSF and throat cultures	Manages existing infection and prevents further spread of infection
Note any seizure activity including onset, frequency, duration and type of movements before, during or after seizure: remove objects/toys from bed, and administer any ordered anticonvulsants	Prevents injury during seizure, which is a complication of meningitis
Administer stool softeners, avoid use of restraints, and reduce crying episodes	Prevents Valsalva's maneuver, which will increase ICP
Position with head elevated up to 30°, and maintain head alignment with sand bag	Decreases intracranial pressure by allowing blood flow from brain by gravity or any obstruction of jugular drainage
Stay with infant/child and speak in a low voice	Provides limited stimulation to infant/child during acute stage of disease

Nursing Process for the Child with Neurological Disorder

Evaluation
- Verbalizes signs and symptoms of complications to report
- Absence of complications associated with the disease
- Resolution of the disease with minimal or no long-term effects
- Monitors neurologic status for changes or deviations from baselines
- Maintains safe environment of resolution of disease and convalescence.

Nursing diagnosis

Knowledge deficit of parent(s) caretaker related to lack of exposure to information **(Table 12.17)**.

Assessment: Request for information about medications, signs and symptoms and behaviors to report, general care during convalescence of infant/child.

Evaluation
- Statements of knowledge of medication regimen, dietary and activity requirements of infant/child
- Appropriate precautions taken to prevent spread or recurrence of infection
- Performs developmental activities related to the age and needs of the infant/child
- Statement of signs and symptoms to report to physician

Table 12.17: Nursing interventions for knowledge deficit of parent(s); caretaker.

Interventions	Rationales
Assess knowledge of disease and method to control and resolve disease; willingness and interest of parent(s) to implement care	Promotes realistic plan of instruction to ensure compliance of medical regimen; prevents repetition of information
Provide information and explanations in clear, understandable language; use pictures, pamphlets, video tapes, model in teaching about disease	Ensures understanding based on readiness and ability to learn; visual aids reinforce learning
Instruct in an administration of medications, including action of drugs, dosages, times, frequency, side effects, expected results, methods to give medication; provide written instructions and schedule to follow, and inform to administer full course of antibiotic to child	Provides information for compliance in medication therapy to prevent or treat infection and seizure activity resulting from the disease; bacterial meningitis is treated with antibiotics, and viral meningitis may be treated with antibiotics until diagnosis is established
Instruct and assist in planning feedings, and/or develop menus to include nourishing fluids, caloric and basic four groups for age group	Promotes optimal nutrition in a progressive manner as tolerated
Inform of importance of adequate rest and activities that provide age-appropriate play and stimulation	Rest important for convalescence, and stimulating activities needed for continued development or to promote stimulation if developmental lag is present
Inform to isolate other children in family for 24 hours, if respiratory infection present or until culture is negative	Prevents transmission of bacteria to others in family
Inform to report elevated temperature, poor feeding or anorexia, irritability or other changes in behavior or level of consciousness, decrease in hearing acuity	Reveals signs and symptoms of presence of or spread of infection

- Adaptation to appropriate care during convalescence within prescribed requirements and limitations
- Maintains follow-up visits to physician as scheduled
- Appropriate growth and development advances for age group.

Neurosensory Deficits

Sensory deficits or impairments lead to auditory and/or visual deprivation that place a child at risk for cognitive, perceptive, communication and socialization development skills. These skills affect the way the child relates to his or her environment, and improper development of the skills can result in disability and disadvantage for the child in achieving long-term goals. Vision disorders are common in children, with the most prevalent problems of a refractive type (myopia or hyperopia). Other visual disorders include amblyopia, strabismus, cataracts, and glaucoma. Trauma from injury with balls or sticks, use of contact lenses, or improper eye care may result in conjunctivitis, keratitis, or loss of an eye, any of which may result in visual loss or even blindness. Auditory disorders are classified as conductive, sensorineural, or mixed conductive-sensorineural, hearing loss causes include damage to the inner ear structures or the auditory nerve from congenital defects; infection; ototoxic drugs; long-term, excessive exposure to noises (sensorineural); or middle ear infection such as otitis media (conductive). Hearing and vision screenings vary with the age of the infant/child and are performed as part of physical assessment of all children. Treatment focuses on the correction and rehabilitation of any actual or potential impairment **(Flowchart 12.1)**.

Nursing Management

A. Essential Nursing Diagnoses and Nursing Process Associated with these Conditions

Nursing diagnosis

Altered growth and development related to effects of physical disability.

Assessment: Delay or difficulty in performing skills (motor, social, expressive) typical of age group, behavior and/or intellectual deficits, poor academic performance, reduced independence in performance of ADL.

(Refer Table 14.4 from chapter 14)

B. Specific Nursing Diagnoses and Nursing Process

Nursing diagnosis

Sensory/perceptual alteration: Auditory related to altered sensory perception, transmission and/or integration of neurologic disease or deficit; altered state of sense organ, inability to hear (partial or complete deafness) **(Table 12.18)**.

Assessment: Change in behavior pattern, anxiety, change in usual response to stimuli, altered communication pattern, auditory distortions, reduced auditory acuity, inappropriate responses.

Evaluation
- Optimizes auditory acuity
- Uses assistive aid to maximize hearing (hearing aid)
- Learns lip-reading and/or signing and uses for communication
- Corrects any language or speech impairment for optimal effect

Nursing Process for the Child with Neurological Disorder

Flowchart 12.1: Pathophysiology of neurosensory deficits.

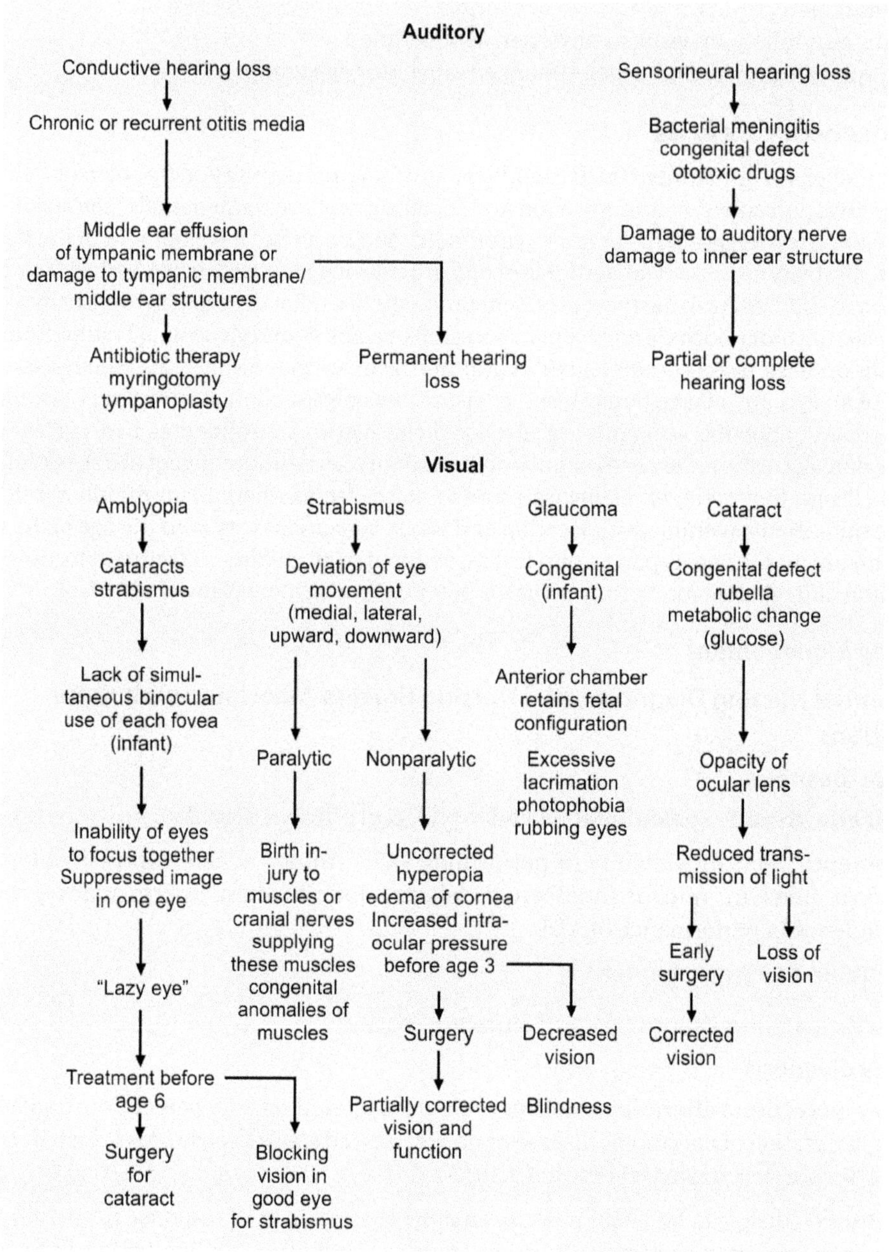

Auditory

Conductive hearing loss → Chronic or recurrent otitis media → Middle ear effusion of tympanic membrane or damage to tympanic membrane/middle ear structures → Antibiotic therapy, myringotomy, tympanoplasty → Permanent hearing loss

Sensorineural hearing loss → Bacterial meningitis, congenital defect, ototoxic drugs → Damage to auditory nerve, damage to inner ear structure → Partial or complete hearing loss

Visual

Amblyopia → Cataracts, strabismus → Lack of simultaneous binocular use of each fovea (infant) → Inability of eyes to focus together, Suppressed image in one eye → "Lazy eye" → Treatment before age 6 → Surgery for cataract

Strabismus → Deviation of eye movement (medial, lateral, upward, downward) → Paralytic / Nonparalytic
- Paralytic: Birth injury to muscles or cranial nerves supplying these muscles, congenital anomalies of muscles
- Nonparalytic: Uncorrected hyperopia, edema of cornea, Increased intraocular pressure before age 3 → Surgery → Partially corrected vision and function / Blocking vision in good eye for strabismus

Glaucoma → Congenital (infant) → Anterior chamber retains fetal configuration → Excessive lacrimation, photophobia, rubbing eyes → Surgery → Decreased vision / Blindness

Cataract → Congenital defect, rubella, metabolic change (glucose) → Opacity of ocular lens → Reduced transmission of light → Early surgery / Loss of vision → Corrected vision

- Maintains independence in learning and activities
- Maintains and/or progresses in developmental tasks
- Participates in play and other social interactions with other
- Attends school regularly
- Adapts to hearing loss
- Utilizes any helpful devices or signaling aids

Table 12.18: Nursing interventions for sensory/perceptual alteration: Auditory.

Interventions	Rationales
Assess history of chronic otitis media, brain infection, use of ototoxic drugs, rubella or other intrauterine infections (viral), congenital defects of ear or nose, presence of deafness in family members, hypoxemia and increased bilirubin levels in low birth weight infants	Provides information about possible risks for conductive or sensorineural hearing loss
Assess for auditory acuity: Infant: Failure to waken to sounds, failure to turn head when sounds is present (use rattle), no response to loud noise, no response to sound made out of visual field Child: Delayed speech development, failure to respond to name or to locate sound, failure to respond to being read to or to sound of music, failure to respond to verbal speech, requesting repeat of message, gesturing instead of speech, shy, timid, inattentive, poor performance in school	Provides information of infant/child ability to hear using techniques that are age-dependent
Perform audiometry or other tests, depending on age of child and preparation of technician	Evaluates degree of hearing acuity and/or loss and type of hearing loss
Face infant/child when speaking, speak distinctly and slowly without shouting to gain child's attention	Provides opportunity to develop lip-reading
Assist with use of hearing aid	Promotes maximum benefit from aid
Encourage use of sign language and as much verbal communication as possible	Promotes communication with others
Provide for play and social interactions, self-care in all activities for age group, continued attendance at school	Promotes independence for age group and security in interacting with peers
Encourage child to read books and practice responding to cues with language development or use of aids or methods learned	Promotes effective communication and corrects or prevents impairments

- Participates in formal rehabilitation program or home training program
- Contact national associations for information and assistance for hearing aids, signing, lip-reading, rehabilitation programs.

Nursing diagnosis

Sensory/perceptual alteration: Visual related to altered sensory perception, transmission and/or integration of neurologic disease or deficit, altered state of sense organ, inability to see (partial or complete loss of sight) **(Table 12.19)**.

Assessment: Change in behavior pattern, anxiety, change in usual responses to stimuli, visual distortions, reduced visual acuity, myopia, hyperopia, lazy eye, cross-eye, cataracts, glaucoma, trauma to eye, frequent injury by walking into objects.

Evaluation

- Provides and functions in safe environment
- Optimizes visual acuity
- Uses assistive aids to maximize vision, development, and independence
- Maintains and/or progresses in developmental tasks
- Attends school regularly
- Adapts to visual loss and maintains activities, play, and social interactions

Nursing Process for the Child with Neurological Disorder

Table 12.19: Nursing interventions for sensory/perceptual alteration: Visual.

Interventions	Rationales
Assess history of rubella or syphilis of mother before birth of child, presence of genetic disorders in the family, excessive oxygen given to infant, congenital conditions that cause blindness, impairment caused by strabismus, cataract or glaucoma	Provides information about risks for or presence of sight impairment or blindness
Assess for risk of trauma to an eye from toys, missiles or projectiles into eye during games or play, excessive sunlight to eyes	Eye trauma caused by accidents is most common cause of blindness in children, and information provides safety education plan to prevent eye injury
Assess for visual acuity: Infant: Failure to follow light or object with eye movement. Failure to fixate on mother's face, Delay in posture and in developmental tasks, Absence of binocularity. Failure to move eyes together Child: Failure to respond to visual stimuli, such as squinting, blinking, rubbing of eyes, eye crossing after 6 months of age, headache after using eyes, failure to initiate eye contact, nystagmus, head tilt, holding reading material close to face, bumps into objects when walking or crawling, poor performance in school	Provides information of infant/child ability to see using techniques that are age-dependent
Perform visual tests for acuity, peripheral vision, and muscle balance depending on age and intellectual development level; include tests for strabismus, amblyopia	Evaluates degree of acuity and/or loss and possible causes, with consideration for improving visual acuity with age
Face infant/child when speaking, explain sounds and what is happening in the environment	Promotes comfort and security with environment
State name when approaching and explain any procedure before starting, use touch if acceptable	Reduce anxiety and sudden, unexpected contact
Assist with use and care of glasses or patching one eye, and encourage wearing of these as prescribed	Promotes independence in use of aids for refractive disorders and strabismus
Provide for age-related toys and social interactions within secure environment	Promotes stimulation and development
Provide well-lit environment and familiar placement of objects orient child to environment	Promotes safety and security in the environment and prevent possible trauma from bumping into furniture or falling
Emphasize the abilities and praise attempts and/or accomplishments	Promotes self-esteem of child

- Administers ophthalmic medications correctly
- Absence of injury to eye, removal of hazards in the environment
- Complies with visual testing schedule
- Participates in rehabilitation or special programs for child.

Seizure Disorders

A seizure is a central nervous system (CNS) condition characterized by an excessive level of neuronal electrical discharges in the brain. It may be idiopathic or chronic and recurrent (epilepsy) or acute acquired and nonrecurrent. Seizures may be partial or generalized, with signs and symptoms dependent on the areas involved and ranging from varying degrees of motor, sensory, and sensorimotor changes and altered consciousness. Partial seizures may be classified as partial or complex-partial. Generalized seizures may be classified as tonic-clinic, absence, a tonic or akinetic, myoclonic, and infantile spasms. Seizures occur at any age in children with epilepsy occurring mostly in children over 3 years of age. Infantile spasms occur in infants between 3–9 months of age. Treatment focuses on prevention of subsequent seizure activity by a medication regimen or surgical removal of a focal lesion, tumor, or hemorrhage. Febrile seizures occur in children between 3 months and 5 years of age, and the younger the age of the child at first episode, the more likely the chance of recurrence. Status epilepticus is characterized by a seizure lasting more than 30 minutes or repeated seizures without regaining consciousness. It is viewed as a medical emergency with the prognosis dependent on the length of the seizure activity and the effect on the brain **(Flowchart 12.2)**.

Nursing Management

A. Essential Nursing Diagnoses and Nursing Process Associated with this Condition

Nursing diagnosis

Ineffective breathing pattern related to neuromuscular impairment, perception, or cognitive impairment.

Assessment: Dyspnea, tachypnea, changes in respiratory depth, cyanosis, cessation of breathing in status epilepticus, obstruction of airway by secretions during a seizure.

(Refer Table 14.2 from chapter 14)

Nursing diagnosis

Altered nutrition: Less than body requirements related to inability to ingest food because of rejection of diet.

Assessment: Weight under ideal for height and frame, poor eating patterns, anorexia, rejection of decrease in protein and carbohydrate and increase of fat in dietary intake.
(Refer Table 14.3 from chapter 14)

B. Specific Nursing Diagnoses and Nursing Process

Nursing diagnosis

High-risk for injury related to internal factors of biochemical regulatory function (seizure, tissue hypoxia), physical trauma (broken skin, altered mobility), psychological changes (orientation) **(Table 12.20)**.

Nursing Process for the Child with Neurological Disorder

Flowchart 12.2: Pathophysiology of seizures.

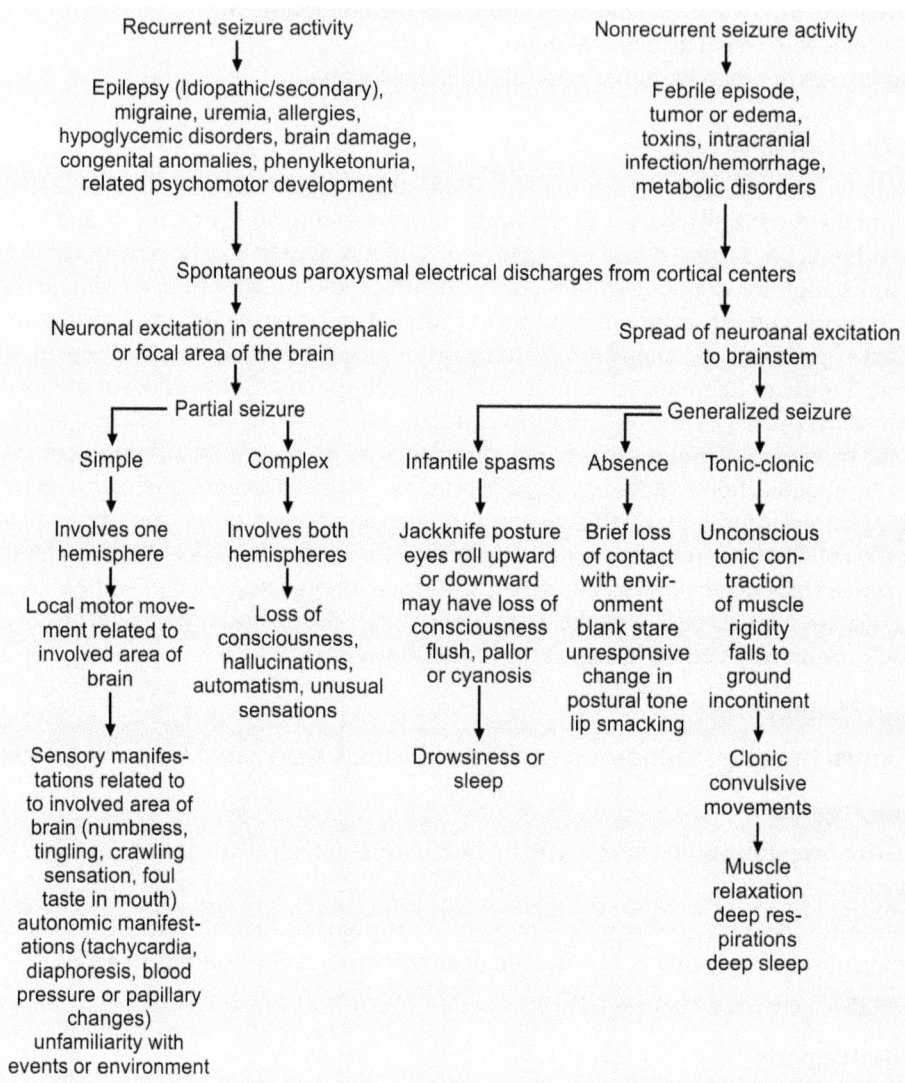

Assessment: Seizure activity with change in consciousness, falls, muscle flaccidity or rigidity, aspiration of secretions, cyanosis, change in sensation in a body part, muscle weakness, presence of aura before seizure.

Evaluation
- Verbalization of understanding of condition and preventive measures to take to comply with medical regimen
- Supports child during seizure with calm, effective actions
- Prevents any injury caused by seizure activity
- Acts to maintain respiratory function and ventilation
- Records and reports seizure activity to physician.

Table 12.20: Nursing interventions for high-risk for injury related to internal factory of biochemical regulatory function (seizure, tissue hypoxia), physical trauma (broken skin, altered mobility), psychological changes (orientation).

Interventions	Rationales
Assess seizure activity including type of activity before, during, and after seizure; movements and parts of body involved (tonic and clonic); site of onset and progression of seizure; duration of seizure; papillary changes; bowel or bladder incontinence, paralysis, sleepiness, alertness, or confusion after seizure; presence of aura	Provides information that prepares environment for prevention of trauma or complications as a result of seizure
Assess skin for color (pallor, flush, or cyanosis), respiratory rate, depth and ease for signs of distress; have oxygen, suctioning equipment on hand	Provides information about possible obstruction or aspiration of secretions if seizures are prolonged and affect ventilation
Maintain side-lying position with side-rails up, bed or crib padded, and articles removed from area near child	Allows for secretions to drain and maintains airway patency; padding protects child from injury during seizure
Avoid attempts to restrain any movements or put anything in child's mouth; provide gentle support to head and arms if harm might result	Restrain may result in fracture and inserting object in mouth increases stimuli
Loosen clothing, assist child to floor if not in bed and place pad under head	Prevents injury from fall
Stay with child during seizure, reorient when awake, and allow to rest or sleep after seizure	Provides support and prevents any injury to child
Administer and evaluate anticonvulsants, obtaining blood levels as ordered	Prevents subsequent seizures, since medications are the most effective prevention of seizures

Nursing diagnosis

Infective family coping: compromised

1. **Related to** situational crisis faced by the parent(s) and family members **(Table 12.21)**.
   Assessment: Preoccupation of significant persons with anxiety, guilt, fear regarding child's disorder, display of protective behaviors by significant persons that are disproportionate to child's needs (too much or too little), recurrence of seizure activity, lack of support by family members to child.
2. **Related to** inadequate or incorrect information or understanding by a primary person and/or significant persons.
   Assessment: Verbalization by significant persons of inadequate knowledge base that interferes with care and support of infant/child.

Evaluation
- Verbalizes and clarifies family's and child's knowledge about seizures and emotional responses to disorder
- Supports child and participates in care by family members
- Verbalizes that improved coping skills practiced by family

Nursing Process for the Child with Neurological Disorder

Table 12.21: Nursing interventions for ineffective family coping: compromised.

Interventions	Rationales
Assess anxiety, fear, erratic behavior, perception of crisis situation by family members	Provides information affecting family ability to cope with infant/child's recurring disorder
Assess coping methods used and effectiveness; family ability to cope with ill member of family, stress on family relationships, developmental level of family, response of siblings, knowledge and attitudes about disorder and health practices	Identifies coping methods that work and need to develop new coping skills; family attitudes and coping abilities directly affect child's health and feeling of wellness; members of family may develop emotional problems when stressed, and ill member may strengthen or strain family relationships
Encourage expression of feelings and questions in accepting, non-judgmental environment, and assist family members in expressing problems and exploring solutions responsibly	Reduces anxiety and enhances family's understanding of infant/child's condition and provides opportunity to express feelings, problems, and problem-solving strategies by whole family
Encourage family involvement in care during hospitalization and after discharge	Provides for reduction of anxiety and fear
Allow for open visitation, encourage telephone calls to hospital by family members	Encourages bonding and assists in coping with infant/child's hospitalization, if unable to stay
Provide place for family members to rest, freshen up	Promotes comfort of family
Suggest social worker referral if needed	Provides support and resources for financial or infant/child's care relief
Give positive feedback and praise family efforts in developing coping and problem-solving techniques and caring for infant/child	Encourages parent(s) and family to participate in care and gain some control over the situation
Assist in establishing short-and long-term goals in maintaining child care and family integration of child into home routine	Promotes inclusion of ill child in family routines and activities

- Verbalizes that adaptations and inclusion of child into family maintained
- Maintains positive and proper behaviors toward child without preferential treatment
- Maintains social responsibilities and health of family
- Secures genetic counseling if appropriate, services of social worker if needed
- Family relationships preserved and stressors minimized, with differences resolved
- Maintains social and school activities of child
- Wears or carries identification information about condition.

Nursing diagnosis

Knowledge deficit of parent(s) and child related to lack of exposure to information about ongoing care **(Table 12.22)**.

Assessment: Expressed request for information about medication regimen, causes of seizures, and when to report to physician.

Table 12.22: Nursing interventions for knowledge deficit of parent(s) and child.

Interventions	Rationales
Assess perceptions and knowledge parent(s) and child about disorder; fears and misconceptions about disorder, nature and frequency of seizures, and factors that initiate seizures	Provides information regarding long-term care of child with a seizure disorder and how to deal with seizures and the stigma attached to them
Instruct in administration of anticonvulsants, including name of drug(s), action of drug(s) and when given in combination, times, frequency, side effects, expected results, methods to give drugs; provide written instructions to follow related to age group and a schedule to follow. Give at most convenient times with meals or at bedtime with as few disruptions in routines and activities as possible give in tablets, liquid extracts, emulsions, or crushed in syrup or jelly. Avoid milk if giving phenytoin or phenobarbital, and supplement vitamin D replace prescription before running out of drug(s), and avoid skipping doses	Promotes compliance to drug regimen, which is the most important treatment to prevent seizure
Instruct parent(s) and child to report lethargy, ataxia, nausea, vomiting, hyperactivity, blood dyscrasia, stomatitis, tremor, nystagmus	Indicates side effects of sedatives and anticonvulsants
Inform parent(s) of need to have blood testing for therapeutic levels, blood count, liver function tests when instructed	Prevents toxicity and other severe side effects of drug therapy by adjusting dosage or changing medication(s)
Inform that seizures may be provoked by omission of medication administration, an illness or infection, too much activity, lack of sleep, excessive alcohol or drug intake, emotional stress, or other caused specific to child	Promotes knowledge and understanding of causes of increased frequency of seizures
Inform parent(s) to supervise child in bathroom, avoid dangerous play and toys, avoid exposure to incidents that trigger seizure, pad areas in bed or wear protective clothing if needed	Provides precautions to prevent injury as a result of a seizure
Inform parent(s) to notify school nurse and teacher of disorder and of actions to take, including telephone number to call	Promotes knowledge and understanding to prevent injury and embarrassment to child
Instruct and assist in planning menus for ketogenic diet to manage seizures	Increases seizure threshold
Inform of any activity restrictions, such as sports, rough play, and need for someone in attendance	Promotes knowledge of activity based on individual child and seizure activity and response to therapy
Alert parent(s) of possible changes in behavior, activity, or personality, or changes in school performance or interactions with family and peers	Indicates effects of anticonvulsants on behavior and learning

Evaluation
- Statements of knowledge of disorder, causes of seizure activity
- Adaptation and compliance of parent(s) and child with medication regimen, including all aspects of dosage and form, time and frequency, side effects
- Complies with recommended visits to physician and laboratory for ongoing care and testing
- Continues with activities, and limits those that are to be avoided because they may be harmful of initiate seizure
- Provides ketogenic diet and varies inclusions according to preference
- Reports signs and symptoms of medication side effects or changes in learning or behavior
- Verbalizes understanding of need for long-term therapy and support for child to comply with medical regime.

Spina Bifida

Spina bifida is a defect of the central nervous system involving the failure of neural tube closure during embryonic development, it may be spina bifida occulta, which is a defect in the closure without the herniation and exposure of the spinal cord or meninges at the surface of the skin in the lumbosacral area, or it may be spina bifida cystica (meningocele or myelomeningocele), which is a defect in the closure with a sac and herniated protrusion of meninges, spinal fluid, and some part of the spinal cord and nerves at the surface of the skin in the lumbosacral or sacral area.

Hydrocephalus is often associated with spina bifida cystica. The neurologic effects area related to the anatomic level and nerves involved in the defect. The effects range from varying degrees of sensory deficits to partial or total motor impairment resulting in flaccidity, partial paralysis of lower extremities, and loss of bladder and bowel control. Spina bifida cystica patients, especially those with myelomeningocele, are commonly afflicted with orthopedic abnormalities that may include hip dislocation, spinal curvatures, and clubfeet. These patients may require assistive devices such as braces. Special crutches, or wheelchairs for mobility. Treatment includes surgical repair of the defect, as well as other anomalies, depending on the severity of the neurologic deficit and may be done during infancy or late. Other treatments focus on prevention of complications, bowel and urinary management, and promotion of optimal growth and development **(Fig. 12.5)**.

Symptoms of Spina Bifida

Spina bifida occurs in three forms, each varying in severity:

Spina Bifida Occulta

This mildest form results in a small separation or gap in one or more of bones (vertebrae) of the spine. Because the spinal nerves usually aren't involved, most children with this form of spina bifida have no signs or symptoms and experience no neurological problems. Visible indications of spina bifida occulta can sometimes be seen on the newborn's skin above the spinal defect, including:
- An abnormal tuft of hair
- A collection of fat
- A small dimple or a birthmark
- Skin discoloration

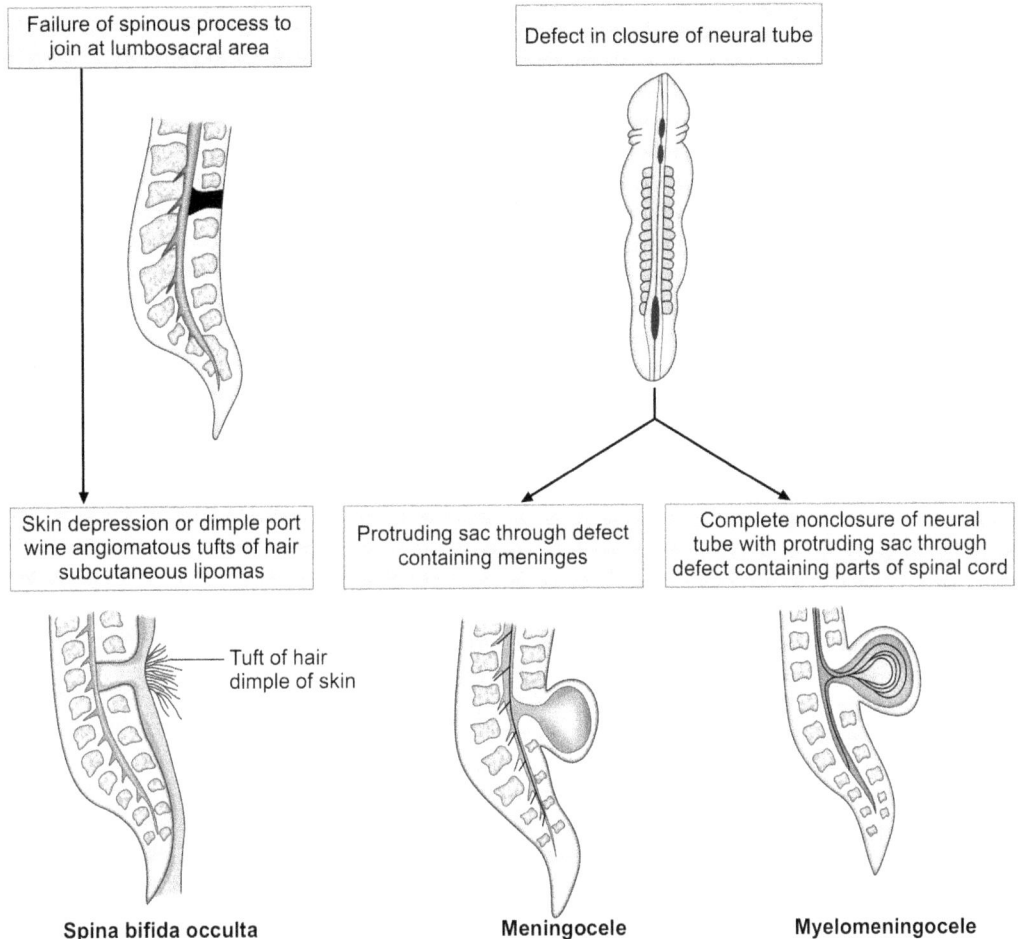

Fig. 12.5: Pathophysiology of spina bifida.

Meningocele

In this rare form, the protective members around the spinal cord (meninges) push out through the opening in the vertebrae. Because the spinal cord develops normally, these members can be removed by surgery with little or no damage to nerve pathways.

Myelomeningocele

In myelomeningocele, the baby's spinal canal remains open along several vertebrae in the lower or middle back. Because of this opening, both the membranes and the spinal cord protrude at birth, forming a sac on the baby's back.

Neurological impairment is common, including:
- Muscle weakness, sometimes involving paralysis
- Bowel and bladder problems
- Seizures, especially if the child requires a shunt
- Orthopedic problems—such as deformed feet, uneven hips and a curved spine (scoliosis).

Nursing Process for the Child with Neurological Disorder

Nursing Management

A. Essential Nursing Diagnoses and Nursing Process Associated with this Condition

Nursing diagnosis

High-risk for impaired skin integrity
1. **Related to** external factors of excretions and secretions.
   Assessment: Urinary and/or fecal incontinence, redness and irritation of perineal and anal areas, disruption of skin in perineal and anal areas, leakage of CSF from sac, rupture of sac, use of diapers.
2. **Related to** external factors of physical immobilization and pressure.
   Assessment: Redness, excoriation at bony prominences or other pressure areas, skin breakdown at pressure points, inability to change position, paralysis.
3. **Related to** internal factors of altered sensation, circulation, and skeletal prominence.
   Assessment: Loss of tactile perception in extremities, pressure on bony prominences, lack of padded protection and massage of bony prominences, improper application of hot or cold.

(Refer Table 12.1)

Nursing diagnosis

Impaired physical mobility related to neuromuscular impairment.

Assessment: Inability to purposefully move within physical environment, including bed mobility, transfer, ambulation, imbalance, impaired coordination, partial or complete paralysis of lower extremities, flaccidity, spasticity, skeletal abnormalities (hip, feet, spine).
(Refer Table 14.19 from chapter 14)

Nursing diagnosis

Altered nutrition: Less than body requirements related to inability to ingest food

Assessment: NPO status following surgery, inadequate swallowing or sucking in presence of ICP, reduced muscle tone, abnormal eating pattern development.
(Refer Table 14.3 from chapter 14)

Nursing diagnosis

Constipation related to neuromuscular impairment.

Assessment: Frequency less than usual, hard-formed stool, palpable mass, inability to maintain normal bowel elimination pattern, poor anal sphincter tone and in ability to feel urge to defecate.
(Refer Table 12.9 from chapter 12)

Nursing diagnosis

Altered growth and development related to effects of disorder or disability before or after surgery.

Assessment: Frequent hospitalizations, delay or difficulty in performing skills typical of age group (motor, social or expressive), inability to perform self-care or self-control activities appropriate for age, behavior and/or intellectual deficits.
(Refer Table 14.4 from chapter 14)

B. Specific Nursing Diagnoses and Nursing Process

Nursing diagnosis

High-risk for infection related to inadequate primary defenses (broken skin), inadequate bladder emptying **(Table 12.23)**.

Assessment: Breaks or leaks in meningeal sac, abrasion or irritation of sac, contamination of sac, or surgical repair by urinary or stool incontinence.

Evaluation
- Maintains sac or surgical wound integrity
- Absence of infection in sac or wound area or CNS

Table 12.23: Nursing interventions for high-risk for infection.

Interventions	Rationales
Assess sac for breaks or leakage of CSF, irritation of sac, redness, swelling, purulent drainage at or around sac area, fever, irritability, nuchal rigidity, cloudy, foul-smelling urine	Provides information about potential for infection of the sac site or meningitis if sac is ruptured, or UTI if present
Maintain the infant in prone position with head lower than buttocks or hips slightly flexed with a pad between the knees; anchor position with sandbags	Reduces pressure on the sac to prevent possible rupture, and prevents rolling on side or back
Apply a moist, sterile dressing over the sac; use sterile saline or antibiotic solution; ointment, if ordered, may be applied	Prevents drying of sac membrane, which could predispose breaking or rupturing of sac and contamination
Reinforce moist dressing with dry, sterile dressing, and change when needed, being careful to avoid damage to sac by removing moist dressing after it has dried	Prevents contamination by capillary action through moisture
Apply a shield over the sac dressing and tape a plastic sheet below the defect; following surgical closure on the defect, apply a transparent occlusive dressing over the area below the sac site	Protects the sac from contamination by urine or feces
Perform handwashing before any care or procedure involving the site before or after surgery, and carry out sterile technique for all sac and wound care	Prevents transmission of microorganisms to site
Maintain cleanliness of anal area, and apply a sterile shield between anus and sac or wound site	Prevents contamination by feces caused by poor anal sphincter control, which allows dribbling and incontinence of stool
Administer antibiotics as ordered	Prevents or treats infection
Following surgical repair of defect, note any changes in wound, including redness, swelling, warmth, drainage, fever	Indicates wound infection
Following surgery cleanse wound with antiseptic, and change dressings when needed, using sterile technique for at least 24 hours	Promotes cleanliness of wound and prevents infection

Nursing Process for the Child with Neurological Disorder

- Protects sac or wound from contamination
- Performs sterile or clean technique in care of sac or wound
- Administers or applies antibiotic therapy systemically or topically
- Reports changes and signs and symptoms of infection to physician
- Complete bladder emptying with assistance and absence of signs and symptoms of infection.

Nursing diagnosis

Hypothermia related to illness and abnormal presence of sac **(Table 12.24)**.

Assessment: Fluid and heat loss from large area of expose sac, cool skin, body temperature lower than normal range.

Evaluation
- Maintains temperature within normal range for age
- Monitors temperature for increases or decreases and report changes.

Nursing diagnosis

Bowel incontinence related to neuromuscular involvement **(Table 12.25)**.

Assessment: Constant dribbling or involuntary passage of stool, reduced anal sphincter tone and control.

Evaluation
- Reduces episodes of bowel incontinence
- Maintains bowel elimination pattern with control over incontinence

Table 12.24: Nursing interventions for hypothermia.

Interventions	Rationales
Assess temperature q2 4h and note lack of stability; assess temperature of extremity	Provides information as to source of changes in temperature, which may be low if infection is present
Place infant in an isolette, or provide radiant warmer based on hypothermia evaluation, keeping sac moist preoperatively	Provides warmth and reduce the heat loss that causes hypothermia

Table 12.25: Nursing interventions for bowel incontinence.

Interventions	Rationales
Assess presence of neurogenic bowel, degree of incontinence, potential for rehabilitation	Provides information about condition for use in plan of establishing bowel elimination routine
Place child on a toilet or potty chair at the same time each day; use stimulation and suppository, if helpful	Establishes a routine for elimination to empty bowel
Maintain fluid intake of up to 2000 mL/day, depending on age; include fiber and roughage in diet at regular times of the day	Promotes bulk for easier and more manageable passage
Apply padding in waterproof undergarments, but avoid use of diapers	Prevents embarrassment for the child if bowel elimination not controlled

Table 12.26: Nursing interventions for altered urinary elimination pattern.

Interventions	Rationales
Assess presence of neurogenic bladder, degree of incontinence, potential for rehabilitation	Provides information about condition for use in plain for establishing urinary elimination routine
Assess urine for cloudiness, foul odor, fever lethargy, dysuria, retention	Indicates urinary bladder infection caused by urinary retention or residue resulting in urinary stasis and medium for bacterial growth
Offer and encourage intake of 30 mL/lb/day, including acid-containing beverages and dietary inclusion of foods high in acid content	Promotes renal blood flow and acidifies urine to prevent infection
Maintain clean genital and anal areas after each elimination episode or as needed if incontinent	Controls introduction of microorganisms into urethra and urinary bladder
Catheterize after urination if indicated and ordered	Moves residual urine if unable to empty bladder completely
Perform scheduled rehabilitation program of placing child on toilet or potty chair at same times each day	Establishes a routine for urinary elimination if this is a possibility
Perform intermittent catheterization q3 4h, if indicated, to resolve incontinence	Ensures emptying of bladder to prevent incontinence and infection
Perform Crede method if indicated	Promotes emptying of bladder
Administer antispasmodic, smooth muscle relaxant, anticholinergic as ordered	Improves bladder storage and continence by increasing bladder capacity

- Prevents embarrassing situations caused by incontinence
- Complies with rehabilitation regimen established to control bowel incontinence.

Nursing diagnosis

Altered urinary elimination patterns related to neuromuscular impairment **(Table 12.26)**.

Assessment: Incontinence, retention, neurogenic bladder with increased or decreased tone (flaccid or spastic), absence of awareness of bladder fullness, passing of urine or inability to stop flow of urine (reflex incontinence).

Evaluation
- Maintains urinary elimination pattern with control over incontinence
- Complies with rehabilitation regimen established to control urinary incontinence
- Performs necessary procedures to attain continence
- Prevents urinary bladder infection
- Prevents embarrassing situations caused by incontinence
- Complies with long-term medication regimen
- Verbalizes changes, signs and symptoms to report to physician.

Nursing diagnosis

Body image disturbance related to biophysical, psychosocial factors of child **(Table 12.27)**.

Assessment: Urinary/bowel incontinence, partial or complete paralysis, recurring hospitalizations, change in social, verbal expression of negative feelings about body and functional disabilities, feelings of helplessness and hopelessness, inability to perform ADL.

Nursing Process for the Child with Neurological Disorder

Table 12.27: Nursing interventions for body image disturbance.

Interventions	Rationales
Assess child for feelings about abilities and disabilities in ADL, social interaction, effect on self-concept	Provides information about potential for independence in thinking and functioning
Encourage independence and maximize functioning with use of aids for bathing, grooming, dressing, eating, mobility, and toileting, and praise any attempts at self care activities	Promotes ADL capability by use of assistive aids as needed depending on disability
Encourage expression of feelings and concerns, and support communication of child with parents and peers	Provides opportunity to vent feelings to reduce anxiety and negative feelings
Provide touching and hugging, age-appropriate activities with other children	Conveys caring and concern for child and enhances socialization
Stress positive accomplishments; avoid negative comments	Enhances body-image and confidence

Evaluation
- Verbalization of improved body-image and sense of well-being
- Participates in ADL with or without assistive aids as needed
- Verbalizes feelings about disabilities in positive terms
- Parent(s) support and care for child and allow for maximal independence.

Nursing diagnosis

Altered family process related to situational crisis of long-term condition of child (Table 12.28).

Assessment: Family system unable to meet physical, emotional needs of its members inability to express or accept wide range of feelings, family unable to deal with or to adapt to chronic condition and disabilities of child in a constructive manner, excessive involvement with child by family members, guilt expressed by family members, lack of support from family and friends, irritability and impatience as a response by family members to child.

Evaluation
- Family has open discussions and identifies problem areas
- Family develops and uses problem-solving techniques to resolve differences
- Family health and social responsibilities met
- Child integrated into family life, with care becoming a part of family routines
- Family displays supportive behaviors for each other and constructive responses to problems
- Family relationships preserved and stressors minimized
- Family secures assistance from community agencies
- Complies with daily care and therapy regimens
- Statements by family members of adjustment and progressive adaptation to child's disabilities
- Verbalization of knowledge of normal growth and development of child and family.

Table 12.28: Nursing interventions for altered family process.

Interventions	Rationales
Assess family ability to cope with child, stress on family relationships, developmental level of family, response of siblings, knowledge of health practices, family role behavior and attitude about long-term care, economic pressures and resources to care for long-term condition	Provides information about family attitudes and coping abilities which directly affect the child's health and feeling of well-being; chronic condition affecting a child in a family may strengthen or strain relationships, and members may develop emotional problems when family is stressed
Assist individual family members to identify stressors and behaviors and to define them in positive terms (bad, indifferent, rebellious)	Defines and explores individual problems that have meaning for entire family
Assess anxiety level of family and child, perception of crisis situation, copying and problem-solving methods used and their effectiveness	Identifies need to develop new coping skills and realistic behaviors in goal setting and interventions necessary for family and child to adapt to crisis
Encourage expression of feelings and provide factual, honest information about care with or without surgical repair, abilities and disabilities	Allows reduction in anxiety and enhances family understanding of condition and child's needs
Assist in identifying helpful techniques to use to problem solve and copy with problem and again control over the situation	Provides support for problem solving and management of situation
Provide anticipatory guidance for crisis resolution	Assists family in adapting to situation and developing new coping mechanisms
If hospitalizations frequent, assign same personnel to care for child if appropriate	Promotes trust and communication with family members
Support and encourage parental and family caretaking efforts	Provides positive reinforcement of roles and reduces stress in family members
Allow family members to express feelings and reaction to appearance and condition of infant/child	Relieves anxiety and concern and allows a show of acceptance for their responses

PRACTICE QUESTIONS

1. Master Manish 6-year's child admitted in pediatric medicine ward with the seizure disorder. Write nursing care plan for the child with seizure disorder by applying nursing process.
2. Baby Pallavi 7-months admitted in pediatric surgical ward with the diagnosis of hydrocephalus. Write pre and postoperative nursing management of the child by applying nursing process.

CHAPTER 13

Nursing Process of the Child with Gastrointestinal Disorder

> **LEARNING OBJECTIVES**
> - To identify the signs and symptoms of a child with gastrointestinal disorder.
> - To frame nursing diagnosis based on the needs of the child.
> - To plan nursing interventions and outcome identification.

INTRODUCTION

The gastrointestinal tract is a common site of disorders and illnesses in infants and children. It begins in the mouth and ends with the anus and is concerned with ingestion, digestion, absorption of nutrients and the elimination of solid waste materials from the body. It consists of the mouth (tongue and teeth), esophagus, stomach, small intestine, pancreas, liver, gallbladder, large intestine, and anus. Alterations in this system include defects in structure and abnormalities causing obstruction which affects ingestion and the transport or movement of nutrients or disturbances caused by inflammation, malabsorption, and maldigestion that results in gastrointestinal dysfunction. Because of the system's multiple functions and overlapping of symptomatology resulting from an alteration in any one function, additional complications may occur. Also, as in the adult, gastrointestinal function is affected by psychological factors (anxiety) and physiological factors (diseases of other systems).

The physiologic and biochemical functions of the system are present at birth to take over digestion, absorption, and elimination that had been performed by the placenta. With growth and maturity of the tract, the system progressively functions within adult parameters.

NURSING PROCESS OF THE CHILD WITH GASTROINTESTINAL DISORDER (IN GENERAL)

1. **Nursing diagnosis:** Fluid volume, risk for deficit; risk factors may include excessive losses through vomiting or diarrhea, inadequate oral intake, possible nil per orals (NPO) status (particularly in the surgical client).
   Goal: Child will be able to maintain adequate fluid volume.
   Intervention: Maintaining fluid balance.
   - Maintain IV line and administer IV fluid as ordered to maintain fluid volume
   - Offer small amounts of oral rehydration solution frequently to maintain fluid volume; small amounts are usually well tolerated by children with diarrhea and vomiting
   - When symptoms have lessened or resolved, reintroduce regular diet to reduce number of stools, provide adequate nutrition, and shorten duration of effects of illness
   - Avoid high-carbohydrate fluids such as Kool-Aid and fruit juice, as they are low in electrolytes, and increased simple carbohydrate consumption can decrease stool transit time

- Assess hydration status (skin turgor, oral mucosa, presence of tears) every 4–8 hours to evaluate maintenance of adequate fluid volume
- Assess adequacy of urine output to assess end-organ perfusion
- Maintain strict intake and output record and weight child daily to evaluate effectiveness of rehydration
- Weigh child daily; accurate weight is one of the best indicators of fluid volume status in children
- Discourage fluids and milk products that contain high levels of sugar during the acute phase of illness, as these products may worsen diarrhea.

Evaluation: Child achieved elastic skin turgor; moist, pink oral mucosa; presence of tears; urine output 1 mL/kg/h or more.

2. **Nursing diagnosis:** Diarrhea may be related to inflammation of small intestines, presence of infectious agents or toxins, possibly evidenced by loose liquid stools, hyperactive bowel sounds or abdominal cramping.
   Goal: Child will be able to experience decrease in diarrhea.
   Interventions: Relieving diarrhea.
   - Maintain clear liquid diet no longer than 24 hours, as prolonged clear liquids will result in continued liquid stools
   - Avoid milk products until diarrhea improves: temporary poor absorption form villus injury follows viral diarrhea
   - Encourage complex carbohydrate foods to bulk up the stools
   - Add fat to carbohydrates to increase intestinal transit time encourages water absorption (bulks up stool).

   Evaluation: Passed bulkier stool as per normal routine.

3. **Nursing diagnosis:** Constipation, related to G1 obstructive lesions, pain on defecation, diagnostic procedures, inadequate toileting or behavioral stool holding, possibly evidenced by change in character or frequency of stools, feeling of abdominal or rectal fullness or pressure, changes in bowel sounds and abdominal distention.
   Goal: Child will be able to pass smooth stools.
   Intervention: Relieving constipation.
   - Palpate for abdominal distention, percuss for dullness, and auscultate for bowel sounds to assess for signs of constipation
   - Encourage adequate fluid intake to soften the stool
   - Administer medications as ordered to keep stool moving on daily basis
   - Encourage activity as tolerated: immobility contributes to constipation
   - The child with stool withholding should sit on the toilet twice daily, preferably after breakfast and dinner, to maximize chances for successful stool passage by taking advantage of the gastro colic reflex
   - For behavioral stool holding, use rewards or stickers to encourage appropriate toileting.

   Evaluation: Child having daily soft bowel movement without pain or straining.

4. **Nursing diagnosis:** Skin integrity, risk for impaired: risk factors include frequent loose stools, poor nutritional status, presence of stoma, acidic gastric contents contact with skin, if gastrostomy present.
   Goal: Infant's skin will be able to remain intact.

Intervention: Maintaining skin integrity.
- Change diapers frequently to limit acidic stool content contact with skin
- Use barrier diaper cream to protect skin
- Assess skin integrity at every diaper change to recognize skin changes early so that corrective measures can begin
- Leave diaper area open to air several times a day if redness is present, so that air can circulate and skin healing can be facilitated
- Use plain water or only mild soap to cleanse the skin with diaper changes to avoid pH changes that contribute to diaper area skin breakdown
- Avoid diaper wipes that contain fragrance or alcohol if the skin is red or has a rash, as both alcohol and perfume cause stinging if used on non-intact skin and can worsen skin breakdown.

For the child with an ostomy:
- Ensure proper fit of the ostomy appliance/pouch to avoid acidic stool contact with skin
- Use a barrier wafer (e.g., stomahesive or DuoDERM) to attach appliance: avoids repeated pulling of adhesive tape from skin
- If redness occurs, use barrier/healing cream or paste on skin around stoma to promote healing and prevent further skin breakdown
- Consult enterostomal therapy nurse as needed to provide additional support

Evaluation: Buttocks skin will be free from rash, excoriation. In the child with an ostomy, skin surrounding stoma will remain intact, free from redness, rash and excoriation.

5. **Nursing diagnosis:** Nutrition: imbalanced, less than body requirements: may be related to inability to ingest, digest, or absorb nutrients; intestinal pain after eating; decreased transit time through bowel; or psychosocial factors, possibly evidenced by lack of appropriate weight gain or growth, weight loss, aversion to eating, poor muscle tone or observed lack of intake.
   Goal: Nutritional status will be maximized.
   Intervention: Maintaining appropriate nutrition
   - Encourage favorite foods (within prescribed diet restrictions if present) to maximize oral intake
   - Administer enteral tube feedings as ordered to maximize caloric intake
   - Add butter, gravy, cheese as appropriate to foods (if allowed with in diet restrictions) to increase caloric intake
   - Encourage high-quality, high-calorie snacks between meals, so as not to interfere with meal intake
   - Document response to feeding to determine feeding tolerance
   - Limit intake of calorie-free beverages: beverages should contain nutrients and calories
   - Consult nutritionist for appropriate diet supplementation recommendations.
   Evaluation: Child gained weight appropriately.

6. **Nursing diagnosis:** Breathing pattern ineffective, risk factors include postoperative immobility, abdominal pain interfering with breathing, use of narcotic analgesics.
   Goal: Child will be able to demonstrate effective breathing pattern.

Intervention: Promoting effective breathing pattern.
- Turn, cough, deep breathe every 2 hours to encourage adequate aeration discourage fluid pooling in lungs, in the infant or children, turn every 2 hours and use precursor or chest physiotherapy to prevent pooling of secretions
- Play games to encourage deep breathing (blow out penlight, blow cotton ball across bedside table with straw, etc.): children are more likely to cooperate with interventions if play is involved
- In the developmentally able child, encourage incentive spirometer use every 2 hours to improve lung aeration
- Demonstrate/encourage use of pillow splinting with coughing to decrease abdominal pain and stress on incision.

Evaluation: Respiratory rate normal for age, absence of accessory muscle use, adequate aeration with clear breath sounds throughout all lung fields.

7. **Nursing diagnosis:** Body image disturbance; may be related to presence of stoma, loss of control of bowel elimination, scars from multiple surgical procedures, or effects of treatment regimen possibly evidenced by verbalization of negative feelings about body, refusal to look at stoma or participate in care.

   Goal: Child or teen will be able to accept change in body image.

   Intervention: Promoting proper body image
   - Observe child's coping mechanisms to reinforce their use in times of stress
   - Acknowledge denial, anger and other feelings as normal to support child/teen through difficult transition
   - Allow child gradual introduction to stoma to ease transition
   - Encourage child/teen to participate in care, as this sense of control will contribute to positive self-esteem.

   Evaluation: Child verbalized adjustment; looking at, touching, caring for body; returning to previous social involvement.

8. **Nursing diagnosis:** Caregiver role strain, risk factors may include infant with congenital defect, child with chronic illness, marginal caregiver coping patterns, long-term stress, complexity and quantity of care child requires.

   Goal: Caregiver will be able to exhibit emotional health.

   Intervention: Easing caregiver role strain.
   - Assess parental behavior to identify role strain
   - Provide emotional support and encourage talking about feelings, fears, and concerns: to promote trust in nurse as a source of emotional support
   - Arrange for and/or encourage respite care for child: provides parent with time away from continual care
   - Consult social services to identify community resources available for caregiver support (home health, support group, etc.)
   - Encourage parent to meet own needs and find personal time to increase energy level and self-esteem, ultimately enhancing the quality of care given.

   Evaluation: Verbalizes concerns calmly, participates in child's care, and demonstrates knowledge of resources.

NURSING PROCESS FOR SPECIFIC GASTROINTESTINAL DISORDER

Appendicitis

Appendicitis is the inflammation of the appendix, a blind sac connected to the end of the cecum. It is caused most commonly by a fecalith (hard feces) and may result in obstruction which leads to ischemia, necrosis, perforation and peritonitis. Surgical removal of the appendix (appendectomy) is performed as treatment for this disorder, preferably before rupture for a positive outcome. Surgery after rupture requires external drainage and management to reduce the spread of peritonitis. The condition occurs more commonly in children over 2 years of age **(Fig. 13.1)**.

Signs and Symptoms of Appendicitis

Symptoms can vary widely among children.

The most common early symptom is continuous tummy pain around belly button (navel) which may move to the lower right side of the tummy (abdomen) and become sharper and more severe. It often hurts the child to move around, and the pain is worse with coughing or walking.
- A low fever
- Loss of appetite

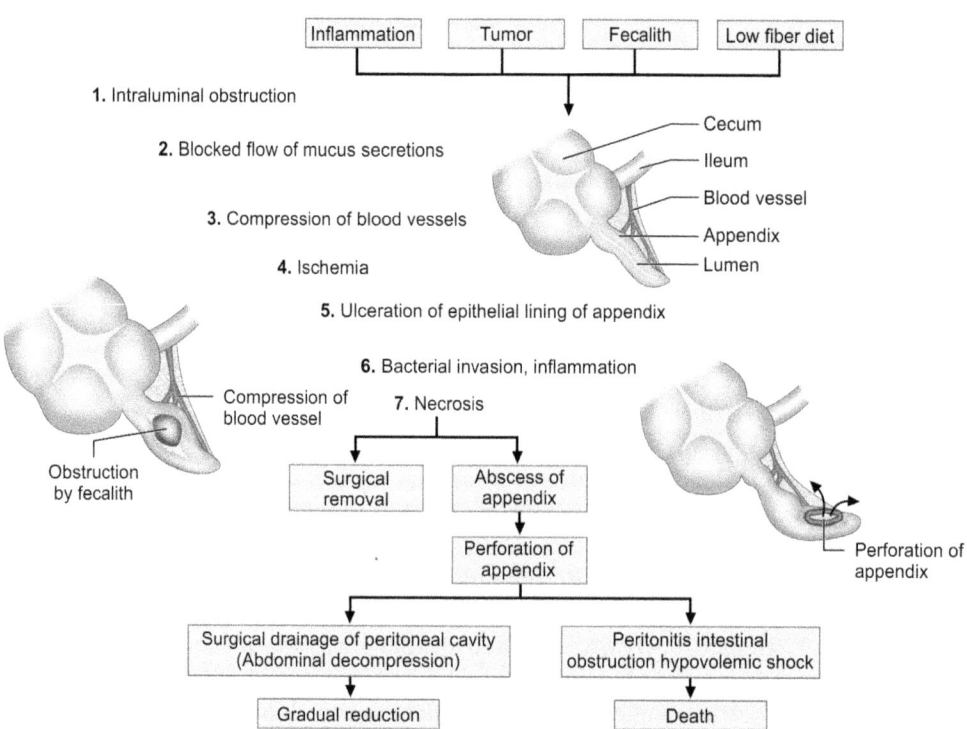

Fig. 13.1: Pathophysiology of appendicitis.

- Nauseas (feeling sick)
- Vomiting
- Constipation or diarrhea.

Nursing Management

A. Essential Nursing Diagnoses and Nursing Process Associated with this Condition

Nursing diagnosis

High-risk for fluid volume deficit related to excessive losses through normal routes; NPO status postoperatively.

Assessment: Vomiting, deviations affecting intake of fluids, elevated temperature, reduced urinary output, diaphoresis.

(Refer Table 14.11 from chapter 14)

Nursing diagnosis

Hyperthermia related to illness (presence of infectious process).

Assessment: Increase in body temperature pulse and respiratory rate, flushing, abrupt rise in temperature with rupture of appendix.

(Refer Table 14.18 from chapter 14)

Nursing diagnosis

Altered nutrition: Less than body requirements related to inability to ingest food.

Assessment: Vomiting, anorexia, nausea, abdominal pain, presence of nasogastric sanction postoperative.

(Refer Table 14.3 from chapter 14)

Nursing diagnosis

Constipation related to less than adequate physical activity.

Assessment: Bed rest following surgery, decreased or absent bowel sounds, frequency less than usual pattern, hard formed stool, abdominal pain.

(Refer Table 14.9 from chapter 14)

B. Specific Nursing Diagnoses and Nursing Process

Nursing diagnosis

Pain related to biological injuring agents; inflammation **(Table 13.1)**.

Assessment: Verbal descriptor of pain, guarding and protective behavior of painful area, irritability, refusal to move or change position, crying, muscular rigidity, clinging behavior, side lying position with knees flexed.

Evaluation
- Preoperative or postoperative pain relieved and/or controlled
- Limits movement or procedures that increase pain
- Child rests comfortably with absence of behavioral responses to pain
- Analgesic therapy administration based on severity of pain and age with desired results.

Nursing Process of the Child with Gastrointestinal Disorder

Table 13.1: Nursing interventions for pain.

Interventions	Rationales
Assess severity of pain, generalized abdominal pain descending to lower right quadrant and localized at McBurney's point with rebound tenderness, reduced bowel sounds; behaviors indicating pain	Provides information symptomatic of appendicitis with pain being the most common presenting complaint; behaviors manifested by pain vary with age with infant responding with crying, facial expression of pain and physical resistance; young children responding with crying loudly, clinging, irritability, uncooperation, rigid position, side lying position with knees flexed up to abdomen, refusal to move
Assess for severity of postoperatives pain	Provides information needed to administer most effective analgesic therapy
Assess for acuteness of abdominal pain that progresses to abdominal rigidity, abdominal distention, tachycardia, shallow respirations, fever, pallor	Indicates rupture of appendix and peritonitis
Administer narcotic or no narcotic analgesic PO or IV preoperatively or postoperatively as ordered	Promotes relief of pain depending on severity age and general condition, NPO status
Avoid palpation of abdomen and unnecessary movements and care procedures of child	Prevents increased pain and possible rupture of appendix
Apply ice packs to abdomen	Provides relief of pain
Place in position of comfort; right side lying or low to semi-Fowler's	Promotes comfort to reduce pain; postoperatively will facilitate drainage if appendix has ruptured and prevent spread of infection
Provides toys, games for quiet play	Promotes diversional activity to distract from pain

Nursing diagnosis

High-risk to infection related to inadequate primary defenses (rupture appendix); invasive procedure (surgery) **(Table 13.2)**.

Assessment: Spread of infection in peritoneal cavity, absent bowel sounds, diffuse abdominal pain followed by an absence of pain, abdominal distention, vomiting, increased pulse and respirations, fever, redness, swelling, drainage at incisional site whether closed by primary intension (appendectomy) or open and draining (ruptured appendix).

Evaluation
- Administration of antibiotic therapy
- Appendectomy incision free of infectious process and healing
- Open incisional area draining and healing
- Dry and clean wound dressings maintained with changes as needed
- Wound isolation precautions maintained until culture is negative for infectious fast agent.

Nursing diagnosis

Anxiety of parent(s) and child related to change in health status of child, hospitalization of child, possible surgery of child **(Table 13.3)**.

Table 13.2: Nursing interventions for high-risk to infection.

Interventions	Rationales
Assess closed incisional site for redness, swelling, pain, drainage, approximation of edges, healing, changes in VS and bowel sounds	Provides information indicating incisional infection
Assess open incisional site for drainage and characteristics, drain placement and potency, need for dressing change	Provides information about effectiveness of wound drainage to prevent abscess formation and spread of peritonitis
Administer antibiotic	Destroys infectious agent based on culture and sensitivities of wound drainage
Position in side lying or semi-Fowler's	Facilitates drainage through wound drain and prevents spread of infection upward in abdomen
Redress incisional wound using sterile technique	Promotes cleanliness of wound and prevents introduction of pathogens
Change dressings on open wound or reinforce as needed, use Montgomery straps to hold dressings in place	Maintains clean, dry dressings and allows for frequent changes without removing taps
Apply warm, wet pack to open incision as ordered	Promotes circulation to the area and reduces inflammation
Irrigate open wound with antibiotic solution as ordered	Cleanses wound and destroys pathogens
Initiate wound isolation precautions	Prevents transmission of infectious agents to or from the child

Assessment: Increased apprehension that condition might worsen and appendix rupture, expressed concern and worry about impending surgery, need for IV, NPO and N/G tube and other treatments and procedures while hospitalized, lack of information about postoperative care.

Evaluation
- Expresses reduction in anxiety about illness, pre and postoperative care and procedures
- Parent(s) verbalize that anxiety decreases as acute phase is resolved
- Child verbalizes or demonstrates decreased anxiety postoperatively
- Verbalizes positive effect of caring for and supporting ill child
- Participates in care and decision making regarding child
- Demonstrates wound care and dressing changes postoperatively and other procedures to enhance wellness and verbalizes comfort with knowledge and performance of postoperative care with reduced anxiety
- States signs and symptoms to report postoperatively.

Cleft Lip/Palate

Cleft lip and/or palate is a defect caused by in utero development by the failure of the soft palate and bony tissue of the maxilla to fuse. They may occur singly or together and often occur with other congenital anomalies such as spina bifida, hydrocephalus, and cardiac defect. Treatment consists of surgical repair, usually of the lip first at 10 weeks of age followed by the palate between 1–3 years of age. The surgical procedures are dependent on condition of the child and physician

Table 13.3: Nursing interventions for anxiety of parent(s) and child.

Interventions	Rationales
Assess source and level of anxiety and how anxiety is manifested; need for information that will relieve anxiety	Provides information about anxiety level and need for interventions to relieve it; sources for the parent(s) include fear and uncertainty about treatment and recovery, guilt for presence of illness and sources for child include separation from parent(s), procedures, fear of mutilation or death, unfamiliar environment; anxiety in the child may be manifested by crying, inability to play or sleep or eat, clinging, aggression
Allow expression of concerns and ask questions about condition, procedures, surgery, recovery by parent(s) and child	Provides opportunity to vent feelings and fears and secure information to reduce anxiety
Communicate with parent(s) and answer questions calmly and honestly; use picture, drawings, and models for explanations to child	Promotes calm and supportive trusting environment
Allow parent(s) to stay with child and encourage to assist in care or open visitation	Allows parent(s) to care for and support child and continue parental role
Give parent(s) and child as much input decisions about care and routines as possible	Allows for more control over situation

preference. Management involves a multidiscipline approach that includes the surgeon, pediatrician, nurse, orthodontist, prosthodontist, otolaryngologist, speech therapist **(Fig. 13.2)**.

Symptoms of Cleft Lip/Palate

A child may have one or more birth defects.
- A cleft lip may be just a small notch in the lip. It may also be a complete split in the lip that goes all the way to the base of the nose.
- A cleft palate can be on one or both sides of the roof of the mouth. It may go the full length of the palate.

Other symptoms include:
- Change in nose shape (how much the shape changes varies)
- Poorly aligned teeth.

Problems that may be present because of a cleft lip or palate are:
- Failure to gain weight
- Feeding problems
- Flow of milk through nasal passages during feeding

Nursing Process of the Child with Gastrointestinal Disorder

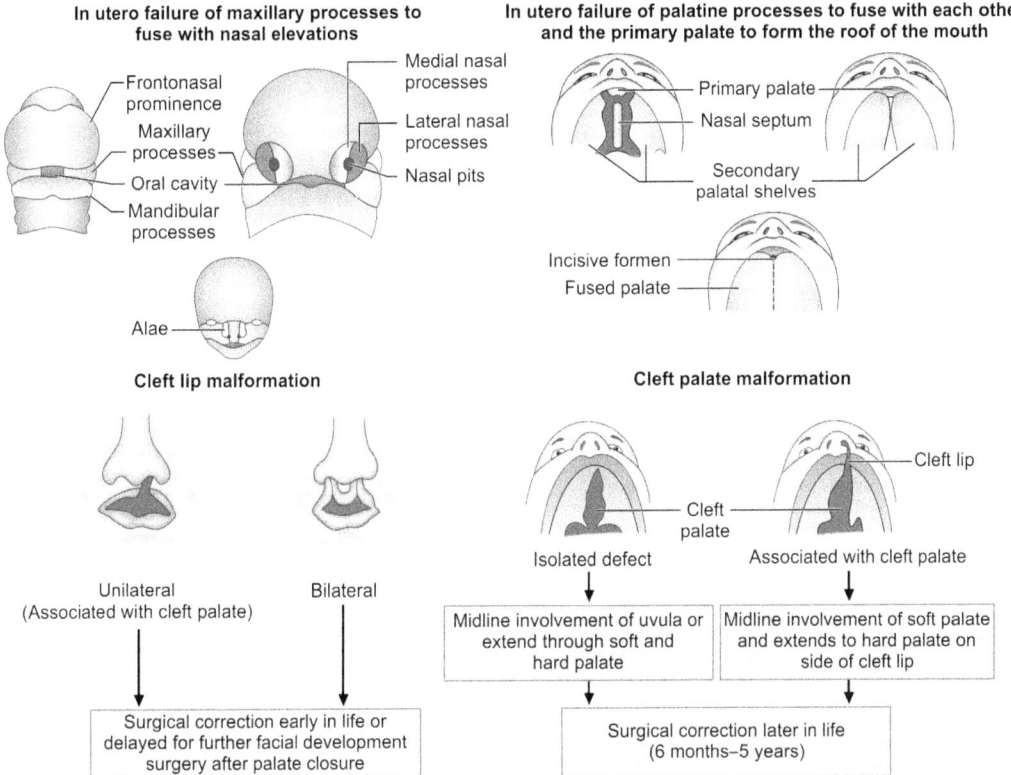

Fig. 13.2: Pathophysiology of cleft lip/cleft palate.

- Poor growth
- Repeated ear infections
- Speech difficulties.

Nursing Management

A. Essential Nursing Diagnoses and Nursing Process Associated with these Conditions

Nursing diagnosis

Altered nutrition: Less than body requirements related to inability to ingest food.
Assessment: Presence of cleft lip/palate, sore, inflamed buccal cavity, inability to suck, weakness of sucking and swallowing muscles.
(Refer Table 14.3 from chapter 14)

Nursing diagnosis

Ineffective airway clearance related to tracheobronchial aspiration of feedings, trauma of surgery.

Assessment: Abnormal breath sounds, dyspnea, tachypnea, cyanosis, changes in rate or depth of respirations, cough with or without sputum postoperative.
(Refer Table 11.1 from chapter 11)

Nursing Process of the Child with Gastrointestinal Disorder

Table 13.4: Nursing interventions for anxiety of parent(s).

Interventions	Rationales
Assess level of anxiety and need for information that will relieve anxiety	Provides information to ally anxiety manifested by the infant's appearance at birth with level increased with the location and extent of the defect (lip and/or palate defect)
Allow expression of concerns and questions about condition, to discuss negative feelings about appearance of infant	Provides an environment conducive to venting of feeling to facilitate adjustment to the infant's defect
Provide an accepting environment and attitude and handle the infant in a gentle caring way	Promotes trust and conveys to parent(s) that infant is a valuable baby deserving of love and caring
Communicate with parent(s) in a calm, honest way, discuss the surgical procedure(s) for correction of the defect(s) using pictures and models and allow to view pictures of children with successful defect repair	Promotes a calm and supportive environment to reduce anxiety and instill hope
Allow parent(s) to stay with infant and encourage to assist in care as appropriate	Reduces anxiety and promotes bonding that may be blocked by infant's appearance
Emphasize the infant's positive features when providing information	Promotes positive feelings for infant

B. Specific Nursing Diagnoses and Nursing Process

Nursing diagnosis

Anxiety of parent(s) related to situational crisis of congenital defect of infant **(Table 13.4)**.

Assessment: Severe reaction to appearance of infant with a facial defect, responses to imperfect infant (shock, denial and grief), expression of guilt, blame and helplessness, feelings of inadequacy and uncertainty, worried and anxious about impending surgery, bonding abandonment of infant or rejection by parents, apprehension about feeding and potential aspirations.

Evaluation
- Express reduction in anxiety as feelings about defect, correction and prognosis are discussed
- Verbalizes positive effect of caring for feeding, and supporting infant
- Demonstrates accepting attitude towards infant with progressive adjustment to appearance of defect and progression in bonding.

Nursing diagnosis

Knowledge deficit related to lack of information about preoperative care **(Table 13.5)**.

Assessment: Request for information about cause of defect(s), feeding techniques, prevention of complications caused by defect(s) preoperatively.

Evaluation
- Verbalizes understanding of defect(s) and preoperative requirements before surgical correction

Table 13.5: Nursing interventions for knowledge deficit related to lack of information about preoperative care.

Interventions	Rationales
Assess parent(s) ability to feed infant with a defect and acceptance of methods used, knowledge cause and type of defect(s), preoperative needs and care, ability of infant to swallow	Provides information about defect which may be inherited or congenital, partial or complete, unilateral or bilateral cleft lip and/or palate; adequate nutritional status and freedom from infection before surgery done
Instruct parent(s) to hold infant while feeding with the head in an upright position, use a nipple or feeding device for feeding, allow feeder to control the flow or the infant to express the formula, apply gentle, steady pressure on the bottom of the bottle and avoid removing the nipple frequently; instruct in feeding method that will be used postoperatively	Holding head upright reduces possibility of aspiration, pressure at the base of the bottle prevents choking or coughing, special nipples or devices are used because the cleft interferes with the ability to suck and liquid often flows into the nose when taken into the mouth, use of a nipple encourages development of sucking muscles
Instruct to feed slowly and in small amounts, burping frequently (tends to swallow air), and extend nipple or feeding device well back into the mouth	Prevents choking, abdominal distention possible flow of liquid into nose or aspirated into lungs causing pneumonia or otitis media or upper respiratory infections
Inform parent(s) that feeding should not last any longer than 20–30 minutes	Prolonged feedings may deplete an infant's energy and cause fatigue
Instruct in use and care of preoperative orthodontic device (plastic palate mold) for infant with cleft palate including removing and cleaning daily, replacing, preventing infant from removing palate	Promotes the alignment of maxilla and more normal speech sounds and prevents food from entering nasal cavity
Instruct parent(s) to cleanse lip, oral cavity and nose with water before and after feeding; apply mineral oil to lips	Prevents infection or skin breakdown with cleft lip or palate
Instruct parent(s) about need to avoid prone position and place child on back or side, use arm restraints, use cup for feeding if palate repair to be done, feed upright if lip repair is to be done for the period preoperatively	Accustom the child to treatments that will be done postoperatively
Inform parent(s) of procedure for correction of defect, medications and procedures done to prepare infant for surgery, what to expect postoperatively	Prepares parent(s) for surgical correction of defect and what to expect during convalescence

- Performs safe, effective feeding techniques and maintains nutritional status and weight gains
- Absence of infection or aspiration (upper respiratory, otitis media)
- Maintains clean cleft lip and/or palate
- Verbalizes understanding of need to carry out care and procedures that will be utilized postoperatively.

Nursing diagnosis

High-risk for injury related to internal physical factor of surgery (broken skin) **(Table 13.6)**.

Assessment: Trauma to suture line, use of protective device, formula or drainage at suture site, improper mouth care and teeth brushing, hands or other objects in mouth redness swelling and drainage form incisional site, crying caused by pain of incision, improper feeding method.

Evaluation
- Absence of trauma to incisional site
- Surgical incision healing without infection or injury
- Facilitates feeding without trauma to suture line
- Provides comfort measures and pain control
- Verbalizes and demonstrates dietary inclusions and restrictions.

Table 13.6: Nursing interventions for high-risk for injury related to internal physical factor of surgery (broken skin).

Interventions	Rationales
Assess suture line for cleanliness, redness, swelling or drainage	Provides information indicating possible infection and need for cleansing away formula or drainage
Assess for respiratory distress following palate surgery	Monitors breathing though a smaller airway caused by edema and breathing through nose
Cleanses suture site of lip repair with gauze or cotton tipped applicator with saline, apply medicated ointment after cleansing as prescribed; rinse mouth with water before and after each feeding	Removes material to prevent inflammation or sloughing and final cosmetic result expected
Place in side lying position, gently aspirate mouth of any secretions; maintain suture at end of tongue if present	Facilitates breathing and prevents aspiration; suture at end of tongue extends tongue to prevent obstruction of airway
Apply warm compresses to suture site on lip if prescribed	Reduces swelling
Provide air humidification or place in mist tent for a short time following surgery	Decreases dry mouth and nasal mucous membranes
Monitor lip protective device taped on operative site	Relaxes the site and prevents tension on sutures caused by facial movement or crying
Provide analgesic therapy for pain, hold, cuddle or rock child, anticipate needs to need to reduce tension on suture line	Promotes comfort and prevents crying caused by pain which creates tension on sature line
Apply soft elbow restraints and remove periodically to perform ROM on arms and allow for some movement and holding; a child may need a jacket restraint to prevent rolling over	Prevents child from touching or injuring operative site
Remove sharp objects or toys, avoid use of forks, straws or other pointed objects	Prevents trauma to mouth and suture line
Feed with a cup or spoon if palate repair done; avoid placing spoon in mouth	Prevents damage to suture line
Accompany child when playing or ambulating	Prevents trauma caused by accidental falls

Table 13.7: Nursing interventions for ineffective family coping; compromised.

Interventions	Rationales
Assess family coping methods used effectiveness, family ability to cope with child that needs long-term care and guidance, stress on family relationships, developmental level of family, perception of crisis situation by family, response of siblings	Provides information identifying coping methods that work and need to develop new coping skills; family attitudes directly affect child's feeling of self-worth, child with special needs may strengthen or strain family relationships
Assess knowledge of long-term treatment of defect(s)	Provides a basis for information needed about therapy
Encourage family members to express problem areas and explore solutions responsibly	Reduces anxiety and enhances understanding; provides opportunity to identify problems and problem solving strategies
Assist family to establish short and long-term goals for child and importance of integrating child into family activities	Promotes involvement and control over situations and maintains parental role
Encourage to follow home routines and meet child's needs with participation of family members	Increases child's sense of security and sense of belonging
Give positive feedback to family and praise family efforts in development of coping and problem solving techniques in caring for child	Encourages family to continue involvement in long-term care

- Demonstrates proper positioning and restraining procedures
- Cleanses suture site properly before and after feeding and when needed.

Nursing diagnosis

Ineffective family coping: Compromised related to inadequate information and temporary family disorganization caused by defect and future correction **(Table 13.7)**.

Assessment: Expression of concern about defect, long-term care required for successful outcome, confirmation of worry about normal growth and development, limited family support and assistance.

Evaluation

- Verbalizes and clarifies child's and family's knowledge about long-term needs and rehabilitation following surgery
- Develops and uses coping skills and problem solving techniques effectively
- Supports and cares for child by family members while meeting own need
- Preserves family relationships and minimizes family stressors with differences resolved
- Implements preventive measures to ensure optimal hearing, speech outcomes
- Progressive adoption and acceptance of long-term disorder and therapy by family
- Contacts community resources for assistance and support.

Gastroenteritis

Gastroenteritis is an acute infectious process affecting gastrointestinal tract caused by bacteria or viruses. Younger children are most commonly affected with specific organisms

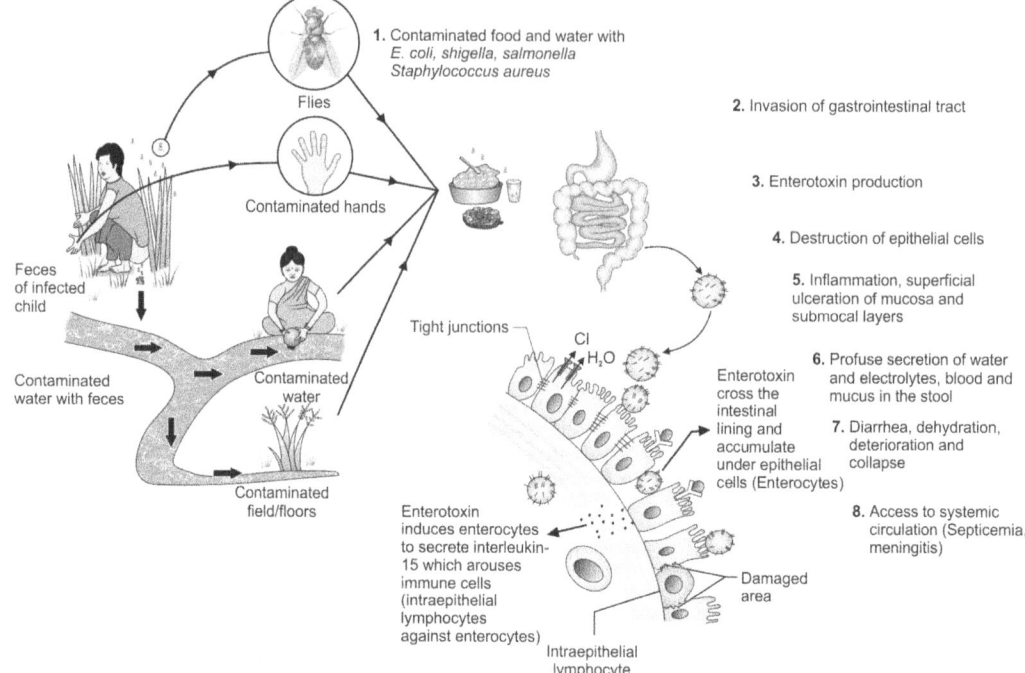

Fig. 13.3: Pathophysiology of gastroenteritis.

found in different age groups. At highest risk are those in daycare centers, schools, and in children with immune system abnormalities. The disease is transmitted by ingestion of contaminated food, water, contaminated hands, linens, equipment and supplies. Its most serious complication is dehydration and electrolyte losses which may lead to metabolic acidosis and death **(Fig. 13.3)**.

Symptoms of Gastroenteritis

Beside the nausea, vomiting, and diarrhea symptoms of gastroenteritis can include a low-grade fever of about 99°.

More serious symptoms include:
- Vomit or stool that contains blood
- Long-duration vomiting, such as more than 48 hours
- Fever that is 101°F or higher
- Abdominal swelling or pain the right lower side of the abdomen
- Dehydration.

Nursing Management

A. Essential Nursing Diagnoses and Nursing Process Associated with this Condition

Nursing diagnosis

High-risk for fluid volume deficit related to excessive losses through normal routes, NPO status.

Nursing Process of the Child with Gastrointestinal Disorder

Assessment: Vomiting, diarrhea, decreased skin turgor, dry skin and mucous membranes, weakness, fever, deceased urinary output, decreased pulse volume, increased pulse rate.

(Refer Table 14.11 from chapter 14)

Nursing diagnosis

High-risk for impaired skin integrity related to external factor of excretions and secretions.

Assessment: Redness, excoriation at anal site and perineum, presence of persistent diarrhea.

(Refer Table 12.1 from chapter 12)

Nursing diagnosis

Altered nutrition: Less than body requirements related to inability to ingest and digest foods.

Assessment: NPO status, nausea, vomiting, diarrhea, weight loss, anorexia, abdominal cramps.

(Refer Table 14.3 from chapter 14)

Nursing diagnosis

Hyperthermia related illness (infectious process).

Assessment: Increase in body temperature above normal range, warm to touch, increased pulse and respirations.

(Refer Table 14.18 from chapter 14)

Nursing diagnosis

Diarrhea related to dietary intake, contaminants, toxins, inflammation and irritation of bowel **(Table 13.8)**.

Assessment: Abdominal pain, cramping, increased frequency, increased frequency of bowel sounds, loose, liquid stools, changes in color, urgency.

Evaluation
- Absence of diarrhea with return to baseline bowel elimination pattern
- Dietary and fluid modifications to treat diarrhea and prevent recurrence of episodes
- Appropriate administration of medications
- Corrects fluid/electrolyte imbalance potential
- Maintains nutritional status and skin integrity
- Maintains enteric precaution measures
- Collects stool specimens for testing
- Relieves discomfort associated with diarrheal episodes
- Verbalizes proper preparation and storage of foods
- Cooperates with follow-up care instructions and reporting of signs and symptoms of potential complications.

B. Specific Nursing Diagnoses and Nursing Process

Nursing diagnosis

Knowledge deficient of parent(s) and child related to lack of information about disease and treatment **(Table 13.9)**.

Table 13.8: Nursing interventions for diarrhea.

Interventions	Rationales
Assess normal pattern of bowel elimination and characteristics of stool (frequency, amount, consistency, presence of blood, pus, mucus, color change); presence of diseases or contact with contaminants, infective organisms, medications being taken	Provides information about baseline parameters for comparison, reason for changes; diarrhea may be acute caused by an inflammation, toxin or a systemic disease and lasts about 72 hours or chronic caused by inflammation, allergy, malabsorption, bowel motility changes or disease and last longer than 72 hours, antibiotic therapy may cause diarrhea as it destroys the normal flora in the bowel
Assess abdomen for distention by palpation and bowel sounds for increases by auscultation	Indicates a distended bowel with fluid and hypermotility of bowel which reduces the amount of material that is absorbed by the bowel mucosa
Assess for temperature elevation, irritability, flaccidity, lack of expression, whiny cry, lethargy, anorexia, vomiting, eyes lacking luster	Provides information about signs and symptoms associated with diarrhea
Assess for fluid loss, weight loss, dry skin and mucous membranes, poor skin turgor, serum potassium, sodium for decreases	Indicates possible dehydration (isotonic, hypotonic, hypertonic) associated with fluid/electrolyte loss from frequent watery stools and vomiting and insensible fluid loss from fever that leads to metabolic acidosis
Obtain stool specimen for laboratory examination for toxins, ova and parasites, number of colonies of infective organisms present; fecal analysis for occult blood, fat content; repeat specimen examination as needed to confirm presence of organisms	Indicates possible cause of diarrhea
Place on enteric isolation and explain reasons why this is necessary until diagnosis is confirmed; maintain precautions if cause is identified as an infective organism; encourage parents and visitors to maintain hand washing before and after visiting or caring for child	Prevents undue anxiety and transmission of disease to others since bacterial and viral infections are the most common causes of diarrheas in children
Place on NPO, administer and monitor IV fluids and electrolytes	Allows bowel to rest and IV replaces lost fluids and electrolytes
Administer oral rehydration fluids q46 hours and increase or decrease depending on hydration status; volume should equal stool losses and as prescribed, and maintenance therapy includes the addition of 1 bottle of plain water for every 2 bottles of rehydration fluid	Provides therapy of choice for mild or moderate dehydration in infants
Gradually reintroduce fluids and solid foods orally; begin with clear fluids followed by full liquid diet and then to dry foods without milk or fats followed by low residue diet; eventually allow a general diet or return to previous pattern of foods/fluids ingested	Allows for graduated, slow return to dietary intake based on decrease or cessation of diarrhea and as stool increases in firmness

Contd...

Contd...

Interventions	Rationales
Administer anti-infective therapy and antidiarrheals	Destroys or inhibits growth of microorganisms; decreases bowel motility in children over 2 years of age
Change diaper frequently as needed in infant, expose buttocks to air and apply skin protective ointment to buttocks and perianal area in infants and anal area in children if irritated and sore; wash area with warm water after each diarrheal episode	Protects skin from excretions and secretions that are irritating and cause excoriation and skin breakdown

Assessment: Request for information about effect and treatment of the disease and prevention of transmission.

Evaluation
- Stool elimination decreases with return to baseline characteristics after instruction
- Disease transmission prevented with instruction ineffective preventive measures

Table 13.9: Nursing interventions for knowledge deficit for parent(s) and child.

Interventions	Rationales
Assess knowledge of causes of types of enteritis, methods to treat and control disease, willingness and interest to implement treatment preventive measures	Promotes effective plan of instruction that is realistic to ensure compliance of medical regimen, prevents repetition of information
Provide parent(s) and child with information and clear explanations in understandable language, include teaching aids and encourage questions	Ensures understanding based on interest and need to know to promote compliance
Inform to avoid food and fluid (NPO) until diarrhea subsides and when allowed begin with rice cereal, bread, weak tea and progress as tolerated	Allows bowel to rest until foods allowed
Inform that abdominal cramping may occur, that diarrhea may occur after eating or if a new food is offered	Reveals symptoms associated enteritis
Instruct to offer fluids (pedialyte) and avoid those fluids high in Na (milk, broth)	Provides and replaces fluids and electrolytes lost in frequent diarrheal stools, Na increases removal of fluid from cells by osmosis
Instruct in collection of stool specimen(s) for culture from other family members and inform to take to laboratory for examination	Reveals identification of specific organism responsible for enteritis as a basis for treatment
Instruct in enteric precautions and effective hand washing	Prevents transmission of organisms
Inform to take temperature by axillary method	Prevents additional irritation to rectum
Instruct to avoid over the counter drugs to treat diarrhea or vomiting	Prevents use of medications that may exacerbate condition
Demonstrate and instruct to insert antiemetic or sedative suppository	Treats vomiting and additional fluid loss and promotes rest
Instruct to measure 1:0 and determine imbalance to report	Prevents possible fluid imbalance complication which leads to dehydration

- Stools free from blood, mucus, infectious organisms
- Absence of fluid and electrolyte imbalance with compliance of instruction
- Nutritional status returned and maintained following instruction.

Hepatitis

Hepatitis is the inflammation of the liver caused by a virus. It includes four different types of viruses: hepatitis A (HAV), hepatitis B (HBV), hepatitis D (HDV) and hepatitis non-A, non-B (NANB). Most common of the types found in children is the hepatitis. A which is transmitted by the fecal-oral route. The incidence in children is increased in those living in crowded housing or attending daycare centers. The disorder is usually self-limiting with resolution within 2–3 months or may develop into chronic hepatitis. Symptomology varies with severity of the disease **(Fig. 13.4)**.

Symptoms of Hepatitis

Symptoms of acute (abrupt onset) hepatitis may include the following:
- Flu-like symptoms
- Jaundice (yellow color in the skin and/or eyes)

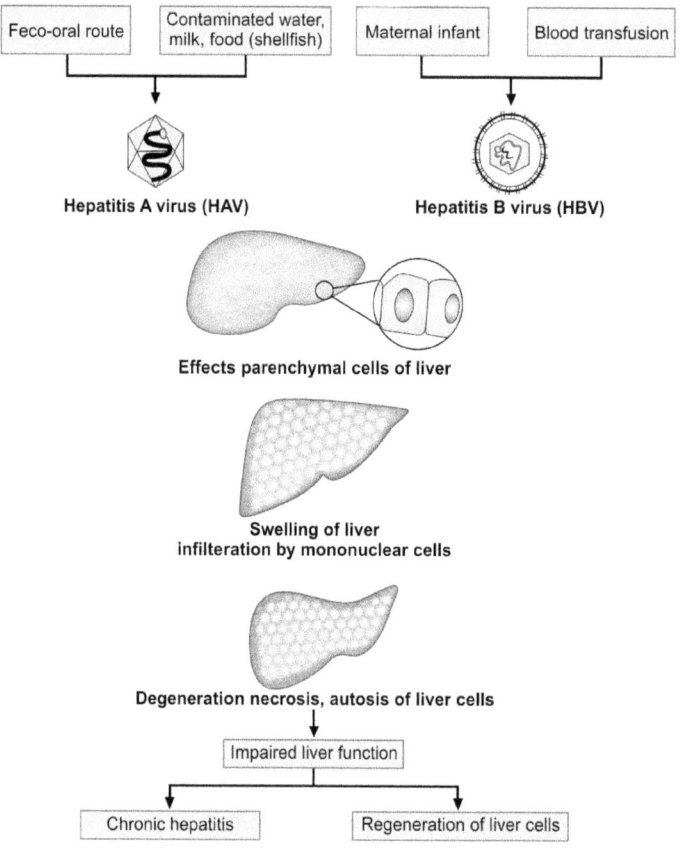

Fig. 13.4: Pathophysiology of hepatitis.

- Fever
- Nausea and/or vomiting
- Decreases appetite
- Not feeling well all over
- Abdominal pain or discomfort
- Diarrhea
- Joint pain
- Sore muscles
- Itchy red hives on skin
- Clay-colored stools
- Dark urine.

Late symptoms include dark-colored urine and jaundice (yellowing of the skin and eyes).

Nursing Management

A. Essential Nursing Diagnoses and Nursing Process Associated with this Condition

Nursing diagnosis

Altered nutrition: Less than body requirements related to inability to ingest, digest food.

Assessment: Anorexia, nausea, vomiting, weight loss, fatigue, abdominal discomfort.

(Refer Table 14.3 from chapter 14)

Nursing diagnosis

High-risk for fluid volume deficit related to excessive losses through normal routes.

Assessment: Vomiting, diarrhea, signs and symptoms of dehydration, gastrointestinal bleeding.

(Refer Table 14.11 from chapter 14)

Nursing diagnosis

High-risk for impaired skin integrity related to external factors of excretions and secretions, internal factor of altered pigmentation.

Assessment: Redness, irritation of perianal area with diarrhea, jaundice with pruritis.

(Refer Table 12.1 from chapter 12)

B. Specific Nursing Diagnoses and Nursing Process

Nursing diagnosis

High-risk for activity intolerance related to generalized weakness, bed rest **(Table 13.10)**.

Assessment: Easy fatigue, malaise, preference for inactivity, deconditioning with bed rest.

Evaluation
- Progresses in activities until baseline achieved
- Complies with activity and rest schedule
- Absence of fatigue and weakness.

Nursing Process of the Child with Gastrointestinal Disorder

Table 13.10: Nursing interventions for high-risk for activity intolerance.

Interventions	Rationales
Assess intolerance to activity and manifestations	Provides information about extent of fatigue
Maintain bed rest while illness is in acute stage but allow for quiet play and progress as condition allows	Allows for time for liver to heal and prevents any further damage
Provide access to needed articles within reach, aids to assist in performing ADL	Preserves energy which improves endurance
Provide increasing activity participation as tolerated on a daily basis	Promotes recovery without compromising energy or causing fatigue

(ADL: activities of daily living)

Nursing diagnosis

Knowledge deficit related to lack of information about transmission of disease **(Table 13.11)**.

Assessment: Request for information about spread of disease, measures to take to prevent spread of disease and possible relapse of condition.

Evaluation
- Verbalizes understanding of disease process and transmission to others
- Performs precautions to prevent transmission of disease to others

Table 13.11: Nursing interventions for knowledge deficit.

Interventions	Rationales
Assess knowledge of disease and isolation precautions to take to prevent transmission	Promotes knowledge and understanding of disease
Instruct parent(s) and child in proper hand wash and inform to perform before meals, after using bathroom	Prevents transmission of microorganisms for type a which is carried via the oral-rectal route
Inform parent(s) and child that toys may become contaminated and that they should not be shared	Prevents transmission to others via handling of toys
Inform of need to use disposable gloves when handling blood, excreta or any other body fluids	Prevents transmission of microorganisms
Instruct parent(s) to use disposable dishes, wash linens in hot soapy water and rinse well and dry, separate child's personal hygiene articles from other members of household	Prevents transmission of microorganisms to others
Inform parent(s) and child of signs and symptoms of disease, how disease is transmitted, dietary inclusions of protein and carbohydrate, activity program and signs and symptoms of disease recurrence (pain, anorexia, fever, nausea and vomiting, jaundice) to report	Provides information about disease and treatments to prevent transmission or relapse
Inform parent(s) of immune globulin available for hepatitis A, if given before exposure or after exposure, if during early incubation period or hyperimmune gamma globulin for hepatitis B, if given after exposure but reserved for those at risk	Provides information about prophylactic measures available
Inform parent(s) and child to avoid over the counter drugs without physician advice	Prevents potential for toxicity, if liver is unable to detoxify drugs

- Acquires passive immunization if at risk
- Absence of reinfection or relapse of disease
- Maintains enteric precautions of strict isolation as indicated by type of hepatitis.

Hernia

A hernia results from a protrusion of abdominal contents through an opening in a weakened musculature. An umbilical hernia is the protrusion of intestine and momentum through the umbilical ring caused by a failure of complete closure after birth. Inguinal hernia is the protrusion of intestine through the inguinal ring caused by a failure of the processus vaginalis to atrophy to close before birth allowing for a hernial sac to form along the inguinal canal. Umbilical hernia usually resolves by 4 years of age; those that have not by school age are corrected by surgery. Inguinal hernia becomes apparent in the infant by 2–3 months of age when intra-abdominal pressure increases enough to open the sac. It is usually associated with a hydrocele. Both are corrected by surgical repair (herniorrhaphy) to prevent obstruction and eventual incarceration of a loop of bowel **(Figs. 13.5A and 13.5B)**.

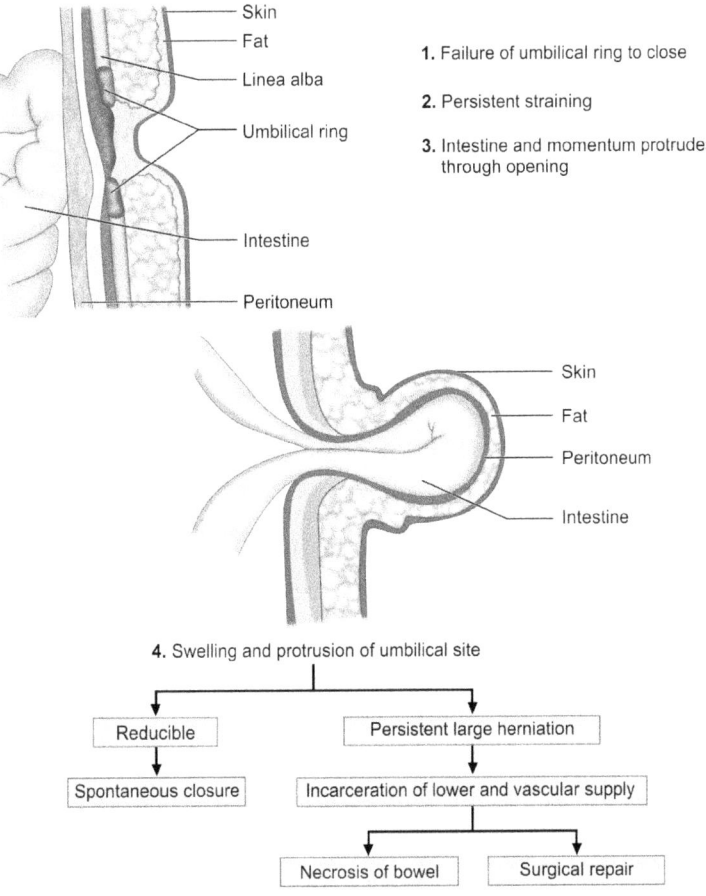

Fig. 13.5A: Pathophysiology of umbilical hernia.

Nursing Process of the Child with Gastrointestinal Disorder

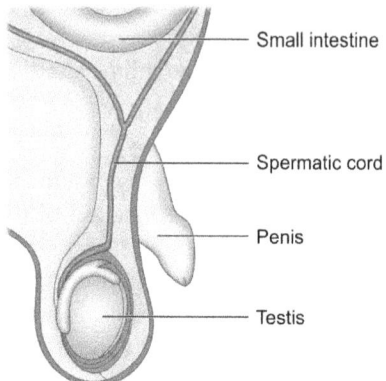

1. In utero failure of upper portion of processus vaginalis to atrophy and close
2. Development of hernial sac along inguinal canal
3. Increased abdominal pressure
4. Abdominal fluid and structures forced into sac
5. Inguinal swelling palpable mass during straining

- Reducible obstruction of intestinal loop when forced into the sac → Surgical repair
- Irreducible incarceration of loop of bowel → Complete obstruction → Gangrene

Fig. 13.5B: Pathophysiology of inguinal hernia.

Symptoms of Hernia

There are usually no symptoms. Some people have discomfort or pain. The discomfort may be worse when you stand, strain, or lift heavy objects. In time, most people will complain about a bump that is sore and growing. If a hernia gets bigger, it may get stuck inside the hole and lose its blood supply. This is called "strangulation."

Nursing Management

A. Essential Nursing Diagnoses and Nursing Process Associated with these Conditions

Nursing diagnosis

Ineffective breathing pattern related to pain, decreased lung expansion.

Assessment: Dyspnea, tachypnea, respiratory depth changes, altered chest excursion.

(Refer Table 14.2 from chapter 14)

Nursing diagnosis

High-risk for fluid volume deficit related to deviations affecting intake of fluids (postoperative status).

Assessment: NPO status, altered intake, signs and symptoms of dehydration, 1:0 imbalance.

(Refer Table 14.11 from chapter 14)

Nursing diagnosis

High-risk for impaired skin integrity related to surgical incision.

Assessment: Disruption of skin surface, invasion of body structures, excreta in diaper contaminating the incisional area.

(Refer Table 12.1 from chapter 12)

B. Specific Nursing Diagnoses and Nursing Process

Nursing diagnosis

High-risk for injury related to internal factor of intestinal obstruction **(Table 13.12)**.

Assessment: Irreducible loop of bowel, incarceration of the bowel with complete obstruction.

Evaluation
- Bowel contents easily reduced from sac with compression
- Absence of signs and symptoms of partial or complete obstruction
- Preventative measures taken to reduce straining and intra-abdominal pressure
- Verbalizes signs and symptoms to report to physician.

Nursing diagnosis

Pain related to biological injuring agent (surgical repair) **(Table 13.13)**.

Assessment: Irritability in infant, crying, moaning, guarding behavior, verbal descriptor of pain, refusal to move, change in facial expression in child, changes in vital signs.

Evaluation
- Postoperative pain relieved or controlled
- Takes measures to prevent pain postoperatively
- Infant/child rests comfortable with absence of behavioral responses to pain
- Analgesics therapy administered based on severity and age with desired results.

Table 13.12: Nursing interventions for high-risk for injury related to internal factor of intestinal obstruction.

Interventions	Rationales
Assess by palpation for umbilical or inguinal swelling that appears when infant cries or when child strains or coughs and ability to reduce swelling with gentle compression if bowel forced into sac	Reveals hernia that is reducible
Assess tenderness at hernia site with abdominal distention, anorexia, irritability and defecation changes	Indicates partial or complete obstruction caused by incarceration and strangulation

Nursing Process of the Child with Gastrointestinal Disorder

Table 13.13: Nursing interventions for pain.

Interventions	Rationales
Assess incisional pain and associated symptoms	Provides information about need for analgesic therapy
Administer analgesic appropriate for severity of pain and age	Relieves pain and discomfort caused by incision
Maintain position of comfort	Promotes comfort and reduces pain caused by strain on incision
Support buttocks when lifting or changing position	Prevents strain and pull on incisional site
Apply ice bag to scrotal area if hydrocele corrected and apply scrotal support if applicable	Promotes comfort by decreasing edema
Provide toys, games for quiet play	Promotes diversional activity to detract from pain

Nursing diagnosis

Knowledge deficit of parent(s) related to lack of knowledge about postoperative care **(Table 13.14)**.

Assessment: Request for information about activity allowed wound care, diet, bathing and comfort measures.

Evaluation
- Verbalizes and demonstrates postoperative including restrictions and progressive return to baselines
- Incision healing, fluid and dietary status maintained, activity monitored according to age
- Verbalizes comfort in caring for infant/child postoperatively
- Absence of postoperative complications or recurrence of hernia.

Table 13.14: Nursing interventions for knowledge deficit of parent(s).

Interventions	Rationales
Assess knowledge of causes of hernia, surgical procedure performed, willingness and interest to implement treatment regimen	Promotes effective plan of instruction to ensure compliance
Provide parent(s) and child as appropriate with information and clear explanations in understandable language, include teaching aids and encourage questions	Ensures understanding based on learning ability and age
Inform to maintain incisional site design until it peels off and to apply diaper, so that it does not cover incision and to change it frequently	Maintains dry and clean incisional site
Inform to give sponge baths until incision heals	Maintains incisional integrity
Hold infant when crying and to feed, activity is not usually restricted; advise child to refrain from lifting, pushing or engaging in strenuous play	Reduces stain on incision and possible recurrence of hernia
Advise parent(s) to increase and progress diet and fluids until baseline achieved	Promotes return to nutritional status without causing gastrointestinal strain on incision

Inflammatory Bowel Disease

Inflammatory bowel disease includes Crohn's disease and ulcerative colitis which have similar signs and symptoms but have different intestinal pathology. Actual cause of either disease is unknown but they are known to be associated with immunologic, nutritional, and infections disturbances with psychogenic factors responsible for severity and exacerbation of the disease. Crohn's disease affects the small and/or large intestine with the terminal ileus the most common site. It involves all layers of the bowel and results in a thickening and eventual obstruction. Lesions from this disease are patchy with areas of normal tissue while lesions from ulcerative colitis are continuous in the affected bowel. Ulcerative colitis also affects the mucosa and submucosa of the large intestine and rectum causing hyperemia and edema which effects absorption of nutrients and eventually a narrowed, inflexible, scarred bowel. Both diseases are characterized by remissions and exacerbations and occur in children of school age but are most commonly found in the adolescence age group **(Fig. 13.6)**.

Symptoms of Inflammatory Bowel Disease

- Cramping pain in the belly
- Ongoing diarrhea
- Blood in stool (feces)

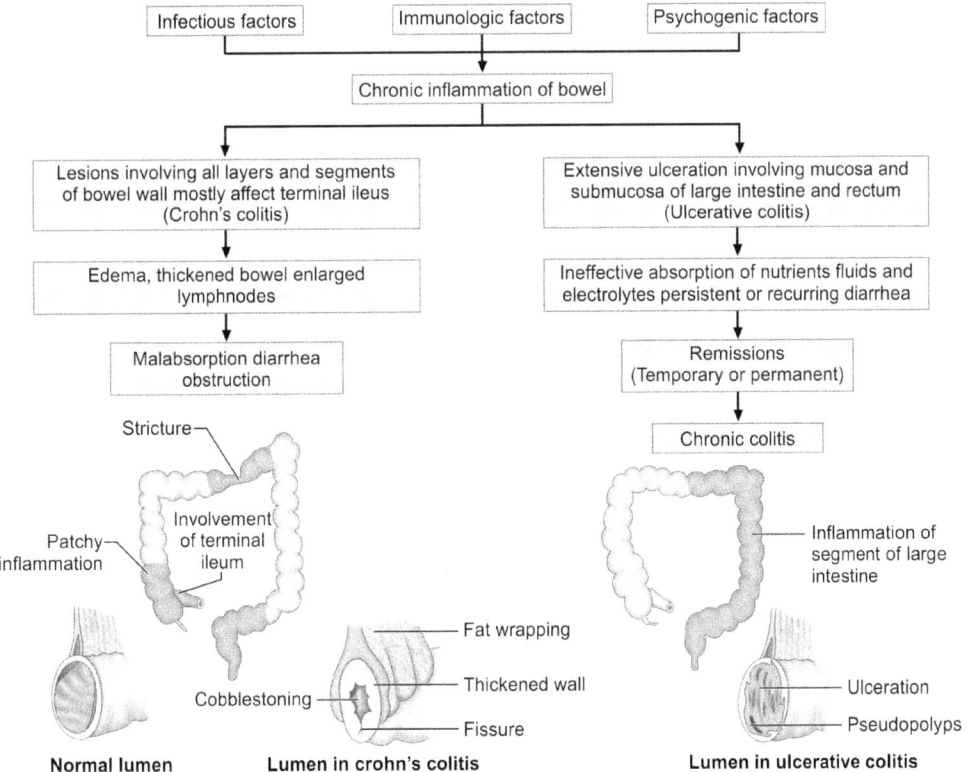

Fig. 13.6: Pathophysiology of inflammatory bowel disease.

- Weight loss
- Slowed growth
- Delayed puberty
- Weakened bones or lower bone density
- Anxiety
- Depression and emotional challenges.

Nursing Management

A. Essential Nursing Diagnoses and Nursing Process Associated with this Condition

Nursing diagnosis

Altered nutrition: Less than body requirements related to inability to ingest and digest food, absorb nutrients.

Assessment: Anorexia, diarrhea, abdominal cramping, weight loss, growth retardation, abdominal distention, possible vomiting.

(Refer Table 14.3 from chapter 14)

Nursing diagnosis

High-risk for fluid volume deficit related to excessible losses through normal routes.

Assessment: Diarrhea, output greater than intake, signs and symptoms of dehydration, electrolyte imbalance (K).

(Refer Table 14.11 from chapter 14)

Nursing diagnosis

Diarrhea related to inflammation, irritation, or malabsorption of bowel, dietary intake.

Assessment: Abdominal pain, cramping, increased frequency, increased frequency of bowel sounds, loose, liquids, watery stools, urgency, changes in color and constituents (blood, mucus), ingestion of high fiber foods.

(Refer Table 13.8 from chapter 13)

Nursing diagnosis

High-risk for impaired skin integrity related to external factor of secretions and excretions, internal factor of extraintestinal skin lesions.

Assessment: Irritation, redness, pain at perianal area, disruption of skin surfaces, chronic and excessive diarrhea.

(Refer Table 12.1 from chapter 12)

Nursing diagnosis

Altered growth and development related to effects of physical disability.

Assessment: Altered physical growth, delay in sexual maturation, delay in bone age, weight loss, school absences during exacerbations.

(Refer Table 14.4 from chapter 14)

Table 13.15: Nursing interventions for pain.

Interventions	Rationales
Assess severity of pain, onset and precipitating factors, location, duration, remissions and exacerbations	Provides information symptomatic of inflammatory bowel disease with pain common in Crohn's disease and less frequent in ulcerative colitis; pain is associated with dietary intake in both diseases
Administer analgesics, antispasmodics and anti-inflammatories and assess effect of medications in relieving discomfort	Relieves pain, bowel activity and the inflammatory process associated with pain
Allow to assume position of comfort	Promotes comfort to reduce pain
Provides toys, TV, book, games for quiet play during painful episodes	Promotes diversional activity to distract from pain

B. Specific Nursing Diagnoses and Nursing Process

Nursing diagnosis

Pain related to biological injuring agents, inflammation and irritation of the bowel **(Table 13.15)**.

Assessment: Abdominal cramping, abdominal distention, intermittent pain aggravated by eating or pain that is constant and aching, verbalization of other pain descriptors, guarding and protective behavior towards abdomen.

Evaluation
- Pain relieved or controlled
- Limits or avoids factors that initiate or increase pain
- Analgesic therapy administration based on severity of pain and age with desired results
- Participates in self-concept (body image), change in health status.

Nursing diagnosis

Impaired adjustment related to disability requiring change in life style, inadequate support systems **(Table 13.16)**.

Assessment: Verbalization of no acceptance of health status change, unsuccessful inability to be involved in problem solving, lack of movement towards independence.

Evaluation
- Modifies lifestyle within limitations
- Maximizes strengths and resources towards acceptance and adjustment of lifestyle changes
- Demonstrates self-care and independence in healthcare
- Accepts responsibility and need for involvement and cooperation by family and child
- Verbalizes progress towards acceptance of health status (including ostomy if present)
- Utilizes social services, dietary consult, community agencies and resources if appropriate
- Complies with medication and dietary regimen.

Nursing diagnosis

Knowledge deficit related to lack of information about long-term medical regimen **(Table 13.17)**.

Table 13.16: Nursing interventions for impaired adjustment.

Interventions	Rationales
Assess for ability of child and family to adapt, willingness of family and child to support medical regimen and need to change lifestyle, ability to problem solve and utilize coping mechanisms	Provides information about ability of family and child to modify lifestyle, make plans of a constructive lifestyle within limits imposed by change in health status
Encourage to identify strengths and roles of family and child, coping mechanisms that have been successful in the past, resources and support groups available	Allows for support needed to manage long-term illness of child
Assist child and family to develop a healthcare regimen by making decisions regarding care, sharing goals and progress, accepting accountability for specific aspects of care	Promotes independence and control over care and situations
Assist child and family to deal with denial behavior and to differentiate between denial of change in health status and denial of limits imposed by change in health status	Permits realistic lifestyle changes that are congruent with health status changes
Maintain a positive, hopeful attitude about lifestyle changes accomplished to promote health	Promotes maximal use of personal resources and acceptance of support system

Assessment: Request for information about medication, dietary regimen, care of colostomy or ileostomy.

Table 13.17: Nursing interventions for knowledge deficit.

Interventions	Rationales
Assess parent(s) and child for knowledge of prescribed medical regimen and postoperative care if applicable	Provides information of learning needs of parent(s) and/or child
Instruct in special nutritional needs including diet that is high in protein and calories and low in fat and fiber	Provides replacement of nutritional losses caused by the disease and to promote metabolic function and energy levels
Inform that mouth care before meals and bland foods should be encouraged if mouth pain is present	Promotes comfort if stomatitis present
Instruct in long-term administration of anti-inflammatories, antispasmodics, folic acid supplement including actions, dosages during acute and chronic stages, frequency, times, side effects, effect of discontinuing a steroid without tapering, signs and symptoms to report	Ensures compliance with medication regimen to reduce exacerbations
Instruct, demonstrate and allow for return demonstration for ostomy care including application and removal of appliance, peristomal skin care, emptying and cleansing of ostomy bag, odor control; continent ileostomy care and catheterization of the pouch	Promotes independence in ostomy care with as normal a return to activities as possible; procedure done, if child does not respond to medical treatment
Inform of nasogastric tube feedings or total parenteral nutrition if required	Provides information about alternate methods of nutritional support during acute state of disease

Evaluation
- Complies with medication and dietary regimen
- Demonstrates safe, effective ostomy care
- Maintains long-term remission.

Intussusception

Intussusception is a telescoping of one section of the bowel into another section resulting in obstruction to passage of the intestinal contents and in inflammation and decreased blood flow to the parts of the walls that are pressing against one another, if left untreated, eventual necrosis, perforation and peritonitis occurs. It occurs in infants most commonly between 3–12 months of age or in children 12–24 months of age. The actual cause is unknown but risk for the condition is increased in children with Meckel's diverticulum, celiac disease, cystic fibrosis, diarrhea or constipation. Surgical correction is done if the obstruction of the involved segment cannot be reduced manually or by barium enema of if bowel becomes necrotic **(Fig. 13.7)**.

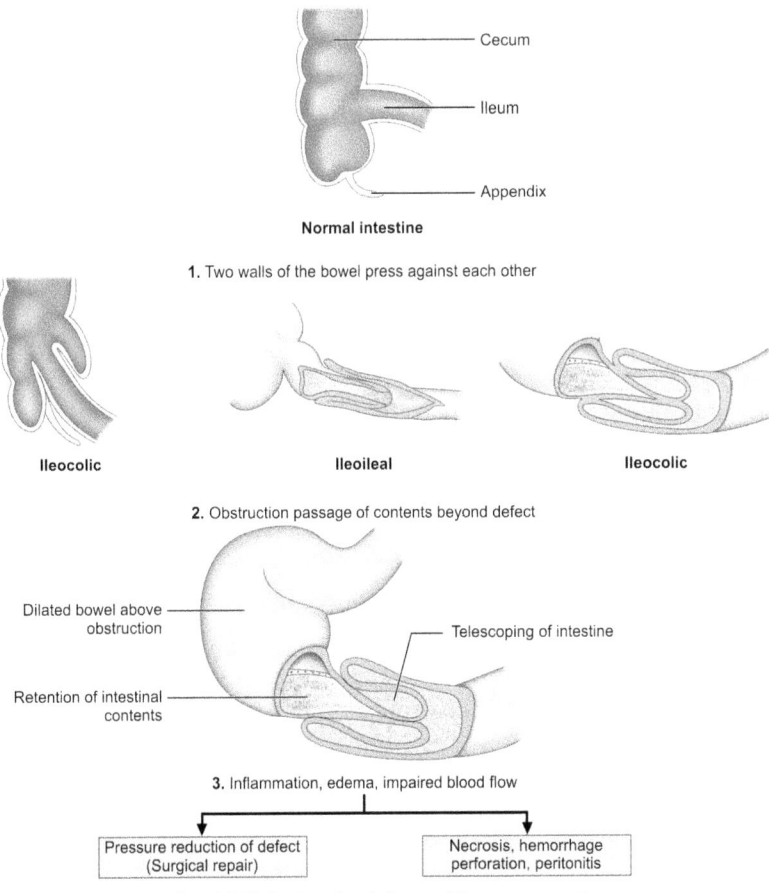

Fig. 13.7: Pathophysiology of intussusception.

Symptoms of Intussusception

The first sign of intussusceptions in an otherwise healthy infant may be sudden, loud crying caused by abdominal pain. Infants who have abdominal pain may pull their knees to their chests when they cry. The pain of intussusceptions comes and goes, usually every 15 to 20 minutes at first. These painful episodes last longer and happen more often as time passes.

Other frequent signs and symptoms of intussusceptions include:
- Stool mixed with blood and mucus (sometimes referred to as "currant jelly" stool because if its appearance)
- Vomiting
- A lump in the abdomen
- Lethargy.

Less common signs and symptoms include:
- Diarrhea
- Fever
- Constipation.

Nursing Management

A. Essential Nursing Diagnoses and Nursing Process Associated with this Condition

Nursing diagnosis

Altered nutrition: Less than body requirements related to inability to ingest and digest foods.

Assessment: Vomiting, abdominal pain, NPO status, N/G tube pre and postoperatively.

(Refer Table 14.3 from chapter 14)

Nursing diagnosis

High-risk for fluid volume deficit related to excessive losses through normal routes.

Assessment: Vomiting, decreased urine output, altered intake with NPO status, signs and symptoms of dehydration or electrolyte imbalance.

(Refer Table 14.11 from chapter 14)

Nursing diagnosis

Constipation related to medications (diagnostic procedure using barium enema).

Assessment: Hard formed barium colored stools, decreased bowel sounds, less frequent passage of stools and flatus, abdominal discomfort.

(Refer Table 12.9 from chapter 12)

B. Specific Nursing Diagnoses and Nursing Process

Nursing diagnosis

High-risk for injury related to internal factor of bowel function **(Table 13.18)**.

Assessment: Severe abdominal pain, bowel obstruction.

Table 13.18: Nursing interventions for high-risk for injury.

Interventions	Rationales
Assess presence of acute abdominal pain with loud crying and drawing knees up to chest which may be episodic, vomiting, passage of a brown stool followed by red, currant jelly-like stool, pallor, irritability	Provides information that indicates that intussusceptions is present which may lead to obstruction and signs of peritonitis if not treated
Assess presence of diarrhea, constipation, episodes of vomiting and colic in older child	Indicates presence of intussusceptions and need for further evaluation
Provide N/G tube attached to suction, IV fluids to decompress bowel and maintain hydration status and maintain patency of therapy	Prevents vomiting and dehydration and prepares child for barium enema procedure to diagnose and reduce the invagination
Note bowel elimination and stool characteristics and ability to eliminate barium following the procedure	Indicates success of the procedure in reducing the affected bowel as the condition may recur within 36 hours
Provide reassurance to parent(s) and allow to accompany child during procedure	Promotes trust and reduces anxiety
Provide information about all care given and allow for opportunity to ask question about procedures	Reduces anxiety

Evaluation
- Invagination reduced by barium enema procedure
- Bowel pattern returned to normal with passage of brown stools
- Absence of signs and symptoms of bowel obstruction
- Monitoring of chronic intussusceptions and reporting signs and symptoms as they occur.

Nursing diagnosis

Knowledge deficit of parent(s) related to lack of information about condition **(Table 13.19)**.

Assessment: Request for information about causes of condition, postoperative or post-procedural care.

Evaluation
- Verbalizes and demonstrates competence in postoperative or post procedural care
- Verbalizes baselines that are expected with the appropriate care
- Return of fluid, dietary, activity within limitations progressively as instructed
- Absence of complications or recurrence of invagination of bowel
- Compliance with monitoring of sign and symptoms indicating a complication that should be reported.

Table 13.19: Nursing interventions for knowledge deficit of parent(s).

Interventions	Rationales
Assess knowledge of condition, causes, treatment regimen following procedure(s), willingness and interest in providing care and compliance with treatment regimen	Promotes development of effective plan of instruction to ensure compliance and wellness

Pyloric Stenosis

Pyloric stenosis is a hypertrophic disorder of the circular muscle of the pylorus in which the pylorus is greatly enlarged and hyperplastic causing progressive narrowing of the canal between the stomach and duodenum. As the canal becomes obstructed over time, associated inflammation and edema results in complete obstruction. The exact cause is unknown although heredity is suspected. The abnormality is most common in young children between 1-6 months of age. Pyloric obstruction is treated successfully with surgical correction (pyloromyotomy) **(Fig. 13.8)**.

Symptoms of Pyloric Stenosis

Forceful projectile vomiting, the baby is usually quite hungry and eats or drinks eagerly. Large amounts of breast milk or formula are then vomited and may go several feet across a room. The milk is sometimes curdled in appearance due to the fact that it remains in the stomach where it is exposed to acid.

Other symptoms include:
- Weight loss
- Dehydration
- Lethargy (lack of energy)
- Fewer bowel movements
- Constipation
- Mild jaundice (yellowish coloring in skin).

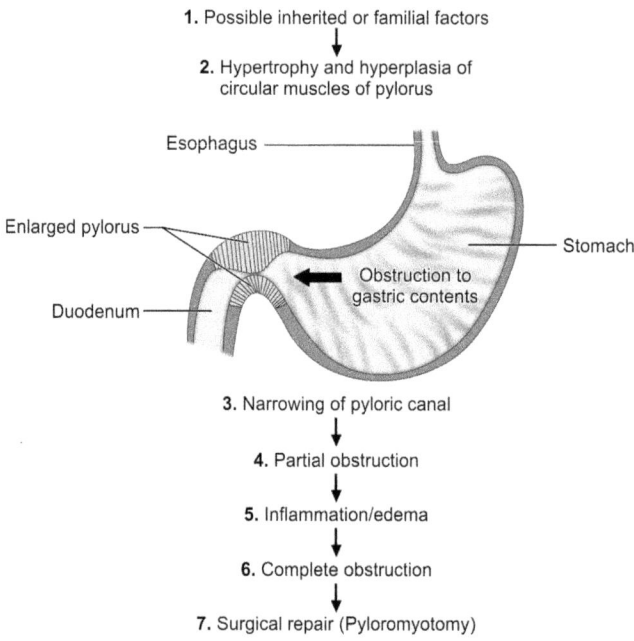

Fig. 13.8: Pathophysiology of pyloric stenosis.

Nursing Management

A. Essential Nursing Diagnoses and Nursing Process Associated with this Condition

Nursing diagnosis

High-risk for fluid volume deficit related to excessive losses through normal routes, NPO status pre and postoperatively.

Assessment: Vomiting with an eventual projectile character, electrolyte losses, signs and symptoms of dehydration, hemoconcentration, decreased urine output.

(Refer Table 14.11 from chapter 14)

Nursing diagnosis

Altered nutrition: Less than body requirements related to inability to ingest, digest food.

Assessment: Excessive vomiting especially after eating, chronic hunger, weight loss, failure to gain weight, diminished stools, abdominal distention, N/G tube pre and postoperatively for stomach decompression.

(Refer Table 14.3 from chapter 14)

B. Specific Nursing Diagnoses and Nursing Process

Nursing diagnosis

High-risk for injury related to internal factor of pyloric obstruction **(Table 13.20)**.

Assessment: Vomiting that increases in severity leading to dehydration, hunger, weight loss and reduction in frequency and amount of bowel elimination.

Evaluation
- Absence of dehydration, electrolyte imbalance
- Adequate nutritional support maintained with vomiting controlled
- N/G and IV tubes patent

Table 13.20: Nursing interventions for high-risk for injury related to internal factor of pyloric obstruction.

Interventions	Rationales
Assess pattern of vomiting, development of projectile vomiting, vomiting that occurs after feeding or hours after feeding weight loss, diminished stools, palpable mass in the epigastrium to the right of the umbilicus, presence of visible gastric peristaltic waves across the epigastrium	Provides information about presence of hypertrophic pyloric stenosis causing obstruction as the canal to the duodenum narrows
Maintain NPO status and N/G tube connected to suction, position with head slightly elevated	Decompresses stomach for 24–36 hours in preparation for surgery
Assess skin for decreased turgor, elasticity, loss of subcutaneous tissue, sunken eyeballs, urinary output	Provides information about the presence of dehydration caused by excessive vomiting
Maintain IV fluids and electrolytes (Na, K, Ca, Cl), glucose for nutritional support	Provides hydration and replaces lost glycogen stores and electrolytes for 24–36 hours in preparation for surgery or when needed
Weight daily at same time on same scale	Reveals losses or gains related to fluid and nutritional

Table 13.21: Nursing interventions for anxiety of parent(s).

Interventions	Rationales
Assess source and level of anxiety and how anxiety is manifested; need for information that will relieve anxiety	Provides information about anxiety level and need for interventions to relieve it; sources for the parent(s) include fear and uncertainty about treatment and recovery, guilt for presence of illness
Allow expression of concerns and ask questions about condition, procedures, recovery surgery by parent(s)	Provides opportunity to vent feelings and fears and secure information to reduce anxiety
Communicate with parent(s) and answer questions calmly and honestly; use pictures, drawings, and models for explanations	Promotes calm and supportive trusting environment
Allow parent(s) to stay with child and encourage to assist in care and feeding or open visitation	Allows parent(s) to care for and support child and continue parental role
Give parent(s) as much input in decisions about care and routines as possible	Allows for more control over situation
Provide consistent care of infant with familiar staff assigned for care	Promotes trust and reduces anxiety

- Preoperative preparation complete with restoration of hydration, electrolytes, depleted protein stores.

Nursing diagnosis

Anxiety of parent(s) related to change in health status of infant, surgical correction of condition (Table 13.21).

Assessment: Increased apprehension and expressed concern and worry about impending surgery, pre- and postoperative care, treatments while hospitalized and complications following surgery.

Evaluation
- Expresses reduction in anxiety about illness pre and postoperative care and procedures
- Parent(s) verbalize that anxiety decreases as acute phase is resolved
- Verbalizes positive effect of caring for and supporting ill child
- Participates in care and decision making regarding child care
- Demonstrates wound care and dressing changes postoperatively and other procedures to enhance wellness and verbalizes comfort with knowledge and performance of postoperative care with reduced anxiety
- State signs and symptoms to report postoperatively
- Complies with a progressive postoperative feeding regimen successfully with weight gain and absence of vomiting.

PRACTICE QUESTIONS

1. Master Vikram 9-years-old undergone hernioplasty and in pediatric surgical ward. Write the postoperative nursing management of the child by applying nursing process.
2. Write pre and postoperative nursing management for a child with appendicitis by using nursing process.

CHAPTER 14

Nursing Process for the Child with Cardiovascular Disorder

LEARNING OBJECTIVES
- To identify the signs and symptoms of a child with cardiovascular disorder.
- To frame nursing diagnosis based on the needs of the child.
- To plan nursing interventions and outcome identification.

INTRODUCTION

The cardiovascular system includes a pumping structure (heart) and a network of vessels (arteries, veins, and capillaries), which work together to circulate oxygen and nutrients to all parts of the body. Any alterations in the function of these structures affect the well-being of the infant/child and cause physical and psychosocial problems for both the affected child and family.

NURSING PROCESS FOR THE CHILD WITH CARDIOVASCULAR DISORDER (IN GENERAL)

1. **Nursing diagnosis:** Decreased cardiac output related to structural defect, congenital anomaly or ineffective heart pumping as evidenced by arrhythmias, edema, murmur, abnormal heart rate or abnormal heart sounds.
   Goal: Child or infant will demonstrate adequate cardiac output.
   Interventions: Increasing cardiac output.
   - Monitor vital signs closely, especially BP and heart rate, to detect increases or decreases
   - Monitor cardiac rhythm via cardiac monitor to detect arrhythmias quickly
   - Observe for signs of hypoxia such as tachypnea cyanosis, tachycardia, bradycardia, dizziness, and/or restlessness to identify this change early
   - Monitor for signs of thrombosis such as restlessness, seizure, coma, oliguria, anuria, edema, hematuria, or paralysis to identify this condition early
   - Administer adequate hydration to decrease possibility of thrombosis formation
   - Cluster nursing care and other activities to allow adequate periods of rest
   - Anticipate child's needs to decrease the child's stress, thereby decreasing oxygen consumption requirement.
   Evaluation: Child improved with elastic skin turgor, brisk capillary refill, demonstrate pink color, pulse and blood pressure within normal limits for age, regular heart rhythm, adequate urinary output.

2. **Nursing diagnosis:** Excess fluid volume related to ineffective cardiac muscle function as evidenced by weight gain, edema, jugular vein distention, dyspnea, shortness of breath, abnormal breath sounds or pulmonary congestion.

Goal: Child will be able to attain appropriate fluid balance.

Interventions: Encouraging fluid loss.

- Weigh daily on same scale in similar amount of clothing, in children weight is the best indicator of changes in fluid status
- Monitor location and extent of edema (measure abdominal girth daily if ascites is present); decrease in edema indicates positive increase in oncotic pressure
- Protect edematous areas from skin breakdown, edema leads to increased risk for alterations in skin integrity
- Auscultate lungs carefully to identify crackles (indicating pulmonary edema)
- Assess work of breathing and respiratory rate (increased work of breathing is associated with pulmonary edema)
- Assess heart sounds for gallop (presence of S3 may indicate fluid overload)
- Maintain fluid restriction as ordered to decrease intravascular volume and workload on the heart. Strictly monitor intake and output to quickly note discrepancies and provide intervention
- Provide sodium-restricted diet as ordered (restricting sodium intake allows better renal excretion of extra fluid
- Administer diuretics as ordered and monitor for adverse effects. Diuretics encourage excretion of fluid, elimination of edema, reduce cardiac filing pressures and increase renal blood flow. Adverse effects include electrolyte imbalance as well as orthostatic hypotension.

Evaluation: Child reduced weight (fluid), edema or bloating decreased, lung sounds cleared and heart sounds normal.

3. **Nursing diagnosis:** Imbalanced nutrition, less than body requirements, related to increased energy expenditure and fatigue as evidenced by weight loss or height and weight below accepted standards.

Goal: Child will be able to improve nutritional intake.

Interventions: Promoting adequate nutrition.

- Determine body weight and length/height normal for age to determine goal to work toward
- Assess child for food preferences that fall within dietary restrictions; child will be more likely to consume adequate amounts of foods that he or she likes
- Weigh child daily or weekly (according to physician order or institutional standard) and measure length/height weekly to monitor for increased growth
- Offer highest-calorie meals at the time of day when the child's appetite is the greatest (to increase likelihood of increased caloric intake)
- Provide increased-calorie shakes or puddings within diet restriction (high-calorie foods increase weight gain), consult with the pediatric dietician to provide optimal caloric intake with in dietary restrictions
- Provide small, frequent feedings to discourage tiring with feeding
- Feed infants with special nipple as needed to decrease amount of energy expended for sucking
- Administer vitamin and mineral supplements as prescribed to attain/maintain vitamin and mineral balance in the body.

Evaluation: Child demonstrated steady increase in weight and length/height, feed without tiring easily.

4. **Nursing diagnosis:** Ineffective tissue perfusion related to inadequate cardiac function or cardiac surgery as evidenced by pallor, cyanosis, edema and changes in mental status, prolonged capillary refill, clubbing or diminished pulses.
   Goal: Child will be able to demonstrate adequate tissue perfusion.
   Interventions: Promoting tissue perfusion.
   - Assess level of consciousness, pulse, BP, peripheral perfusion, and skin color frequently to determine baseline and ongoing improvement
   - Administer cardiac glycosides or vasodilators as ordered to promote cardiac output necessary for proper perfusion
   - Monitor pulse oximetry and arterial blood gas results to assess ability to appropriately oxygenate
   - Supplement oxygen as needed to provide oxygen to organs for proper functioning
   - Monitor hemoglobin and hematocrit to identify blood loss
   - Strictly assess intake and output to determine adequacy of renal perfusion position with head of bed elevated to decrease blood volume returning to heart
   - Change position every 2–4 hours to promote circulation and avoid skin breakdown in areas of poor perfusion

   Evaluation: Child attained state of alert, not restless or lethargic, developed pink color, decrease in edema, normal perfusion and strong pulses.

5. **Nursing diagnosis:** Risk for delayed growth and development related to effects of cardiac disease and necessary treatments, inadequate nutrition or frequent separation from care givers secondary to illness.
   Goal: Child will be able to attain development appropriate for age.
   Interventions: Promoting appropriate development.
   - Promote adequate caloric intake to stimulate growth and provide adequate energy
   - Provide age-appropriate developmental activities to stimulate development
   - Consult with the physical or occupational therapist or child life specialist to determine activities most appropriate for the child within the constraints of the child's illness
   - Schedule daily activities to allow for essential rest periods for energy conservation
   - Encourage parents, teachers, and playmates to be sensitive to child's self-image, using positive comments, to improve the child's self-concept
   - As energy allows, encourage participation in all activities as feasible to allow the child to feel normal.

   Evaluation: Evidence of cognitive and motor function within normal limits (individualized for each child).

6. **Nursing diagnosis:** Risk for infection related to need for multiple invasive procedures of cardiac surgery as evidenced by break in skin integrity, decreased hemoglobin or inadequate nutritional intake.
   Goal: Child will be free from infection.
   Interventions: Preventing infection.
   - Maintain strict hand hygiene to prevent spread of infectious organisms to the child
   - Assess temperature to detect elevation early in course of infection

- Avoid contact with persons with known infections to prevent risk of becoming ill
- Ensure appropriate immunization including pneumococcal and influenza vaccinations to prevent development of common childhood illness
- Administer prophylactic antibiotics prior to all dental procedures, surgery and many invasive procedures to prevent sub-acute bacterial endocarditis
- Encourage good dental hygiene to reduce the risk of endocarditis.

Evaluation: Vital signs within normal limits, white blood cell count normal, cultures negative, child exhibit no signs or symptoms of infection.

7. **Nursing diagnosis:** Interrupted family process related to crisis associated with heart disease, frequent need for testing and hospitalizations or stresses associated with care demands, as evidenced by inadequate parental coping, frequent separations of parent and child.
   Goal: Family will be able to maintain functional system of support.
   Interventions: Promoting family processes.
   - Provide ongoing support to the child and family to help them cope
   - Encourage parents and family members to verbalize concerns related to child's illness, diagnosis and prognosis; allows the nurse to identify concerns and areas where further education may be needed, demonstrates family-centered care
   - Allow families to grieve over the loss of a 'perfect' child; parents must work through those grief feelings so they can be fully 'present' for this chronically ill child. Explain therapies procedures, child's behaviors, and plan of care to parents; understand the child's current status and plan of care helps decreases anxiety
   - Encourage parents to be involved in care, allows parents to feel needed and valued and gives them a sense of control over their child's health
   - Identity support system for family and child, helps nurse identify needs and resources available for coping. Educate family and child on additional resources available to help them develop a wide base of support
   - Encourage parents to seek genetic counseling to provide them with the information required to make an informed decision about having another child.

   Evaluation: Demonstrate adequate coping, adoption of roles and functions and decreased anxiety; parents are involved in child care, ask appropriate questions, express fears and concerns, and can discuss child's care and condition calmly.

8. **Nursing diagnosis:** Activity intolerance related to ineffective cardiac muscle function, increased energy expenditure, or inability to meet increased oxygen or metabolic demands as evidenced by squatting positions, shortness of breath, cyanosis or fatigue.
   Goal: Child will be able to increase activity level as tolerated.
   Interventions: Promoting activity.
   - Assess level of fatigue and activity tolerance to determine baseline for comparison
   - Note extent of dyspnea, oxygen requirement, or color change with exertion to provide baseline for comparison
   - Cluster care activities, allowing rest periods in between, to conserve child's energy
   - Work with the parent and child to determine a mutually satisfactory daily schedule to allow adequate rest and energy conservation
   - Instruct family and child in prescribed activity restrictions to prevent fatigue while allowing some activity

- In the infant, avoid long periods of crying or prolonged nipple feeding (expends excessive calories)
- Provide neutral thermal environment to avoid increased oxygen and energy needs associated with excessive heat or cold.

Evaluation: Child participates in play and activities (specify particular activities and level as individualized for each child).

NURSING PROCESS FOR SPECIFIC CARDIOVASCULAR DISORDERS

Congenital Heart Defects

Congenital heart defects are abnormal malformations of the heart that involve the septums, valves, and large arteries. They are classified as acyanotic defects, in which a left-to-right shunt is present allowing a mixture of oxygenated and unoxygenated blood to enter the systemic circulation. The most common consequences of these defects in children are cyanosis and congestive heart failure (CHF), although defects that cause cyanosis may not always do so, and those that do not cause cyanosis may do so in some situations.

Common cyanotic defects include Tetralogy of Fallot and transposition of great vessels. Tetralogy of Fallot involves four defects that include pulmonic stenosis (PS), ventricular septal defect (VSD), right ventricular hypertrophy, and an aorta that overrides the VSD. Transposition of great vessels is a condition in which the aorta arises from the right ventricle instead of the left ventricle, and the pulmonary artery arises from the left ventricle instead of the right ventricle, causing a reversal of the normal position of these arteries **(Fig. 14.1)**.

Acyanotic defects include coarctation of aorta, patent ductus arteriosus and ventricular septal defect. Coarctation of the aorta is the narrowing of the aorta proximal to the ductus arteriosus (preductal), distal to the ductus arteriosus (postductal) or level with the ductus arteriosus (juxtaductal). The position of the narrowing during fetal development determines circulation to the lower body and development of collateral circulation. Patent ductus arteriosus is the failure of the structure needed for fetal circulation to close after birth. Ventricular septal defect is the incomplete development of the septum that separates the right and left ventricles, and it often accompanies other defects **(Fig. 14.2)**.

Congenital heart defects vary in severity, symptoms, and complications, many of which depend on the age of the infant/child and the size of the defect. Treatment may include management with medications, or open heart surgery to repair or resect or to a temporarily correct the defect until the child is older and growth takes place.

Nursing Management

A. Essential Nursing Diagnoses and Nursing Process Associated with these Conditions

Nursing diagnosis

Decreased cardiac output related to structural factors of congenital heart defect **(Table 14.1)**.

Assessment: Hypertension, bounding pulse, tachycardia, electrocardiogram (ECG) changes, arrhythmias, fatigue, dyspnea, oliguria, cyanosis or absence of cyanosis, murmur, decreased peripheral pulsed, widened pulse pressure, squatting or knee-chest position.

Nursing Process for the Child with Cardiovascular Disorder

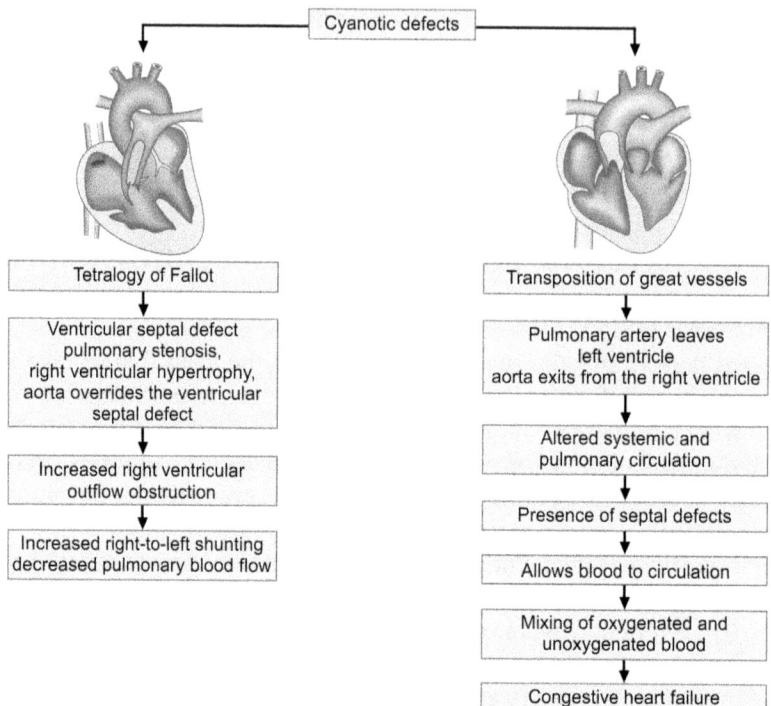

Fig. 14.1: Pathophysiology of congenital heart defects—cyanotic defects.

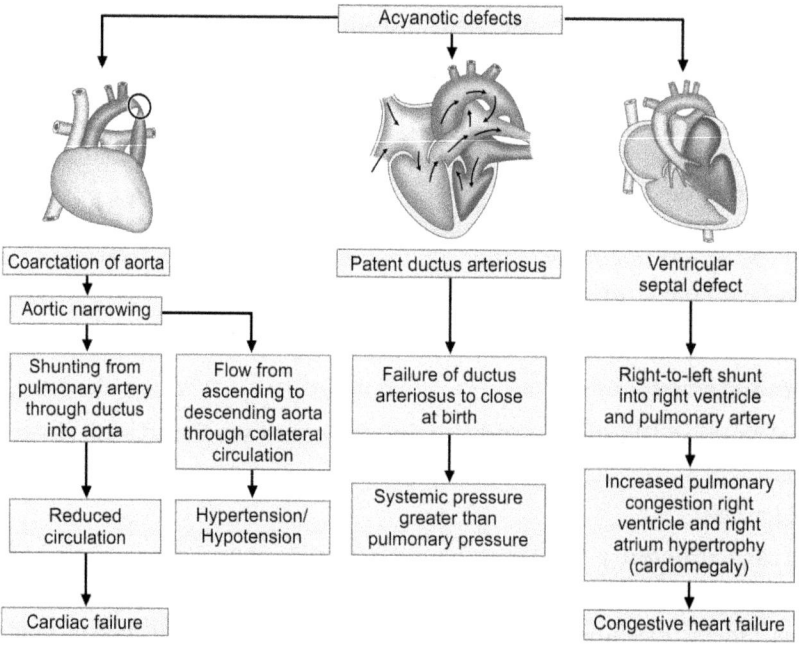

Fig. 14.2: Pathophysiology of congenital heart defects—acyanotic defects.

Table 14.1: Nursing interventions for decreased cardiac output.

Interventions	Rationales
Access cardiac output by monitor-heart rate (apical and peripheral pulses) for 1 minute, noting quality, rate, rhythm, intensity, pulse deficit; use radial site with gentle palpation in child over 2 years of age, and use apical site with stethoscope	Cardiac output is the amount of blood pumped from the heart in 1 minute and is determined by multiplying the heart rate by the stroke volume (amount of blood ejected with 1 contraction), which depends on heart contractility, preload and after load; pulse easily obliterated by compression
Assess blood pressure using proper size cuff; diaphragm on stethoscope of proper size; Doppler method, or electronic device. Approximate cuff width sizes are 4–6 cm for infant, 8–9 cm for child 2–10 years of age	Doppler method transmits audible sounds through a transducer in the cuff caused by ultrasound frequency caused by blood flow in the artery; the used of oscillometry transmits pressure changes through the arterial wall to the pressure cuff which are detected by an indicator that prints out the readings for BP and pulse
Assess BP when infant/child is at rest	Crying or other activity can increase BP 5–10 mm Hg; BP elevations that are considered abnormal are >110/70 in 3–6 years old, >120/75 and >130/80 in 10–13 years old
Assess existence of arrhythmias per ECG tracings	Device that measures and records the heart's electrical activity and provides information about heart rate and rhythm, hypertrophy, effects of electrolyte imbalances, conduction problems and cardiac ischemia
Administer cardiac glycosides, vasodilator; monitor for digoxin toxicity by symptoms of anorexia, nausea, vomiting, bradycardia, arrhythmias and digoxin level within 0.8–2.0 µg/L range (therapeutic level) potassium level; take apical pulse for 1 minute before administering digoxin, and withhold if pulse below desired level for age of child	Vasodilators decrease pulmonary and systemic vascular resistance, which decrease afterload and BP; cardiac glycoside strengthens and decreased the heart rate, which decreases the workload of cardiac performance; decreased potassium level enhances risk for digoxin toxicity
Position for comfort and chest expansion in Flower's, provide quiet environment, pace any activity to allow for rest	Promotes ease of breathing and rest, reduces stress and workload of the heart
Monitor temperature	Pulse increased at rate of 8–10/minutes with every degree of elevation on temperature
Attach cardiac monitor to infant/child, if prescribed	Reveals changes in heart rate and respirations

(BP: blood pressure; ECG: electrocardiogram)

Evaluation

- Vital signs maintained within baseline parameters for age and sex maintained
- Compliance and accurate administration of medications with desired effect achieved
- Provides stress-free environment with adequate rest for infant/child

- Adequate cardiac function maintained with urinary output, breathing, nutritional status, activity tolerance within normal parameters
- Absence of dysrhythmias noted on ECG.

Nursing diagnosis

Ineffective breathing pattern related to decreased energy and fatigue, pulmonary complications **(Table 14.2)**.

Assessment: Dyspnea, hypoxia (blue baby), tachypnea, abnormal arterial blood gases (ABGs), cyanosis.

Evaluation
- Return of respiratory status to baseline parameters for rate, depth, and ease
- Optimal breathing pattern and ventilation
- Breath sounds clear with optimal airflow
- Effective breathing effort and improved chest expansion
- Anxiety reduced or minimized
- Control of respirations and factors that affect them absence of upper or lower respiratory infectious process.

Nursing diagnosis

Altered nutrition: Less than body requirements related to inability to ingest, digest, or absorb nutrients because of biological factors **(Table 14.3)**.

Assessment: Poor feeding, fatigue, slow growth, lack of interest in food, prolonged impaired cardiac function decreasing perfusion to gastrointestinal organs.

Evaluation
- Maintains nutritional status for growth and development
- Complies with and tolerates daily intake of nutrient requirements (caloric and basic 4) for optimal health
- Promotes nutritional intake via method in accordance with disease limitations, presence of gastrointestinal symptoms
- Return to baseline parameters of gastrointestinal function related to ingestion, digestion absorption
- Absence of anorexia, nausea, vomiting, diarrhea, bowel distention, weight loss
- Offers feedings/meals appropriate for specific age and disorder
- Administers nutrients via IV, tube feedings, feeding device safely and with desired results
- Verbalizes caloric and special nutritional needs for infant/child, methods of preparation and storage, factors that encourage and discourage food intake
- Promotes optimal environment for nutritional health
- Maintains acceptable weight for height and frame.

Nursing diagnosis

Altered growth and development related to effects of acute or chronic illness or disability **(Table 14.4)**.

Assessment: Altered physical growth, delay or difficulty in performing motor or social skills typical of age, dependence and isolation.

Table 14.2: Nursing interventions for ineffective breathing pattern.

Interventions	Rationales
Assess respirations for rate (count for one full minute), depth and ease, presence of tachypnea (50–80/minutes), dyspnea and use of accessory muscles and, respiratory rhythm, nasal flaring, periods of apnea	Reveals rate and type of respirations (baselines or deviations) that are related to age and size of the infant/child and presence of anxiety and disease processes, changes in patterns indicate the acuteness of a condition and the respiratory function that result from infection and obstruction; retractions that become severe are responses to a decrease in intrathoracic pressure that may extend to suprasternal area if lung consolidation is severe, nasal flaring occurs as the work of breathing increases
Assess configuration of chest by palpation; auscultate for breath sounds that indicate air movement restriction (absent or diminished, crackles or rhonchi)	Reveals an increased anteroposterior ratio common in children with chronic respiratory disease that results from hyperexpansion of the airways
Assess skin for pallor or cyanosis, distribution and duration of cyanosis (nailbeds, skin, mucous membranes, circumoral)	Reveals presence of hypoxemia causing cyanosis from an uneven distribution of gases and blood in the lungs, and alveolar hypoventilation caused by airway obstruction, weakness of muscles used in respirations
Assess for cough, pain when coughing, characteristics of cough and sputum, ability to mobilize and bring up secretions when amounts increase	Cough is an indication of a respiratory condition and if excessive may cause chest pain and interfere with respirations, accumulation of mucus in airways affects respiration if obstruction is present
Position with head elevated or seated upright with head on pillows; position on side if more comfortable	Facilitates chest expansion and respiratory efficiency by reducing pressure of abdominal organs on diaphragm; position of comfort is age related and dependent on degree of dyspnea
Perform deep breathing exercises and upper body exercises	Strengthens intercostals and abdominal muscles, and diaphragm, which enhances breathing and prolongs expiratory phase
Pace activities and exercises, and allow for rest periods and energy conservation	Prevents changes in respiratory pattern brought about from exertion and fatigue
Monitor blood gas levels and provide supplemental oxygen via hood, tent, cannula, or face mask as needed if hypoxia results from inadequate breathing pattern and ventilation; if an infant is apneic, provide access at bedside at all times	Maintains oxygen level in blood to maintain tissue and organ function, amount and type of oxygen administration dependent on hypoxia and changes in mentation
Administer bronchodilator via oral, subcutaneous, or aerosol therapy; antibiotics or sedatives (cautiously) via oral therapy, if respiratory efficiency is not reduced; anti-asthmatics and steroids via oral or aerosol therapy	Relieves bronchospasms that affect respirations (tachypnea, rhonchi), prevents or treats infection, promotes rest and reduces anxiety to enhance breathing; prevents asthmatic attack and reinforces body defenses against allergic reactions

Nursing Process for the Child with Cardiovascular Disorder

Table 14.3: Nursing interventions for altered nutrition: less than body requirements.

Interventions	Rationales
Assess history of food intake (24 hours recall, amounts formula or breast milk), financial and cultural influences, vitamin/mineral supplement, food allergies	Provides information needed to evaluate nutritional pattern, habits and adequacy (deficiency or excess)
Assess appetite changes (poor or excessive), presence of illness and diagnosis, effect of nutrition on skin, hair, eyes, mouth, head, muscles, behavior	Indicates health status and effect of illness which requires an increase in nutritional needs and appetite and may result in malnutrition
Assess height and weight, head circumference, skin fold thickness and arm circumference and compare with previous values and standard charts	Provides anthropometric information about body's fat and protein content and general nutritional status
Assess difficulty in sucking, swallowing, chewing, gag reflex, teeth, oral mucous membrane, lips, and palate for abnormalities, presence of oral pain or infection	Provides information about ability to ingest foods or formula necessary for normal growth and development; inadequate dental care, oral inflammatory disorders, congenital defects (cleft lip/palate) interferes with feeding
Assess presence of nausea, vomiting and if spitting up, projectile, related to activity or intake or tension/stress, characteristics of vomitus (bloody, bile, digested or undigested food), frequency and persistence, amount, associated conditions (diarrhea, fever, headache, motion sickness, anger, conflict with parent)	Provides information about emesis which affects nutrition and is controlled by the vomiting center in the medulla. Causes include blockage of the pylorus, reflux from incompetent esophageal sphincter, gastroenteritis, duodenal and gastric spasm, increased ICP, bowel obstruction, drugs and allergens; persistent losses may lead to fluid and electrolyte imbalance
Assess abdominal girth, stool characteristics (odor, appearance), presence of diarrhea, bowel sounds for increased motility	Provides information about ability to absorb foods; stool may be bulky and fatty in cystic fibrosis if bile flow obstructed and fats are not digested; diarrhea may cause carbohydrate malabsorption as motility increases and moves nutrients through the bowel before absorption takes place
Place infant/child in position of comfort for feeding/meals, hold infant in arms or upright as condition indicates (cleft defect), child in sitting position at table within easy reach of food and with appropriate sized utensils	Provides most appropriate position to enhance movement of formula/solid food by gravity and peristalsis and to prevent vomiting and/or aspiration
Offer feedings/meals as near usual to normal routine as possible; provide amounts (small when indicated) and frequency (infant feedings q4h and progress to 3 meals/day) with introduction of solid foods at proper age: if ill, spread over 6 meals/day	Promotes feedings/meals that are similar to established pattern and adjusted to special needs caused by specific illness or increased metabolic demand (fever, infection, chronic illness, malnutrition)
Request parent to bring foods from home and serve in age appropriate quantities; allow child to eat in a community setting with other children	Promotes appetite and increased independence and familiar types and preparation of foods

Contd...

Nursing Process for the Child with Cardiovascular Disorder

Contd...

Interventions	Rationales
Offer age appropriate food consistency and foods that are not irritating to oral, stomach, bowel mucosa, thicken formula with cereal when necessary; modify other foods specific to disorder	Promotes ingestion and retention of foods and prevents exacerbation or increased severity of gastrointestinal disorders
Maintain NPO status if prescribed, provide infant with no nutritional sucking	Provides rest of gastrointestinal tract needed because of vomiting, diarrhea, preoperative preparation
Initiate and monitor IV administration of nutrients as prescribed, maintain strict 1:0	Provides short-term fluid and nutritional support via peripheral vein in those who are unable to ingest or retain nourishment (vomiting, diarrhea, postoperative care)
Initiate and monitor IV total parenteral nutrition as prescribed	Provides long-term fluid and nutritional support via a right atrial catheter in a large vein in those who are nutritionally deficient as a result of a chronic disease (Crohn's disease) or negative nitrogen balance
Insert and secure nasogastric tube and initiate and monitor tube feedings as prescribed; initiate and monitor feedings and insertion site of gastrostomy if present	Provides nutritional support for those with persistent weight loss, unable to chew, swallow, suck, who nutrients while ill but with intact digestive and absorption activity
Avoid excessive handling of an infant after feeding; and limit child's activity immediately after feeding	Prevents possible vomiting from increased stimuli
Administer vitamin/mineral supplements, digestive enzymes, antispasmodics, antibiotics	Provides or replaces necessary substances that may be deficient if absorption impaired or be the cause of impaired digestion, absorption; reduces peristalsis and infections process effecting nutritional status
Consult with dietician if needed	Provides support for the infant/child's special dietary needs

Evaluation
- Demonstrates growth and developmental advances appropriate for age and condition
- Resolves growth and developmental deficits for optimal cognitive, psychomotor, psychosocial functioning
- Complies with activities that enhance stimulation, independence, and developmental progression
- Secures appropriate testing for diagnosis and treatment of growth and development problems.

B. Specific Nursing Diagnosis and Nursing Process Associated with these Conditions

Nursing diagnosis

Activity intolerance related to generalized weakness imbalance between oxygen supply and demand **(Table 14.5)**.

Table 14.4: Nursing interventions for altered growth and development.

Interventions	Rationales
Assess height and weight, head circumference, skin fold thickness and arm circumference and compare with previous values and standard charts	Provides anthropometric information about body's fat and protein content and general nutritional status
Provide or arrange for growth and development assessment with the administration of tools such as Denver Developmental Screening Test (DDST-T), Denver II, Revised Denver Prescreening Developmental Questionnaire (R-PDQ), Denver Articulation Screening Exam (DASE)	Identifies developmental level or any lag in development to assist in plan of care or therapy; information should included age, expected gross and fine motor development, language and social development, psychosocial and psychosexual development, inter-personal skills, cognitive and moral and spiritual development
Reassess developmental levels at intervals appropriate for illness or other problem	Provides evidence of progress to evaluate program to correct any growth and developmental deficit
Provide consistent caretaker and care depending on age and abilities, encourage to participate in goal setting, decision making, participation in care	Promotes trust and progress in development promotes independence, needed for control and development
Provide visual, auditory, tactile stimulation, including mobiles with or without color, music, toys, books, television, games or other age-related activities; hold child and rock or pat on back, talk to child	Promotes stimulation needed to maintain developmental status
Provide time for child, either quiet or talking, to play with other children, time for parent(s) that remain in hospital to interact with child	Promotes independence and development or maintenance of motor skills to prevent regression
Initiate referral to child development expert if appropriate	Provides source of assistance to ensure proper age-related development

Table 14.5: Nursing interventions for activity intolerance.

Interventions	Rationales
Assess level of fatigue, ability to perform ADL and other activities in relation to severity of condition	Provides information about energy reserves and response to activity
Assess dyspnea on exertion, skin color changes during rest and when active	Indicates hypoxia and increased oxygen need during energy expenditure
Allow for rest periods between care, disturb only when necessary for care and procedures	Promotes rest and conserves energy
Avoid allowing infant to cry for long periods of time, use small nipple for feeding	Conserves energy
Provide toys and games for quiet play and diversion appropriate for age of child, allow to limit own activities as much as possible	Promotes growth, diversion, and physical and mental development
Provide optimal environmental temperature	Avoids hot or cold extremes, which increases oxygen and energy needs

(ADL: activities of daily living)

Table 14.6: Nursing interventions for high-risk for infection.

Interventions	Rationales
Assess temperature, IV site if present, increased WBC, increased pulse and respirations	Provides information indicating potential infection
Provide adequate rest and nutritional needs for age	Protects against potential infection by increasing body resistance and defenses
Wash hands before giving care	Prevents transmission of microorganisms to infant/child
Avoid allowing those with infections to have contact with infant/child	Prevents transmission of infectious agents to infant/child with compromised defenses
Administer antibiotic therapy	Preventive measure administered as prophylaxis
Use sterile technique for IV maintenance if present	Prevents contamination, which causes infection

(WBC: white blood cell)

Assessment: Presence of circulatory/respiratory problem, verbal complaint of fatigue or weakness, needs to rest after short period of play. Abnormal heart rate of blood pressure response to activity, exertional dyspnea.

Evaluation
- Controls activities that are fatiguing
- Maintains rest and activity schedule
- Engages in activities appropriate for age and energy level.

Nursing diagnosis

High-risk for infection related to chronic illness **(Table 14.6)**.

Assessment: Debilitated condition, IV site contamination, susceptibility to bacterial endocarditis, immobility, change in vital signs.

Evaluation
- Measures taken to prevent exposure to infection
- Absence of infection.

Nursing diagnosis

High-risk for injury related to internal factor of cardiac function from congenital defects and medication administration **(Table 14.7)**.

Assessment: Digoxin toxicity (vomiting, dysrhythmia), congestive heart failure (tachycardia, dyspnea, fatigue, restlessness, cough, cyanosis, orthopnea, edema, weight gain, neck vein distention, decreased BP, cardiomegaly), hypoxemia, possible cardiac surgery.

Evaluation
- Correctly administers prescribed medications with absence of side effects
- Verbalizes signs and symptoms of complications to report
- Takes apical pulse correctly
- Expresses feelings regarding possible need for surgery

Nursing Process for the Child with Cardiovascular Disorder

Table 14.7: Nursing interventions for high-risk for injury.

Interventions	Rationales
Assess for risk of drug toxicity, cardiac complication of heart failure	Early identification of signs and symptoms of complications allows preventive measures and adjustments to be made
Assess for possibility of open heart surgery, need for diagnostic tests and procedures	Allows for preparation and support of parents(s) and infant/child
Administer digoxin or indomethacin in correct dosages, check dosages, take apical pulse for a full minute before administering digoxin, assess for drug responses	Promotes safe administration of cardiotonic to decrease and strengthen heart rate (digoxin) or, to promote closing of ductus (indomethacin)
Assist and support family's feelings and decision regarding surgery	Provides needed support to allay anxiety and promote caring attitude

- Intervenes to relieve cyanotic episodes
- Verbalizes understanding of procedures and tests to be done.

Nursing diagnosis

Ineffective family coping: Compromised related to situational and developmental crises of family and child **(Table 14.8)**.

Assessment: Family expresses concern fear and anxiety about infant/child's disease and condition.

Evaluation

- Optimal health of family members, caretaker maintained
- Statements that anxiety reduced and coping techniques utilized effectively

Table 14.8: Nursing interventions for ineffective family coping: compromised.

Interventions	Rationales
Assess anxiety level, erratic behaviors (anger, tension, disorganization), perception of crisis situation	Information affecting ability of family to cope with infant/child's cardiac condition
Assess coping methods used and effectiveness	Identifies need to develop new coping skills if existing methods are ineffective in changing behaviors exhibited
Assess level of anxiety need for information and support	Provides information about need for interventions to relieve anxiety and concern
Encourage expression of feelings and provide factual information about infant/child	Reduces anxiety and enhance family's understanding of condition
Assist in identifying and using techniques to cope with and solve problem and gain control over the situation	Provides support for problem solving and management of situation
Provide anticipatory guidance for crisis resolution and allow for grieving process	Assists family in adapting to situation and developing new coping mechanisms

- Maintenance of social contacts of family
- Reduction of overprotective behaviors in infant/child care
- Statements of adjustment and progressive adaptation to special physical and behavioral needs
- Ability of family to adopt a positive view of infant/child's condition and need for normal growth and development
- Appropriate growth and development advances for age group
- Uses behavior modification techniques.

Congestive Heart Failure

Congestive heart failure is the inability of the heart, due of ineffective contractions, to maintain the workload necessary to pump blood throughout the circulatory system of the body. In children, cardiac heart failure occurs as a result of changes associated with congenital heart defects, such as those resulting in left-to-right shunts (volume overload) or obstructive lesions with in the heart (pressure overload), of cardiomyopathy affecting the myocardium or dysrhythmias (decreased contractility), or of disorders such as anemia, sepsis (high cardiac output needs). In adults, heart failure is classified as right- or left-sided and presents a different set of signs and symptoms, but in infants and children, failure of one side causes failure in the other side. Normally, any predisposing problem that blocks the effective flow of blood causes the heart to respond by compensatory mechanisms that maintain the work load of the heart. Congestive heart failure occurs when the compensatory mechanisms are not able to maintain the work load of the heart and the body tissues and organs are deprived of oxygen and nutrients they need to function properly **(Flowchart 14.1)**.

Symptoms of Congestive Heart Failure

Breathing
- Fast breathing during rest or exercise
- Shortness of breath or heavy breathing

Fatigue
- Feeling more tired than usual
- Need to take frequent rest breaks while playing with friends
- Falling asleep when feeding or becoming too tired to eat

Growth and Bodily Changes
- Lack of appetite; if child is an infant, she may take longer to feed, or may not want to be fed
- Child seems to stop growing
- Visible swelling of the legs, ankles, eyelids, face and sometimes abdomen

Feeling Sick
- Nausea
- Abdominal pain
- Vomiting
- Cough and feeling of congestion in her lungs
- Sweating

Nursing Process for the Child with Cardiovascular Disorder

Flowchart 14.1: Pathophysiology of congestive heart failure.

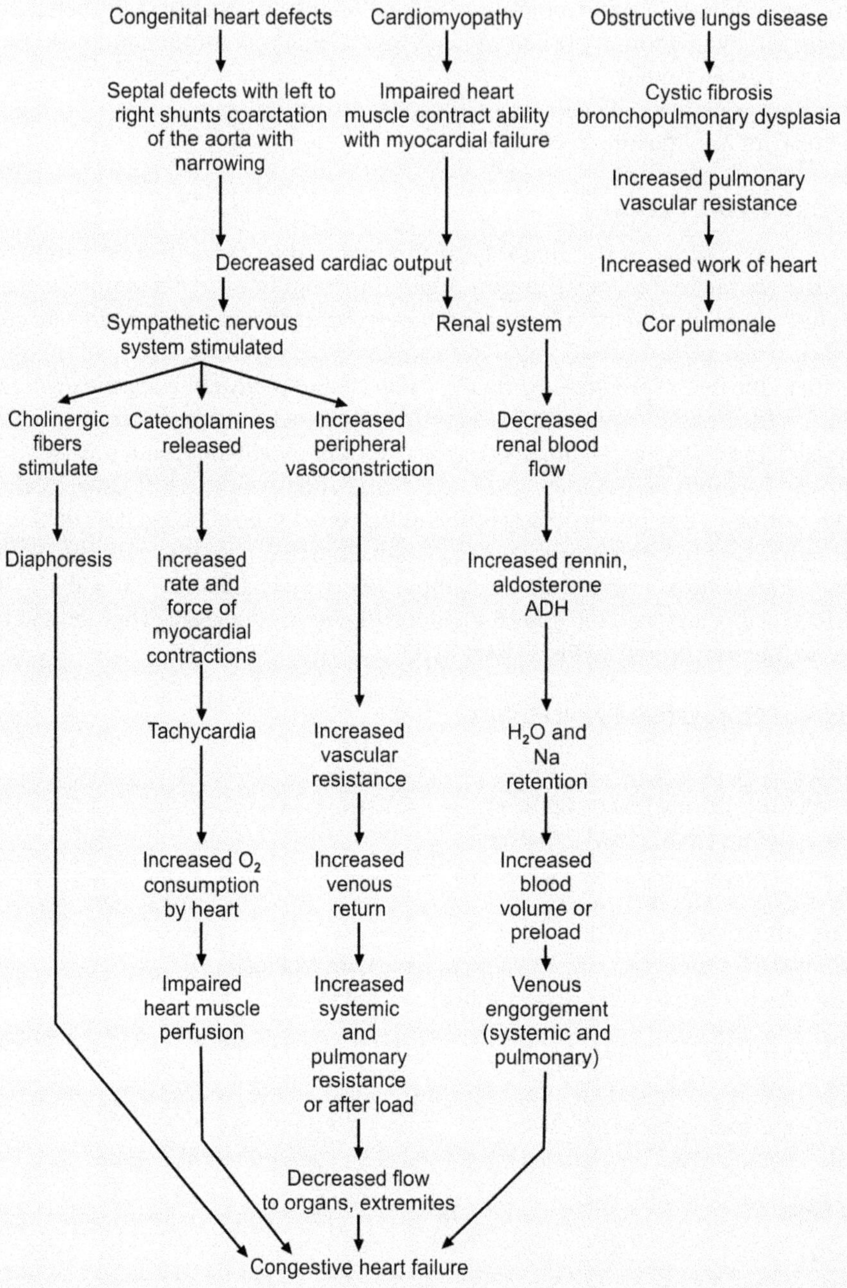

Nursing Management

A. Essential Nursing Diagnoses and Nursing Process Associated with this Condition

Nursing diagnosis

Decreased cardiac output related to mechanical factors of alterations in preload, after load, and inotropic changes in heart.

Assessment: Fatigue; oliguria; decreased peripheral pulses; pale, cool extremities; tachycardia; decreased BP; gallop rhythm, dyspnea, crackles.
(Refer Table 14.1)

Nursing diagnosis

Ineffective breathing pattern related to decreased lung expansion, pulmonary congestion.

Assessment: Dyspnea, tachypnea, orthopnea, cough, nasal flaring, respiratory depth changes, altered chest excursion, use of accessory muscles with retractions, abnormal arterial blood gases, wheezing, crackles, grunting, cyanosis.
(Refer Table 14.2)

Nursing diagnosis

Fluid volume excess related to compromised regulatory mechanisms **(Table 14.9)**.

Assessment: Edema (periorbital, peripheral), effusion, weigh gain, dyspnea, orthopnea, crackles, changes in respiratory pattern, blood pressure changes, oliguria, jugular vein distention, hepatomegaly, restlessness and anxiety, altered electrolytes, change in mental status.

Evaluation
- Absence of edema, signs, and symptoms associated with fluid accumulation in organs
- Blood pressure, pulse, respirations within normal parameters for age and sex
- 1:0 ratio remains within normal amounts
- Weight maintained with absence of sudden increases or decreases
- Correct administration of prescribed medications with expected results
- Compliance with reduced fluid intake, and optimal scheduling of sodium and potassium intake unless potassium depleted with use of diuretics.

Nursing diagnosis

Sleep pattern disturbance related to internal factor of illness **(Table 14.10)**.

Assessment: Interrupted sleep, fatigue, lethargy, restlessness, irritability.

Evaluation
- Verbalizes amount of sleep needed for infant/child specific to age
- Adequate number of hours of sleep daily appropriate for age
- Establishment of age-related nap and bedtime rituals
- Verbalizes plan of approaches to take to solve sleep problems
- Takes appropriate actions to resolve nightmares and sleep problems
- Absence of sleep problems, manifestations of sleep deficits.

Nursing Process for the Child with Cardiovascular Disorder

Table 14.9: Nursing interventions for fluid volume excess.

Interventions	Rationales
Assess presence of edema in periorbital tissue or dependent areas, such as extremities, when standing; in sacrum and scrotum when in lying position; or generalized in an infant, neck vein distention in child	Increased sodium and water retention result in increased systemic vascular pressure and fluid overload, which lead to edema; gravity determines the site of dependent edema
Monitor weight twice a day or as needed on same scale, at same time, and with same clothing	Weight gain is an early sign of fluid retention
Assess for pleural effusion by presence of dyspnea, tachypnea, crackles, orthopnea, ascites; for hepatomegaly by measuring abdominal girth	Indication of gross fluid retention which causes impaired organ function (pulmonary and systemic venous congestion), is associated with some cardiac or renal conditions
Assess for oliguria, increased specific gravity, electrolyte imbalances	Indicates decreased renal perfusion, which activates the rennin-angiotensin-aldosterone mechanism, resulting in water, sodium, and potassium retention
Administer diuretic therapy early in the day (for child), and monitor resulting diuresis by accurate 1:0 and weight	Diuretics prevent resorption of water, sodium, and potassium by tubules in the kidneys, resulting in excretion of excess
Note and document 1:0 (including losses from breathing and diaphoresis) and intake from all fluids IV or orally taken with medications and meals; if child not toilet trained, weight diaper to calculate output at 1 g = 1 mL	Intake and output ratio should normally be 2:1 or 0.5–1 mL/kg/h
Restrict fluid intake by removing availability of fluids; schedule over 24 hours with most given during the day hours, using small cups and allowing older child to keep track of daily amounts.	Supports need for additional loss of fluid based on age and using possible limit of 65 mL/kg/24 h as a guideline
Limit sodium intake by removing salt shaker, foods high in salt	Sodium intake should be limited to 2 g/day or 1–2 mEq/kg/24 h as a guideline
Maintain bed rest, and position and support any edematous body parts; change position q2h or as needed	Protects and supports edematous parts from pressure and trauma

Nursing diagnosis

High-risk for fluid volume deficit related to medication (diuretics) **(Table 14.11)**.

Assessment: Output greater than intake, weight loss, hypokalemia, hypernatremia.

Evaluation
- Absence of fluid and electrolyte imbalance, adequate circulating fluid volume
- Absence/presence of risk for dehydration
- Correct calculation and administration of fluids in proportion to losses

Table 14.10: Nursing interventions for sleep pattern disturbance.

Interventions	Rationales
Assess sleep patterns and changes, nap times and frequency, sleep problems, pattern of awakenings and reason	Provides information about fulfilment of sleep needs related to age requirements; infants need 10–20 hours/24 hours with a routine and sleep through the night by 5 months of age; toddlers need 12 hours/night and 2 naps, gradually changing to 10 hours/night and 1 nap; preschoolers need 10 hours/night with or without a nap, school aged children need 10 hours/night; wakenings may be caused by anxiety, nightmares, and the absence of good sleep habits, which may create sleep problems
Assess presence of temperature elevation, restlessness caused by pain, dyspnea, other signs and symptoms of an illness	Provides possible reasons for restlessness, wakenings, and sleep/rest deficit
Assess for fatigue, irritability, weakness, yawning	Results of sleep deficit of deprivation, over activity
Place infant on abdomen for sleep (especially after feeding), avoid waking or interrupting sleep for feeding or care procedures	Provides comfort for sleep without interruptions
Offer snack and one toy at bedtime, playing tapes of music	Promotes comfort and familiar bedtime pattern
Allow time for quiet play before bedtime	Avoids over stimulation before bedtime
Provide soothing comfort if child has a nightmare and explain bad dream, stay until child returns to sleep	Provides security and explanation, encouraging child to sleep without fear
Promote naps during day if such routine has been established	Follows usual age dependent nap/rest pattern
Provide environment that is quiet, calm, and warm; proper clothing, covers, and diaper change as needed	Promotes sleep and/or rest periods
Avoid painful procedures prior to bedtime when possible	Decreases stimuli which prevent rest and sleep
Encourage parent to stay with child at night if possible, or hold, rock, or stroke child until asleep	Promotes sleep and relaxation with a familiar person giving care

- Progressive return to baseline fluid intake PO
- Maintains NPO status when needed
- Administers IV fluids, electrolytes as prescribed safely and accurately without complications
- Encourages compliance and independence in adequate fluid intake.

Nursing diagnosis

Altered tissue perfusion: Cardiopulmonary, peripheral related to hypervolemia, prolonged cardiac failure **(Table 14.12)**.

Table 14.11: Nursing interventions for high-risk for fluid volume deficit.

Interventions	Rationales
Assess fluid losses, sources, amounts, and effects urinary output (should be 1–2 mL/kg/h; weigh diapers for infant and calculate as 1 mL/g) vomiting (include spitting up); diarrhea (include watery or bloody); stoma drainage (liquid); nasogastric aspirate (suctioning); insensible losses (respirations, diaphoresis from body temperature or ambient temperature); wound drainage; hemorrhage (fluid volume reduced); injury (burns)	Provides information about body fluid losses and depletion which leads to serious consequences in the infant/child and is included compared to intake causes include failure to absorb or reabsorb water, reduced intake or NPO status, excessive renal excretion, inappropriate ADH secretion, increased temperature or respirations, overuse of diuretic therapy improper fluid replacement
Assess intake and accurately compare to losses q2–8h for 1:0 determination and balance oral intake (liquids, fluid content of foods/formula, foods that become liquid at body temperature, fluids given with medications) parenteral (IV, IM, TPN) enteral (NG), gastrostomy tube feedings	Provides strict 1:0 to determine positive or negative balance and potential for fluid deficit/dehydration. Mild dehydration: less than 50 mL/kg fluid loss, Moderate dehydration: 50–90 mL/kg, Severe dehydration: about 100 mL/kg
Assess weight naked on same scale daily in morning or before breakfast	Determines losses related to fluid deficit and potential for dehydration. • Mild dehydration: Loss of 5% in infant, 3% in older child • Moderate: Loss of 10% in infant, 6% in older child • Severe: Loss 15% in infant, 9% in older child
Assess for presence of dehydration q2–8h including decreased urinary output, poor skin turgor testing, dry skin and mucous membranes, gray or mottled color to skin, reduced or absent tears and saliva, sunken, soft eyeballs, sunken fontanels in infants, increased specific gravity and serum osmolality, blood urea nitrogen, hematocrit, thirst in the older child, vital signs changes (tachycardia, lowered blood pressure, postural changes in blood pressure)	Reveals signs and symptoms of dehydration and hydration status; dehydration occurs when output exceeds intake and is classified as isotonic dehydration (water and electrolyte deficits equal), hypertonic dehydration (water loss is greater than sodium loss), hypotonic dehydration (sodium loss is greater than water loss)
Assess for presence of electrolyte depletion and possible cause	Reveals signs and symptoms of electrolyte imbalance which are related to specific diseases provides information regarding fluid/electrolyte imbalances, kidney function and risk acidosis or alkalosis
Potassium (K): Muscle weakness and cramping, irritability, fatigue, hypotension, arrhythmias	K: Excessive urinary output, diuretic therapy, vomiting, diarrhea, NG aspirate (functions in neural transmission in smooth, skeletal and cardiac muscle)
Sodium (Na): Nausea, abdominal cramps, weakness, dizziness, apathy	Na: Excessive water loss via any route, fever, diaphoresis, vomiting diarrhea NG aspirate, fistula or wounds (functions to control movement of fluid between fluid compartments)

Contd...

Contd...

Interventions	Rationales
Calcium (Ca): Tingling sensation of fingers, toes, hypotension, muscle irritability, tetany	Ca: Renal insufficiency, loss through gastrointestinal route, inadequate Ca intake or vitamin D deficiency (functions to prevent metabolic acidosis)
Assess urinalysis, electrolyte panel, serum and urine osmolality, blood urea nitrogen, creatinine, arterial blood gases as indicated	Provides information regarding fluid/electrolyte imbalances, kidney function and risk of acidosis/alkalosis
Encourage increased oral fluid intake in proportion to losses; provide a varied selection of beverages (sweet tea, diluted juice, decarbonated soda) and allow child to request preferences; start with rapid replacement for 4–6 hours and continue over 24 hours for maintenance therapy as tolerated: Infant: 150 mL/kg/day Toddler: 120 mL/kg/day Preschool: 100 mL/kg/day Schoolage: 75 mL/kg/day	Provides replacement of lost fluids if able to retain PO; child requires 750–2000 mL/day fluids depending on age and weight and calculation of losses
Provide pedialyte for infant, alternate formula feedings with water feedings if appropriate	Promotes fluid and electrolyte replacement and prevents risk of dehydration and electrolyte deficits
Maintain NPO status, prepare child and initiate IV fluid therapy with solution selection, rate and amount based on type and cause of dehydration; a possible schedule is to administer ½ of deficit during 8–16 hours and ½ over next 16–24 hours with maintenance volume calculated for continuation of therapy	Provides immediate replacement and ongoing prevention of losses to child who is unable to ingest fluids PO, is dehydrated, or suffers from gastric distention
Use infusion pump or volume control chamber for IV with a pediatric infusion set with a long tubing; restrain body parts as needed	Provides regulated and accurate fluid rate and volume with a micro drip IV infusion set (60 gtt/mL); long tubing allows for movement in bed and proper restraining and monitoring for safe IV administration
Monitor IV hourly for amount, site infiltration, tube patency or displacement; change fluid bag and tubing q24h, use a transparent occlusive dressing over site, correct operation of infusion pump, movement restricted by restraints	Ensures safe fluid administration; allow for range of motion (ROM) of restrained parts, prevents complication of IV therapy
Provide non-nutritive sucking for infant, hold and cuddle child, mouth care (spray water into mouth) for oral dryness, petrolatum to lips	Provides support and comfort to infant/child

Contd...

Nursing Process for the Child with Cardiovascular Disorder

Contd...

Interventions	Rationales
During IV therapy, note presence of headache, cramps, vomiting, crackles, muscle twitching, lethargy, decreased urine output	Indicates overhydration
Discontinue IV when fluids are tolerated orally; begin with small amounts of clear fluids, gradually increase in amounts and frequency as tolerated including jello, popsicles, low salt soup, baby food for infants	Resumes oral fluid intake when condition improves; oral intake may be resumed as soon as 5–10 hours after surgery
Employ play at developmental level including games, use of straws, small cup (medicine or animal image cup)	Promotes oral intake of fluids when child is ill and does not fulfill fluid goals
Place water and cup in room and allow to take frequent sips; praise child for drinking the fluids	Promotes adequate intake of fluids and promote independence
Allow child to participate in the fluid selection and scheduling, to record intake using symbols or checks with colors	Promotes independence and control over the situations and enhance compliance

Table 14.12: Nursing interventions for altered tissue perfusion–cardiopulmonary, peripheral.

Interventions	Rationales
Assess organ functional abilities in relation to disease and its effect on a particular system	Interrelationships of systems cause an overlapping of signs and symptoms associated with tissue perfusion causing changes in elimination, oxygenation, nutrition, and mental function
Assess pulse, blood pressure, presence of peripheral pulses, capillary refill time, skin color and temperature, urinary output, mentation, anorexia, gastric distention	Provides information about cardiac output, which, if decreased, will reduce blood flow and tissue perfusion
Provide O_2 by hood, cannula, or face mask, depending on age and at rate determined by ABGs	Provides oxygen to organs for proper functioning
Administer vasodilator, cardiac glycoside	Promotes cardiac output, slows and strengthens heart rate for a more efficient pump action and increased return flow of blood to the heart and decreased heart workload
Position change q2-4h to avoid pressure on susceptible body parts, perform ROM if needed	Promotes circulation and prevents breakdown of tissue from further perfusion decreases associated with pressure
Position in Fowler's at height of comfort, if respiratory status compromised by pulmonary perfusion	Decreases blood volume returning to heart by pooling of blood in lower dependent part of the body

Assessment: Edema, dyspnea, change in color, temperature of extremities (mottled, cold), decreased peripheral pulses, effusion, changes in BP, tachypnea, orthopnea, tachycardia, cough.

Evaluation
- Return of vital signs to normal ranges for age and sex
- Organ function within normal parameters
- Extremities warm, normal color with equal palpable pulses—arterial blood gases (ABGs) within normal levels
- Resolution of hypoxemia
- Urinary output at baseline levels
- Absence of abdominal distention with adequate nutritional intake.

B. Specific Nursing Diagnoses and Nursing Process

Nursing diagnosis

Anxiety (parent[s], child) related to threat of death, deterioration of health status, threat of change in environment (hospitalization) **(Table 14.13)**.

Assessment: Parent-increased apprehension that condition might worsen into life-threatening situation, increased concern and worry about possible hospitalization, increased tension and uncertainty, chronic worry, child-unhappy and sad attitude; withdrawn or aggressive behavior; somatic and fatigue complaints; failure to thrive and participate in school, play, or social activates.

Evaluation
- Verbalized that anxiety reduced by parent(s)
- Expresses increased comfort in caring for ill child/infant
- Symptoms of anxiety in the child decreasing or controlled.

Table 14.13: Nursing interventions for anxiety (parent[s], child).

Interventions	Rationales
Assess level and manifestations of anxiety in parent(s) and child	Provides information needed for interventions and clues to severity of anxiety
Allow expression of fears and concerns and time to ask questions about disorder and what to expect	Provides opportunity to vent feelings and secure information to reduce anxiety
Provide supportive, nonjudgmental environment and individualized, consistent care	Promotes trust and reduces anxiety
Hold and cuddle infant	Promotes comfort and security
Allow parent(s) to stay and open visitation and telephone communication; encourage to participate in care and to plan care similar to usual home patterns	Reduces anxiety by allowing presence and involvement in care and provides familiar persons and routine for child
Keep parent(s) informed of changes in condition, progress made	Promotes understanding and reduces anxiety about whether child is improving

Nursing Process for the Child with Cardiovascular Disorder

Table 14.14: Nursing intervention for activity intolerance.

Interventions	Rationales
Assess level of fatigue, responses to activity	Provides information about change in vital signs and energy level
Allow for rest periods between care, disturb only when necessary and then perform care and treatments during one period of time	Promotes rest, conserves energy, and reduces heart work load
Avoid allowing infant to cry for long periods of time; use small nipple for feeding and feed frequently, slowly, and in small amounts	Conserves energy and prevents fatigue
Provide meals for child frequently and in smaller amounts	Conserves energy
Provide toys and quiet, age-appropriate play	Allows for play without depleting energy reserves
Provide optimal environmental temperature	Extremes of temperature increase oxygen and energy needs, which increase work of heart

Nursing diagnosis

Activity intolerance related to imbalance between oxygen supply and demand **(Table 14.14)**.

Assessment: Abnormal heart rate or blood pressure response to activity, exertional dyspnea, fatigue, weakness, respiratory/circulatory problem.

Evaluation
- Controls activities that are fatiguing and cause symptoms
- Maintains rest and activity schedule
- Engages in stimulating activities appropriate for age and energy level.

Nursing diagnosis

Knowledge deficit of parent(s), child related to lack of information about disorder and treatments/care **(Table 14.15)**.

Assessment: Verbalization of need for information about disease, medications, dietary restrictions.

Evaluation
- Verbalizes knowledge of disease process, causes and risk factors
- Adapts and complies with dietary, fluid restrictions
- Caretaker and family support for medical regimen
- Correctly administers medications and verbalizes side effects and symptoms of digitalis toxicity, hypokalemia
- Verbalizes signs and symptoms of congestive heart failure and importance of reporting to physician.

Hypertension

Hypertension in children is reflected by the consistent readings of the systolic and/or diastolic blood pressure at the level of or above the ninety-fifth percentile for age and gender. It may be primary or secondary. Hypertension in children is of particular concern because of its close

Table 14.15: Nursing interventions for knowledge deficit of parent(s), child.

Interventions	Rationales
Assess knowledge of disease, causes and methods to prevent or control condition, willingness and interest to implement care to reduce work of heart, ability and readiness to learn	Promotes plan of instruction that is realistic to ensure compliance of medical regimen, prevents repetition of information
Provide information about disorder causes and risk factors; use clear, understandable language, pictures, pamphlets, models, videotapes, anatomical doll in teaching	Ensures understanding and aids in reinforcement of learning
Instruct and assist in planning menus that include sodium restriction, fluids if prescribed, additional calories.	Allows input, control over planning for sodium and fluid restriction may be needed to prevent fluid retention, additional calories provided for higher metabolic needs
Instruct in administration of cardiac glycosides and diuretics, including dosage, frequency, route, side effects to report, expected results	Ensures correct administration of drugs to prevent heart failure and drug toxicity
Instruct in taking pulse for 1 minute and allow return demonstration	Apical pulse taken before administration of cardiac glycoside
Inform of effects of disorder on infant/child (growth and physical development)	Disorder slows growth and development for age
Inform of need to report infection or changes in breathing, pulse, irritability, restlessness, edema, temperature (increase), or weight	Reduction in body defenses predisposes to infectious process, signs and symptoms reported to prevent progressive heart failure

association to hypertension in those adults who were hypertensive as children. That children with an increased blood pressure usually do not display any overt symptoms has led to the inclusion of blood pressure determinations as part of routine examination in those 3 years and older. Children under 3 years, who have been diagnosed with a heart condition are also tested **(Flowchart 14.2)**.

Symptoms of Hypertension

There are a few presenting features that should raise the possibility of hypertension:

Neonates
- Failure to thrive
- Convulsion
- Irritability or lethargy
- Respiratory distress
- Congestive cardiac failure

Older Children
- Headaches
- Fatigue
- Blurred vision
- Epistaxis
- Sleep-disordered breathing

Nursing Process for the Child with Cardiovascular Disorder

Flowchart 14.2: Pathophysiology of hypertension.

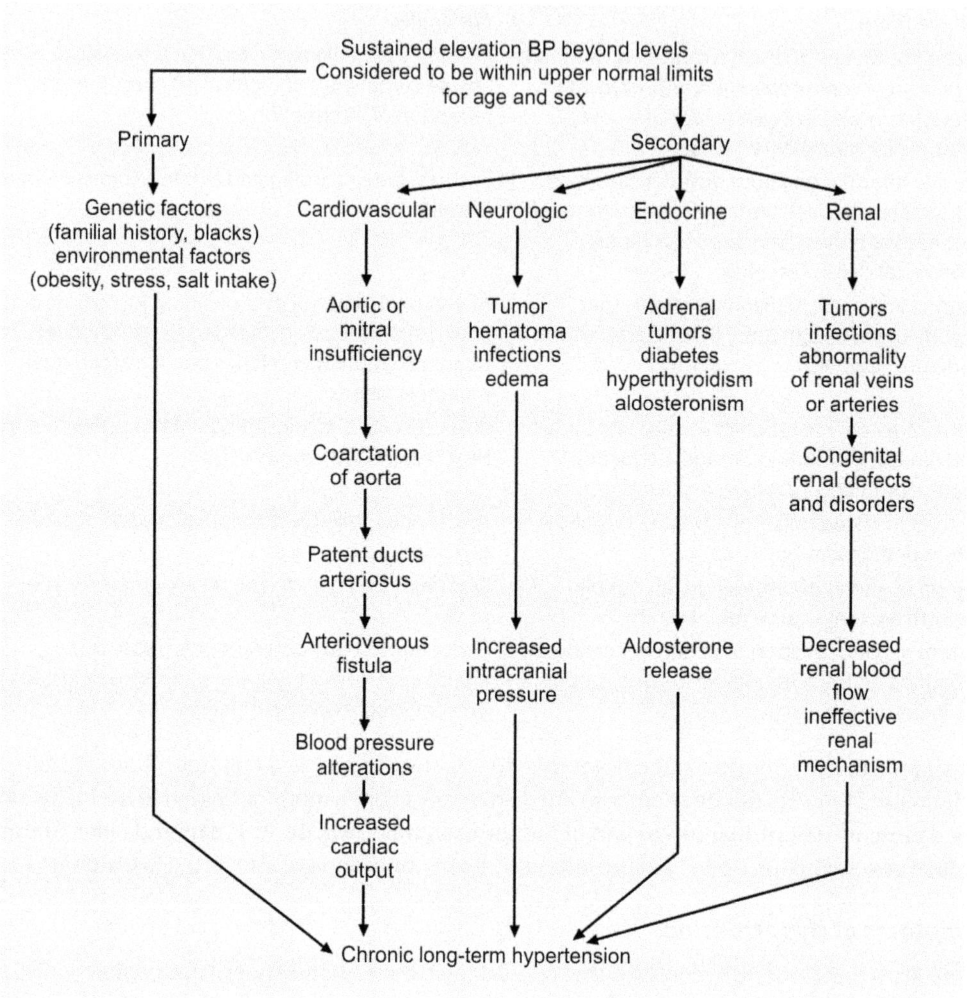

Sustained elevation BP beyond levels considered to be within upper normal limits for age and sex

Primary
- Genetic factors (familial history, blacks)
- environmental factors (obesity, stress, salt intake)

Secondary

- **Cardiovascular**: Aortic or mitral insufficiency → Coarctation of aorta → Patent ducts arteriosus → Arteriovenous fistula → Blood pressure alterations → Increased cardiac output
- **Neurologic**: Tumor hematoma infections edema → Increased intracranial pressure
- **Endocrine**: Adrenal tumors, diabetes, hyperthyroidism, aldosteronism → Aldosterone release
- **Renal**: Tumors, infections, abnormality of renal veins or arteries → Congenital renal defects and disorders → Decreased renal blood flow ineffective renal mechanism

→ Chronic long-term hypertension

If the condition is found, enquiry should be made for certain features in the child's history:
- Prematurity.
- Bronchopulmonary dysplasia.
- History of umbilical catheterization.
- Head or abdominal trauma.
- Familial diseases—for example, neurofibromatosis, hypertension and multiple endocrine neoplasia, especially if associated with pheochromocytoma.
- History of pyelonephritis may have been missed—ask about pyrexia of unknown origin, as urinary tract infection in children is not always overt.
- Medication may have a pressor effect—for example, children on steroids, those taking amphetamines for attention deficit hyperactivity disorder, and those abusing drugs.
- Ask about diet, looking for high salt intake.

Nursing Management

A. Essential Nursing Diagnoses and Nursing Process Association with this Condition

Nursing diagnosis

Fluid volume excess related to compromised regulatory mechanisms, excessive sodium intake.

Assessment: Edema, weight gain, intake greater than output, blood pressure changes, altered electrolytes.

(Refer Table 14.9)

Nursing diagnosis

Altered tissue perfusion: Renal related to interruption in renal, arterial, or venous flow.

Assessment: Edema, oliguria, hypertension.

(Refer Table 14.12)

Nursing diagnosis

High-risk for fluid volume deficit related to medications (diuretic).

Assessment: Increased urinary output, sudden weight loss, hypokalemia, dry skin and mucous membranes.

(Refer Table 14.11)

B. Specific Nursing Diagnoses and Nursing Process

Nursing diagnosis

High-risk for injury related to internal regulatory function **(Table 14.16)**.

Assessment: Uncontrolled hypertension; neurologic status (blurred vision, headache, irritability, dizziness, papilledema); future renal heart, circulatory problems.

Table 14.16: Nursing interventions for high-risk for injury.

Interventions	Rationales
Assess BP using a Doppler method on an infant and proper size cuff on child, noting proper application of cuff, position, and extremity used; obtain readings when infant/child is at rest q2h	Provides accurate systolic and diastolic readings to establish a pattern of elevations, although no definite readings are used to diagnose hypertension in children
Assess for headache, dizziness, nose-bleed, visual changes	Indicates increased BP, although symptoms in children are varies and some or none of the symptoms may be present
Provide quiet environment and reduce activities, stress, and stimuli	Helps in reducing BP
Administer antihypertensive and diuretics as prescribed	Drug therapy is given when BP does not respond to nonpharmacologic methods of reducing it; control is manages with the use of one drug and cautious addition of another drug, depending on side effects produced and achieved reduction of BP

Table 14.17: Nursing interventions for knowledge deficit for parent(s), child.

Interventions	Rationales
Assess knowledge of disease, causes and methods to control disease, willingness and interest to implement long-term care	Promotes plan of instruction that is realistic to ensure compliance of medical regimen, prevents repetition of information
Provide information and explanations in clear language; use pictures, pamphlets, videotapes, models in teaching about disorder, causes and risk factors	Ensures understanding based on readiness, aids reinforce learning
Instruct and assist in planning dietary menu that includes restrictions that help reduce BP	Weight reduction and restricted sodium, fat, and cholesterol intake may be part of the medical regimen
Instruct in an activity and exercise plan specific to child's needs and interests (swimming, cycling)	Assists in weight reduction and contributes to lowering BP
Instruct in relaxation techniques, such as breathing, biofeedback	Reduces stress that raises BP
Inform of importance of follow-up visits to physician	Provides early detection of complication and evaluation of therapy
Inform of long-term nature of medical regimen and potential for cardiac, cerebral, and renal damage or complications that result from noncompliance	Provides rationale for acceptance of long-term care
Inform of availability of stress, weight reduction, or nutritional counseling	Provides specialized guidance if needed to ensure compliance and success

(BP: blood pressure)

Evaluation

- Blood pressure within normal ranges for age and sex
- Correct administration of prescribed medications
- Absence of signs and symptoms associated with elevated BP
- Continues monitoring of BP
- Verbalization of signs and symptoms, side effects to report.

Nursing diagnosis

Knowledge deficit of parent(s) child related to lack of information or experience about disease and treatment **(Table 14.17)**.

Assessment: Verbalization of need for information about nonpharmacologic treatments.

Evaluation

- Verbalization of knowledge of disease process, causes, and risk factors
- Adaptation and compliance with dietary restrictions
- Daily participation in aerobic exercises, individualized activities
- Family participation in stress reduction and support for medical regimen
- Maintains schedule for physician visits
- Weight loss achieved until average for age, height, and frame reached

Flowchart 14.3: Pathophysiology of rheumatic fever.

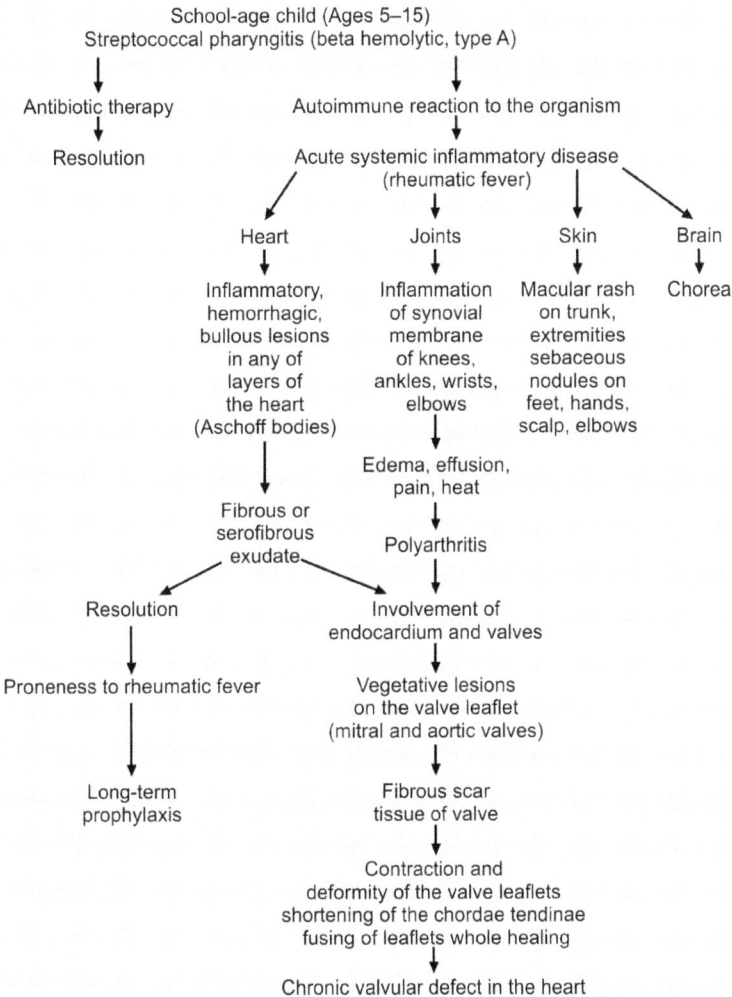

- Practices stress reduction techniques
- Seeks out counseling services if needed for weight loss.

Rheumatic Fever

Rheumatic fever is an autoimmune disease responsible for cardiac valve disease of rheumatic heart disease. It is associated with infections caused by the group A streptococcal upper respiratory infection. It is prevented by treatment of the infection with appropriate antibiotic therapy before further complications can occur. Once diagnosed, children are susceptible to recurrent episodes of rheumatic fever, and long-term prophylactic therapy (5 years) is given following the acute phase. The Jones criteria offered by the American Heart Association are used as guidelines for diagnosis of rheumatic fever **(Flowchart 14.3 and Fig. 14.3)**.

Nursing Process for the Child with Cardiovascular Disorder

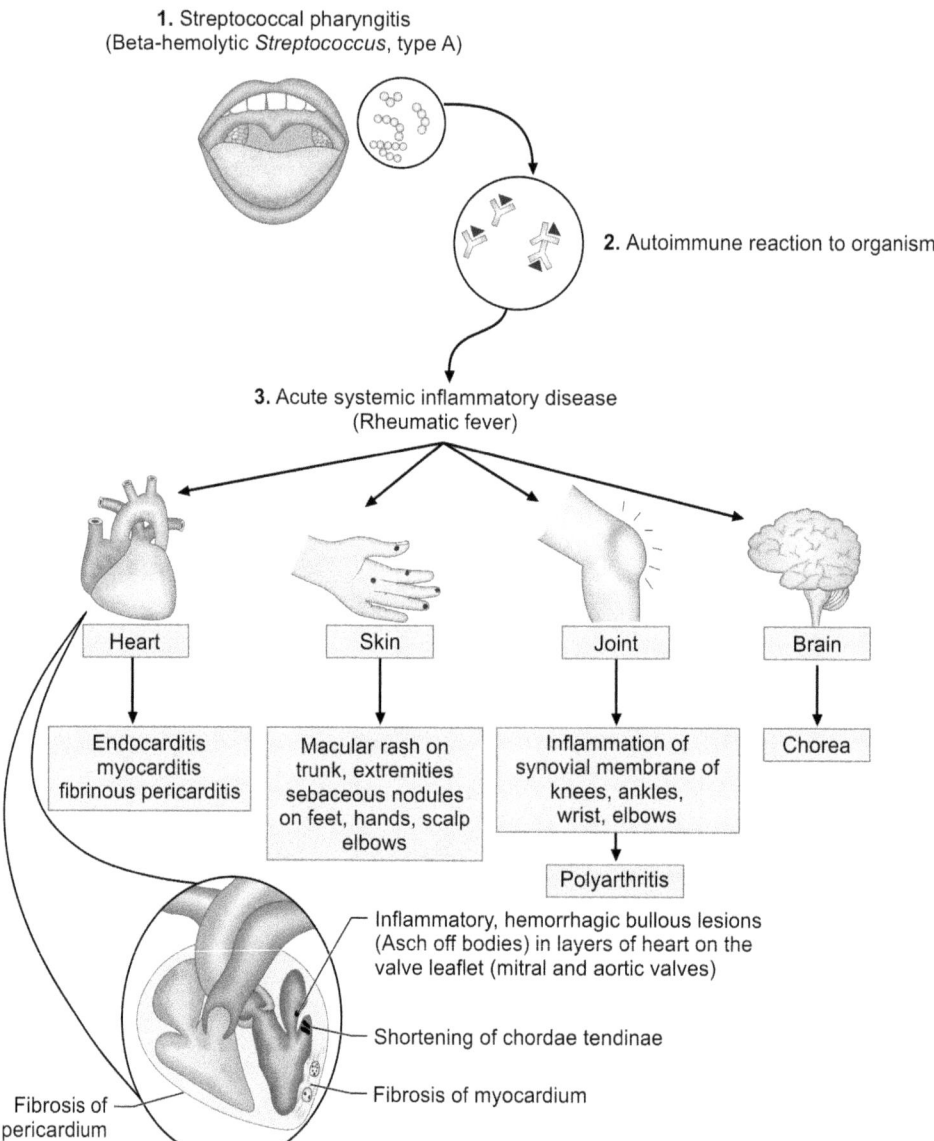

Fig. 14.3: Pathophysiology of rheumatic fever.

Symptoms of Rheumatic Fever

Major Criteria

- **Polyarthritis:** A temporary migrating inflammation of the large joints, usually starting in the legs and migrating upwards.
- **Carditis:** Inflammation of the heart muscle (myocarditis) which can manifest as congestive heart failure with shortness of breath, pericarditis with a rub, or a new heart murmur.

- **Subcutaneous nodules:** Painless, form collections of collagen fibres over bones or tendons. They commonly appear on the back of the wrist, the outside elbow, and the front of the knees.
- **Erythema marginatum**
- **Sydenham's chorea (St. Vitus' dance):** A characteristic series of rapid movements without purpose of the face and arms.

Minor Criteria
- Fever of 38.2–38.9°C (100.8–102.0°F)
- **Arthralgia:** Joint pain without swelling (cannot be included if polyarthritis is present as a major symptom)
- Raised erythrocyte sedimentation rate or C reactive protein
- Leukocytosis
- ECG showing features of heart block, such as a prolonged PR interval (cannot be included if carditis is present as a major symptom)

ECG normal upper range:
- PR interval:
    - 3–12 years: 0.16 second
    - 12–14 years: 0.18 second
    - 17 years: 0.20 second
- Previous episodes of rheumatic fever or inactive heart disease

Other signs and symptoms
- Abdominal pain
- Nose bleeds
- **Preceding streptococcal infection:** Recent scarlet fever raised antistreptolysin O or other streptococcal antibody titer, or positive throat culture.

Nursing Management

A. Essential Nursing Diagnoses and Nursing Process Associated with this Condition

Nursing diagnosis

Hyperthermia related to illness of inflammatory disease **(Table 14.18)**.

Assessment: Low-grade increase in body temperature above normal range.

Evaluation
- Absence of temperature elevation above baseline for age
- Takes temperature q2–4h by proper method and route if child is ill
- Keeps log of temperature readings and associated signs and symptoms to report
- Administers antipyretic correctly and safely, and notes temperature is decreased; limits 24 hours doses to safe levels and frequencies
- Reduces temperature with cooling compresses or baths as appropriate
- Maintains environmental temperature at acceptable level
- Clothes child in cool, comfortable clothing and provides light covering
- Maintains hydration by increasing intake to meet losses caused by fever
- Reports temperature elevations, with associated symptoms if present, that persist over 24 hours to physician.

Nursing Process for the Child with Cardiovascular Disorder

Table 14.18: Nursing interventions for hyperthermia.

Interventions	Rationales
Assess temperature via rectal or axillary methods in infant and young child, oral in older child; check for malaise or lethargy and compare to normal ranges for age or low grade or high elevations associated with specific microorganisms or diseases	Provides information about temperature changes caused by high susceptibility to fluctuations in infants and young children, since their regulatory function is unstable (regulated in the hypothalamus); temperature in infant and young child responds to infection with higher and more rapid elevations, they may become overheated as environmental temperatures changes or from activity, crying, and emotional upsets, since regulating mechanism is immature until age 8
Assess temperature q1–2h for any sudden temperature elevation or increase in illness	Sudden, high temperature elevation may induce a seizure
If temperature reaches 102°F rectally, administer antipyretic in form appropriate for infant or child and ability to swallow if throat sore; observe time intervals of 4–6 hours and total 24 hours dose; limit to 24–48 hours (5 doses/24 hours), if possible	Reduces temperature (lowers set point); prevents possible toxicity caused by accumulation if given too often, since half-life of drug is 1–3.5 hours; may be administered by tablet, liquid, chewable, suppository; dosage based on temperature level and body weight
Maintain environmental temperature of 72°F and provide lightweight clothing and blanket	Assists in reducing temperature and promotes comfort as body temperature responds to changes in environmental temperatures
Provide tepid (90°F) sponge bath for 30 minutes, dry each body part after sponging, cover to prevent shivering/chilling; monitor temperature during and 30 minutes after sponging: sponging may be limited to moist compresses on forehead, hand, feet, back of neck or wrapping child in cool, moist towels	Reduces temperature by conduction of heat from the body to treat hyperthermia, limited sponging may be administered for fever; chilling results in vasoconstriction, allowing decreased blood circulation to the skin surface for cooling
Provide additional fluid orally or IV depending on condition of the infant/child	Maintains hydration when fluids are lost through fever or hyperthermia
Provide warmth to body if chilling occurs by raising environmental temperature, increasing clothing, giving warm bath	Treats chilling, which increases metabolic requirements, especially in those with cardiovascular or neurologic system conditions
Promote rest and provide a stress-free environment, hold and rock infant/child if needed	Increases metabolic requirements if crying and activity increases, as this elevates the temperature

Nursing diagnosis

Altered nutrition: Less than body requirements related to inability to ingest food because of biological factors.

Assessment: Anorexia, fatigue, weight loss, abdominal pain.

(Refer Table 14.3)

Nursing diagnosis

Impaired physical mobility related to pain and discomfort **(Table 14.19)**.

Table 14.19: Nursing interventions for impaired physical mobility.

Interventions	Rationales
Assess muscle tone, strength, mass; joint mobility, pain, stiffness, swelling; ability to move and activity level in performing ADL	Provides information about musculoskeletal condition and function
Assess bed rest status, activity restrictions, imposed immobility by braces, casts, traction, splints	Maintains rest during acute stages to promote healing and restoration of health
Assess sensory (diminished sensation and numbness) and motor (gait and balance) function of extremities; presence of paralysis, fracture, surgical correction of musculoskeletal abnormalities	Provides information about conditions or treatments that affect mobility
Assess physical effects of immobilization on body systems; constipation, skin breakdown, urinary retention, hypercalcemia, loss of muscle strength, contractures, circulatory stasis, stasis of pulmonary secretions, anorexia, renal calculi, decreased metabolism and energy, loss of nerve innervations	Prevents complications of immobility by monitoring and intervening when needed; mobility provides important contributions to development and physical health
Assess psychologic effects of immobilization; reduced body image, inability to reduce stress, loss of stimuli, loss of independence and mastery, anxiety, regressive behavior, anger and aggression, passive and submissive behavior, crying, irritability, temper tantrums	Provides information about behavior and deprivation resulting from immobilization which prevents children from dealing with feelings and expression of anxiety and tensions
Avoid restriction in activities unless ordered; encourage and allow for as much movement as possible in performing daily activities; administer analgesic before activity	Promotes mobility and activity synonymous with health and life; allows for autonomy and control for normal development
Encourage all age-appropriate activities that facilitate mobility, allow infant to crawl	Promotes mobility according to limitations of illness and provides outlet for frustration of imposed immobility
Provide quiet play and progress in ambulation by scheduling dangling at bed side, standing with support, ambulation with support with increase daily and praise for all attempts regardless of progress	Maintains large and small muscle strength as condition permits
Transport/transfer infant/child by Hoyer lift, stroller, wheelchair, bed outside of room/hospital	Provides stimulation by interacting in a different environment in absence of mobility
Provide and apply brace, splint; use of aids including wheelchair, crutches, supportive reading, eating, and other aids for ADL as needed	Promotes independence and support in mobility and activities
Maintain body alignment if on bedrest, reposition q2h or as needed; use a drawing for child to follow for position and where to lie in bed	Prevents contractures and physical deformity and preserves joint function

Contd...

Contd...

Interventions	Rationales
Coordinate rest with periods of mobility	Prevents fatigue and conserves energy
Perform muscle strengthening exercises, passive stretching exercises, joint mobilizing exercises if ordered or as appropriate	Preserves muscle strength or prepares for use of crutches or other mobility aids
Apply special shoes, splint or appliance for day or night use	Maintains position at night and prevents deformity and allows for locomotion by increasing gait efficiency during day use
Prepare for physical and/or occupational therapy during recuperative period as ordered	Promotes and maintains optimal function and mobility of child

(ADL: activities of daily living)

Assessment: Joint pain of polyarthritis. Decreased muscle control and strength, clumsiness, uncoordination, sudden and aimless movement of extremities, bed rest protocol.

Evaluation
- Maximum mobility and participation in ADL according to developmental level
- Correct application and use of appliances, aids, devices to promote mobility and activities
- Absence of complications of immobility
- Compliance with exercise regimen, rest, and energy preservation
- Perform play activities for diversion, development, and mobility
- Comply with physical and/or occupational therapy schedule
- Maintain bed rest of activity restrictions if appropriate with gradual return of mobility and self-care activities.

B. Specific Nursing Diagnoses and Nursing Process

Nursing diagnosis

Pain related to biological injuring agents, arthralgia **(Table 14.20)**.

Assessment: Verbal description of pain, guarding and protective behavior of painful joints, edema, redness, heat at affected joints.

Evaluation
- Joint pain relieved and/or controlled
- Compliance with medication regimen for pain and inflammation compliance with methods to protect joints from pain
- Limits movement and activity that cause discomfort.

Nursing diagnosis

High-risk for infection related to chronic recurrence of disease **(Table 14.21)**.

Assessment: Noncompliance with long-term medication regimen, evidence of exacerbation of signs and symptoms of disease, risk of development of complication of valve damage.

Evaluation
- Compliance with antibiotic regimen daily or monthly
- Notification of dentist regarding history of the disease and therapy

Nursing Process for the Child with Cardiovascular Disorder

Table 14.20: Nursing interventions for pain.

Interventions	Rationales
Assess severity of pain, joints involved, level of joint movement	Provides information regarding pathologic changes in joints; joint involvement is reversible, usually affecting large joints, such as knees, hips, wrists, and elbows; an increase in numbers of affected joints occurs over a period of time
Assess behavior changes, such as crying, restlessness, refusal to move, irritability, aggressive or dependent behavior	Nonverbal responses to pain that are age-related as child or infant may be unable to describe pain, and fear, and anxiety associated with pain causes changes in behavioral responses
Administer analgesic and anti-inflammatory agent, and inform child that the medication will decrease the pain; administer a sustained action analgesic before bedtime or 1 hour before anticipated movement	Relieves pain, edema in joints and promotes rest and comfort
Maintain bed rest during the acute stage of disease	Promotes comfort and reduces joint pain caused by movement
Elevate affected extremities above level of heart	Promotes circulation to the heart to relieve edema
Change position q2h while maintaining body alignment	Prevents contractures and promotes comfort
Move gently and support body parts; minimize handling of affected parts as much as possible	Prevents additional pain to affected parts
Apply bed cradle under outside covers over painful parts	Prevents pressure on painful joints
Provide toys, games for quiet, sedentary play	Provides diversional activity to distract from pain

Table 14.21: Nursing interventions for high-risk for infection.

Interventions	Rationales
Assess compliance to prescribed antimicrobials; daily oral administration or monthly intramuscular injections	Long-term antibiotic therapy (as long as 5 years) as a preventive measure creates compliance difficulty, and need for IM injections may be necessary in order to ensure compliance
Assess for chest pain, dyspnea, cough, tachycardia during sleep, friction rub, gallop during acute stage of disease	Signs and symptoms of carditis, which may lead to endocarditic causing vegetation that becomes fibrous at the valve area that is at increased risk with repeated infections
Administer antibiotic therapy during acute phase of disease	Inhibits cell wall synthesis of microorganisms, destroying causative agent

Nursing Process for the Child with Cardiovascular Disorder

- Reporting of any symptoms to physician
- All preventive measures taken to avoid recurrence of disease.

PRACTICE QUESTIONS

1. A toddler is admitted in pediatric intensive care unit after corrective surgery of tetralogy of fallot (TOF). Write the nursing care management of the toddler by using nursing process.
2. Master Ram 6-year-old admitted with CHF in pediatric medicine ward. Write the nursing care plan for the child using nursing process.

CHAPTER 15

Nursing Process for the Child with Renal Disorder

> **LEARNING OBJECTIVES**
> - To identify the signs and symptoms of a child with renal/urinary disorder.
> - To frame nursing diagnosis based on the needs of the child.
> - To plan nursing interventions and outcome identification.

INTRODUCTION

The urinary tract includes the upper tract (kidneys and ureters) and lower tract (urethra and bladder). The kidneys regulate fluid and electrolytes, body pH, and excretion of the end products of protein metabolism (urea). This in accomplished by urine formation and tubular, reabsorption and secretion in response to the body's requirements for water and electrolyte balance. Another kidney function is the production of enzymes (erythropoietin stimulating factor and rennin) which act to stimulate red blood cell production in the bone marrow and produce angiotensin to increase blood pressure and stimulate aldosterone production. The urinary bladder and urethra provide for the storage and drainage of urine after passage from the kidneys via the ureters. Disease involving the upper and lower urinary tract are common in children and affect urinary excretion by causing inflammation, damage and scarring of tissue and dysfunction of the organs or structures of the organs. These structural or functional abnormalities may obstruct urine flow and cause renal disorders although obstruction in children may also be a result of a congenital malformation and lead to chronic renal damage and failure. Although the system functions the same as an adult, the functional deficiency in the infant's/child's kidney ability to concentrate urine effects its handling of fluid and electrolyte fluctuations and increases proneness to dehydration states when the body is stressed by disease. With growth and maturity of the system, the renal/urinary organs progressively function within adult parameters.

NURSING PROCESS FOR THE CHILD WITH RENAL DISORDER

1. **Nursing diagnosis:** Activity intolerance related to generalized edema, anemia or generalized weakness as evidenced by verbalization of weakness or fatigue, elevated heart rate, respiratory rate or blood pressure with activity, complaint of shortness of breath with play or vactivity.
   Goal: Child will be able to display increased activity tolerance.
   Interventions: Promoting activity.
   - Encourage activity or ambulation per physician's orders; early mobilization results in better outcomes
   - Observe child for symptoms of activity intolerance such as pallor, nausea, light headedness or dizziness or changes in vital signs to determine level of tolerance

- If child is on bed rest, perform range-of-motion exercises and frequent position changes, as negative changes to the musculoskeletal system occur quickly with inactivity and immobility
- Cluster nursing care activities and plan of periods of rest before and after exertional activities to decrease oxygen need and consumption
- Refer the child to physical therapy for exercise prescription to increase skeletal muscle strength.

Evaluation: Child desire to play without developing symptoms of exertion.

2. **Nursing diagnosis:** Excess fluid volume related to decreased protein in the bloodstream, decreased urine output, sodium retention, possible inappropriate fluid intake or altered hormone levels inducing fluid retention as evidenced by edema, bloating, weight gain, oliguria, azotemia or changes in heart and lung sounds.
Goal: Child will be able to attain appropriate fluid balance.
Intervention: Encouraging fluid loss.
   - Weigh child daily on same scale in similar amount of clothing; in children, weight is the best indicator of changes in fluid status
   - Monitor location and extent of edema (measure abdominal girth daily if ascites present): decrease in edema indicates positive increase in oncotic pressure
   - Auscultate lungs carefully to determine presence of crackles (indicating pulmonary edema)
   - Assess heart sounds for presence or absence of gallop (increased work of breathing is associated with pulmonary edema)
   - Maintain fluid restriction as ordered to decrease intravascular volume and workload on the heart
   - Strictly monitor intake and output to quickly note discrepancies and provide intervention
   - Provide sodium-restricted diet as ordered (restricting sodium in the diet allows for better renal excretion of extra fluid)
   - Administer diuretics as ordered and monitor for side effects of those medications. Diuretics encourage excretion of fluid and elimination of edema, reduce cardiac filling pressures and increase renal blood flow. Side effects include electrolyte imbalance as well as orthostatic hypotension.

Evaluation: Child reduced weight, edema or bloating, decreased lung sounds cleared and heart sounds normal.

3. **Nursing diagnosis: Imbalanced nutrition:** Less than body requirements related to anorexia and protein loss as evidenced by weight, length/height and/or body mass index (BMI) below average forage.
Goal: Child will be able to improve nutritional intake.
Intervention: Promoting adequate nutrition.
   - Determine body weight and length/height normal for age, to determine goal to work toward
   - Assess child for food preferences that fall within dietary restrictions, as the child will be more likely to consume adequate amounts of foods that he or she likes
   - Weigh daily or weekly (according to physician order or institutional standard) and measure length/height weekly: to monitor for increased growth

- Offer highest calorie meals at the time of day when the child's appetite is the greatest (to increase likelihood of increased caloric intake)
- Provide increased calorie shakes or puddings within diet restriction (high calorie foods increase weight gain)
- Administer vitamin and mineral supplements as prescribed to attain/maintain vitamin and mineral balance in the body.

Evaluation: Child weight increased steadily.

4. **Nursing diagnosis: Imbalanced nutrition:** More than body requirements related to increased appetite secondary to steroid therapy as evidenced by weight greater than 95th percentile for age or recent increase in weight.
   Goal: Child will be able to demonstrate balanced nutritional intake.
   Intervention: Encouraging appropriate nutritional intake.
   - Determine ideal body weight and BMI for age to determine goal to work toward
   - Consult dietitian for guidance in planning nutrient-rich diet in context of restrictions
   - Evaluate for emotional/psychological reasons for overeating to address these concerns
   - Formulate a contract with the child to involve him/her in the planning process and encourage compliance with the plan
   - With the child, plan for daily exercise/activity to expend excess calories
   - Instruct the child/parent about appropriate nutrient-rich foods to choose within the constraints of diet and fluid restrictions to provide basis for ongoing diet management at home
   - Weigh child twice weekly on same scale to determine progress toward goal.

   Evaluation: Child maintained current weight.

5. **Nursing diagnosis:** Impaired urinary elimination related to urinary tract infection or other urologic condition, or other factors such as ignoring urge to void at appropriate time as evidenced by urinary retention or incontinence, dribbling, urgency or dysuria.
   Goal: Child will be able to maintain continence.
   Intervention: Promoting adequate urinary elimination.
   - Assess the child's usual voiding pattern and success within that pattern to determine baseline
   - Develop a schedule for bladder emptying to encourage voiding in the toilet
   - Maintain adequate hydration, as dehydration irritates the bladder
   - Avoid constipation, as constipation is associated with inability to adequately empty bladder
   - Teach parents to restrict child's fluid intake after dinner to avoid bedwetting
   - Ensure child voids prior to going to bed avoid bedwetting
   - Teach bladder-stretching exercises as prescribed per physician to increase bladder capacity.

   Evaluation: Child voiding in the toilet.

6. **Nursing diagnosis:** Urinary retention related to anatomic obstruction, sensory motor impairment or dysfunctional voiding as evidenced by dribbling, inadequate bladder emptying.
   Goal: Child will be able to empty bladder adequately.
   Intervention: Promoting successful bladder emptying.
   - Assess child's ability to adequately empty bladder via history focused on character and duration of lower urinary symptoms to establish baseline

- Assess for history of fecal impaction or encopresis, as alterations in bowel elimination may have a negative impact on urinary elimination
- Assess for bladder distention by palpation or urinary retention by post-void residual obtained via catheterization
- Maintain adequate hydration to avoid irritating effects of dehydration on the bladder
- Schedule voiding to decrease bladder over distention
- In the child with significant urinary retention, teach parents/child the technique of clean intermittent catheterization, which allows for regular complete bladder emptying.

Evaluation: Usual urine output is 0.5 mL/kg/h.

7. **Nursing diagnosis:** Distributed body image related to anatomic differences, short stature or effects of long-term corticosteroid use as evidenced by verbalization of dissatisfaction with the child's or adolescent's looks.
   Goal: Child or adolescent will be able to display appropriate body image.
   Intervention: Promoting body image.
   - Acknowledge feelings of anger over body changes and illness: venting feelings is associated with less body image disturbance
   - Support the child's or teen's choices of comfortable, fashionable clothing that may disguise anatomic abnormalities and dialysis tubing
   - Involve the child and especially the teen in the decision-making process, as a sense of control of their own body will improve body image
   - Encourage children or teens to spend time with others their own age, who have short stature or other effects of renal disorders: a peer's opinions are often better accepted than those of persons in authority, such as parents or healthcare professionals.

   Evaluation: Child looks at self in mirror and participates in social activities.

8. **Nursing diagnosis:** Knowledge deficit related to lack of information regarding complex medical condition, prognosis and medical needs as evidenced by verbalization, questions or actions demonstrating lack of understanding regarding child's condition or care.
   Goal: Child and parents will be able to verbalize accurate information and understanding about condition, prognosis and medical needs.
   Intervention: Educating the child and parents.
   - Assess child's and parent's willingness to learn: child and parents must be open to learning for teaching to be effective
   - Provide parents with time to adjust to diagnosis: will facilitate adjustment and ability to learn and participate in child's care
   - Teach in short sessions; many short sessions are found to be more helpful than one long session
   - Repeat information: allows parents and child time to learn and understand
   - Individualize teaching to the parent's and child's level of understanding (depends on age of child, physical condition, memory) to ensure understanding
   - Provide reinforcement and rewards to facilitate the teaching/learning process
   - Use multiple modes of learning involving many senses (written, verbal, demonstration, and videos) when possible: child and parents are more likely to retain information when presented in different ways using many senses.

   Evaluation: Child and parents demonstrate knowledge of condition and medication, and demonstrate therapeutic procedures the child requires.

NURSING PROCESS FOR SPECIFIC RENAL DISORDERS

Chronic Renal Failure

Chronic renal failure (CRF) is the progressive deterioration of kidney function that reaches 50% or more loss or a creatinine level of less than 2 mg/dL. Causes include congenital kidney and urinary tract abnormalities in children less than 5 years of age, glomerular and hereditary kidney disorders in children 5-15 years of age. The disease involves all body systems as abnormalities include water, Na, Ca losses, K, P, Mg increases, reduced Hgb, Hct that result in metabolic acidosis, anemia, growth retardation, hypertension, and bone demineralization. Eventually, if untreated, uremic syndrome develops as the kidneys are not able to maintain fluid and electrolyte balance. End stage renal disease is the term applied when the kidneys are no longer able to clear wastes from the body, eventually the disease terminates in death unless kidney transplantation or dialysis is performed **(Flowchart 15.1)**.

Chronic Renal Failure Symptoms

- Poor appetite
- Vomiting
- Bone pain
- Headache
- Stunted growth
- Malaise
- High urine output or no urine output
- Recurrent urinary tract infections
- Urinary incontinence
- Pale skin
- Bad breath
- Hearing deficit
- Detectable abdominal mass
- Tissue swelling
- Irritability
- Poor muscle tone
- Change in mental alertness.

Nursing Management

A. Essential Nursing Diagnoses and Nursing Process Associated with this Condition

Nursing diagnosis

Fluid volume excess related to compromised regulatory mechanism.

Assessment: Edema, water and Na retention, weight gain, clothes begin to feel tight, decreased urinary output, facial puffiness, altered electrolytes, shortness of breath, crackles, hypertension, vascular congestion.

(Refer Table 14.9 from chapter 14)

Nursing Process for the Child with Renal Disorder

Flowchart 15.1: Pathophysiology of chronic renal failure.

```
Congenital           Glomerular          Hereditary           Renal vascular
and urinary          disease             disease              disorder
malformation            ↓                   ↓                    ↓
   |              Chronic pyelo-         Nephritis         Vascular thrombosis
   |                nephritis         Polycystic kidney    Hemolytic-uremic
   |              Chronic glomerulo-  Nephrotic syndrome      syndrome
   |                nephritis              ↓                    ↓
   |                   ↓
   └──────→ Progressive and irreversible destruction ←──────┘
                        of nephrons
                             ↓
                    Loss of kidney function
                             ↓
                 Reduced glomerular filtration rate
           ┌──── progressive intolerance to fluid/electrolyte ────┐
           |           excesses or restrictions                    |
           ↓                    ↓                ↓                  ↓
  Retention of protein    Inability to con-   Electrolyte      Inability to
  metabolism by-product   centrate urine      imbalance        excrete H ion
           ↓              Inability to filter      ↓                ↓
   Increased BUN          albumin          Hypernatremia      Acid-base
   increased creatinine        ↓           Hypocalcemia       imbalance
           |              Water and sodium Hyperphosphatemia        ↓
           |                retention      Hyperkalemia       Metabolic
           |                   ↓                ↓             acidosis
           |                 Edema
           |           vascular congestion
           |                   ↓
           └──────────→ Renal dialysis ←──────────────────────┘
                          ↓       ↓
              Kidney transplantation  Uremic syndrome
                                         ↓
                              Renal osteodystrophy
                        Hypertension/congestive heart failure
                           Anemia/gastrointestinal bleeding
                              Pneumonia/pulmonary edema
                                 Peripheral neuropathy
                                    Hyperthyroidism
                                  Hyperparathyroidism
                              Delayed puberty/retarded growth
                               Anorexia/vomiting/diarrhea
                                Retinopathy/pruritus/pallor
                                     Hyperglycemia
```

(BUN: blood urea nitrogen)

Nursing diagnosis

Altered nutrition: Less than body requirements related to inability to ingest foods, absorb nutrients and vitamins/minerals.

Assessment: Anorexia, nausea, fatigue, weight loss, limited K, P and protein food intake, poor absorption of Ca, iron by intestines, growth retardation.

(Refer Table 14.3 from chapter 14)

Nursing diagnosis

Hyperthermia related to illness (renal failure).

Assessment: Frequent infections, increase in body temperature above normal range that is recurrent, malaise.

(Refer Table 14.18 from chapter 14)

Nursing diagnosis

High-risk for impaired skin integrity related to internal factor of chronic renal failure.

Assessment: Dryness, pruritus, uremic frost, sallow color, disruption of skin surfaces from scratching.

(Refer Table 12.1 from chapter 12)

Nursing diagnosis

Altered growth and development related to effects of physical disability (renal failure).

Assessment: Altered physical growth, delay in sexual maturation, frequent absences from school and disruptions in socialization, inability to participate in activities, frequent hospitalizations.

(Refer Table 14.4 from chapter 14)

B. Specific Nursing Diagnoses and Nursing Process

Nursing diagnosis

Activity intolerance related to general weakness **(Table 15.1)**.

Assessment: Complaints of fatigue on exertion, preference for quiet play, lack of energy.

Evaluation
- Conserves energy and minimizes fatigue
- Participation in activities within capabilities and disease restrictions
- Balances activity with rest periods.

Nursing diagnosis

High-risk for infection related to chronic disease **(Table 15.2)**.

Assessment: Changes in respiratory pattern, productive cough with yellow or other abnormal color, adventitious sounds, elevated temperature, cloudy, foul smelling urine, dysuria, urgency, frequency.

Table 15.1: Nursing interventions for activity intolerance.

Interventions	Rationales
Assess degree of weakness, fatigue, ability to participate in activities (active and passive)	Provides information about effect of activities on fatigue and energy reserves
Schedule care and provide rest periods following an activity and allow child to set own limits in amount of exertion tolerated when feasible	Promotes independence and control of situations as the presence of a chronic disease may encourage dependency
Provide for quiet play, reading, TV, games during times of fatigue	Provides diversion, stimulation and requires minimal energy expenditure

Nursing Process for the Child with Renal Disorder

Table 15.2: Nursing interventions for high-risk for infection.

Interventions	Rationales
Assess temperature, respiratory and urinary system changes as disease progresses	Provides information about presence of infection caused by progressive chronic disease and its deteriorating effect on all systems
Administer antibiotic therapy as ordered in doses related to decreased renal function	Prevents or treats infection
Perform handwash, medical or surgical asepsis during procedures or care as appropriate	Prevents transmission of pathogens to child
Secure urine or sputum cultures for analysis	Identifies presence and type of microorganism responsible for infection and specific sensitivities to antibiotic therapy

Evaluation
- Absence of infections
- Controls transmission of pathogens to child
- Participates in measure to prevent infections.

Nursing diagnosis

Body image disturbance related to biophysical and psychosocial factors **(Table 15.3)**.

Assessment: Verbal and nonverbal responses to change in body appearance, disruptions in school attendance and participation in school activities and socialization, negative feelings about body, multiple stressors and changes in daily living.

Evaluation
- Verbalizes improved body image and sense of well-being
- Participates in school and social activities as appropriate
- Verbalizes feelings about special needs in positive terms
- Supports positive body image and promotes adjustment to chronic illness.

Nursing diagnosis

Anticipatory grieving related to perceived potential loss of child by parent(s); perceived potential loss of physiopsychosocial well-being by child **(Table 15.4)**.

Table 15.3: Nursing intervention for body image disturbance.

Interventions	Rationales
Assess child for feelings about abilities, chronic illness, difficulty in school and social situations, stature, inability to keep up with peers	Provides information about status of self-concept and special needs
Encourage expression of feelings and concerns and support communication with parent(s), teachers, and peers	Provides opportunity to vent feelings and reduce negative feelings about change in appearance
Stress and state positive activities and accomplishments, avoid negative comments	Enhances body image and confidence

Table 15.4: Nursing interventions for anticipatory grieving.

Interventions	Rationales
Assess stage of grief process, problems encountered, feelings regarding long-term illness and potential loss of child	Provides information about stage of grieving as time to work through the process varies with individuals; the longer the illness, the better able the parent(s) and family will be able to move toward acceptance
Provide emotional and spiritual comfort in an accepting environment and avoid conversations that will cause guilt or anger	Provides for emotional needs of parent(s) and assists them to cope with ill child without adding stressors that are difficult to resolve
Allow for parental and child responses and expression of feelings	Allows for reactions necessary to work through grieving
Assist to identify and use effective coping mechanisms and to understand situations over which they have no control	Promotes use of coping mechanisms over long period of time of illness; chronic disease causes physical and emotional stress on family members which may be positive or negative

Assessment: Expression of distress of potential loss, inevitable kidney failure, kidney dialysis, premature death of child.

Evaluation
- Verbalizes understanding of grief process and responses
- Shares feelings with professionals and other members of family
- Identifies and use coping skills that assist in adaptation and acceptance of chronic illness and deterioration
- Performs normal parental tasks/interventions with child
- Verbalizes hope after diagnosis is made and prospect of dialysis and kidney transplant is explained

Nursing diagnosis

High-risk for injury related to internal factor of regulatory mechanism (renal failure) (Table 15.5).

Assessment: Complications of impaired renal function, hypertension, anemia, metabolic acidosis, osteodystrophy, neurologic manifestations, uremic syndrome if disorder untreated.

Evaluation
- Controls systemic complications with medical regimen
- Complies with follow-up supervision of renal function
- Administers medications accurately and reports adverse effects if present
- Verbalizes and promotes therapy to prevent uremic syndrome.

Glomerulonephritis

Acute glomerulonephritis is the inflammation of the structures of the kidney known as the glomeruli. These structures are responsible for the filtration of body fluids and waste products that compose the urine which is eliminated from the body by excretion. The kidney involvement

Nursing Process for the Child with Renal Disorder

Table 15.5: Nursing interventions for high-risk for injury related to internal factor of regulatory mechanism (renal failure).

Interventions	Rationales
Assess blood pressure for increases and administer antihypertensive and diuretics as ordered singly or in combination	Provides data regarding hypertension evident in advanced renal disease
Assess I:O, electrolyte panel, BUN, and creatinine and administer diuretics as ordered for excessive water retention	Provides indication of renal function affecting output with water and electrolyte retention as disease progresses and nephrons are destroyed
Assess RBC, HCT, Hb and administer iron and transfusion of packed red blood cells as ordered	Provides indication of anemia caused by the reduced production of erythropoietin by the failing kidneys and inadequate intake of iron in a restricted diet
Assess bone pain and deformities affecting ambulation and activities and administer supplemental vitamin D, calcium and alkalizing agents	Provides indication of osteodystrophy caused by a calcium/phosphorus imbalance resulting in bone demineralization and growth retardation; kidney disease results in the inability to synthesis vitamin D needed to absorb Ca; acidosis causes dissolution of alkaline salts of bone and phosphate is increased and calcium decreased as glomerular filtration is reduced
Assess presence of acidosis by pH, bicarbonate losses and administer alkalizing agents	Provides indication of impending metabolic acidosis caused by the inability of failing kidneys to excrete metabolic acids that are by-products of metabolism; the hydrogen ion is retained and bicarbonate is lost as the tubules are unable to reabsorb it
Assess for sensory loss, confusion, and changes in consciousness	Reveals possible changes in neurologic status as kidney function deteriorates and uremic syndrome appears

(BUN: blood urea nitrogen; RBC: red blood cell; HCT: hematocrit; Hb: hemoglobin)

usually follows an infection caused by the type A, beta-hemolytic *Streptococcus*, which sets up an antigen-antibody reaction. The disease primarily affects the schoolage child of 6-7 years of age and occurs about 10 years following an upper respiratory disorder but not always identified with an infection. Glomerulonephritis results in retention of water and sodium (edema), reduced circulatory volume (hypovolemia) and circulatory congestion, hypertension, changes in urinary output and urine characteristics **(Fig. 15.1)**.

Symptoms of Glomerulonephritis

- Dark brown-colored urine (from blood and protein)
- Sore throat
- Diminished urine output
- Fatigue
- Lethargy
- Increased breathing effort
- Headache
- High blood pressure

Nursing Process for the Child with Renal Disorder

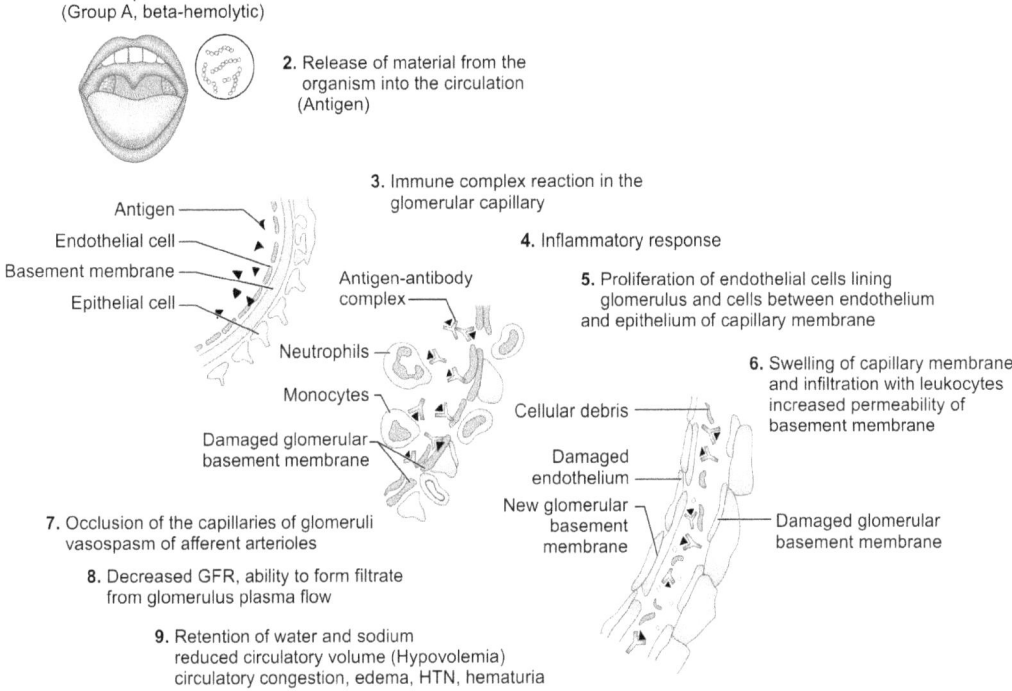

Fig. 15.1: Pathophysiology of glomerulonephritis.

- Seizures (may occur as a result of high blood pressure)
- Rash, especially over the buttocks and legs
- Weight loss
- Joint pain
- Pale skin color
- Fluid accumulation in the tissues (edema).

Nursing Management

A. Essential Nursing Diagnoses and Nursing Process Associated with this Condition

Nursing diagnosis

fluid volume excess related to compromised regulatory mechanism.

Assessment: Dependent edema, periorbital edema, pleural effusion, puffiness in the face, moderate blood pressure increases, intake greater than output, weight gain, azoturia, crackles decreased Hb and HCT, altered electrolytes, decreased urinary output.

(Refer Table 14.9 from chapter 14)

Nursing diagnosis

altered nutrition: Less than body requirements related to inability to ingest food.

Assessment: Anorexia, fatigue, nausea, vomiting, malaise.

(Refer Table 14.3 from chapter 14)

Nursing Process for the Child with Renal Disorder

Table 15.6: Nursing interventions for activity intolerance.

Interventions	Rationales
Assess weakness, fatigue, ability to move about in bed and participate in play activities	Provides information about energy reserves during the acute phase of the disease and acceptance of bed rest status
Schedule care and provide rest periods following any activity in a quiet environment	Provides adequate rest and reduces stimuli and fatigue
Maintain bed rest during the acute stage, disturb only when necessary	Conserves energy and decreases production of waste materials which increases work of the kidneys
Provide for quiet play, reading, TV, games as symptoms subside	Provides diversion, stimulation and requires minimal energy expenditure

Nursing diagnosis

altered tissue perfusion (cerebral) related to hypovolemia, hypertensive encephalopathy, cerebral ischemia.

Assessment: Severe hypertension during acute state headache, changes in mentation, restlessness, lethargy, double vision, seizure activity.

(Refer Table 14.12 from chapter 14)

Nursing diagnosis

High-risk for impaired skin integrity related to internal factor of edema, altered circulation.

Assessment: Bed rest, impaired tissue perfusion, pressure on skin and bony prominences pink or redness of skin, disruption of skin from IV infusions.

(Refer Table 12.1 from chapter 12)

B. Specific Nursing Diagnoses and Nursing Process

Nursing diagnosis

Activity intolerance related to generalized weakness, bed rest **(Table 15.6)**.

Assessment: Expressed weakness and fatigue, anemia, lethargy.

Evaluation
- Conserves energy and minimizes fatigue and weakness
- Engages in activities progressively within capabilities and disease restrictions.

Nursing diagnosis

High-risk for infection related to chronic disease **(Table 15.7)**.

Assessment: Persistent streptococcal infections.

Evaluation
- Absence of streptococcal infection (nephritogenic)
- Controls transmission of the streptococcal microorganism
- Complies with medication regimen.

Nursing Process for the Child with Renal Disorder

Table 15.7: Nursing intervention for high-risk for infection.

Interventions	Rationales
Assess temperature, chills, sore throat, cough (presence or recurrence)	Indicates persistence of streptococcal infection
Obtain throat culture for analysis and sensitivities	Identifies streptococcal microorganism and sensitivity to specific antibiotic therapy
Administer antibiotic therapy to child and to family members if ordered	Destroys microbial agents by preventing cell wall synthesis and prevents transmission to family members
Provide for disposal of used articles properly	Prevents transmission of microorganisms to others or re-infection

Nursing diagnosis

high-risk for injury related to internal factor of regulatory mechanism (renal function) (Table 15.8).

Assessment: Complications of impairs renal function, hypertension, cardiac failure, renal failure.

Evaluation

- Absence of complications of acute disease
- Complies with medication, activity, dietary regimen
- Complies with follow-up supervision of renal function.

Table 15.8: Nursing interventions for high-risk for injury related to internal factor of regulatory mechanism (renal function).

Interventions	Rationales
Assess BP, pulse, respirations q4h; monitor BP qlh if diastolic is more than 90, pulse and respirations qlh if tachycardia, tachypnea or dyspnea present	Provides information about complication of hypertension which may lead to encephalopathy, pulse and respirations which change with heart failure and pulmonary edema
Assess changes in 1:0, urinary albumin, extent of edema, decreased urinary output, headache, pallor, electrolyte balance	Indicates signs and symptoms of possible renal failure
Administer antihypertensive, diuretic therapy, cardiac glycoside and monitor for expected results	Provides therapy for complications if a more severe renal impairment is present
Limit fluids if output is reduced; allow intake of the amount lost via urine and insensible losses	Prevents further fluid retention and edema in the presence of renal damage
Limit Na, K in diet and encourage a diet that includes increased carbohydrate and fat content	Provides nutrition during the acute period with limitation of K during oliguria, Na with presence of edema, protein limitation if oliguria is prolonged
Note behavior changes including lethargy, irritability, restlessness associated with hypertension and administer anticonvulsive if ordered	Indicates need for safety precautions associated with seizure activity as a result of cerebral changes

Hypospadias/Epispadias

Hypospadias and epispadias are congenital defects in which the urethral orifice in the male is located along the ventral surface or dorsal surface of the penis shaft respectively. Hypospadias may be associated with chordee (ventral curvature of the penis), a band of fibrous tissue in place of normal tissue. Epispadias is less common and may be associated with varying degrees of severity. Treatment of both involves surgical correction of the defect usually between 6-12 months of age without the presence of chordee or in stages between 1-2 years or as late as 3-4 years of age to release the chordee, to extend the urethra length and to construct a new meatal orifice. Repair and correction is important to prevent adverse effect on body image by the difference in appearance and function and anxiety associated with concerns abut sterility or sexual dysfunction **(Fig. 15.2)**.

Symptoms of Hypospadiasis/Epispadiasis

Symptoms of Hypospadiasis

- Abnormal appearance of foreskin and penis on exam
- Abnormal direction of urine stream
- The end of the penis may be curved downward.

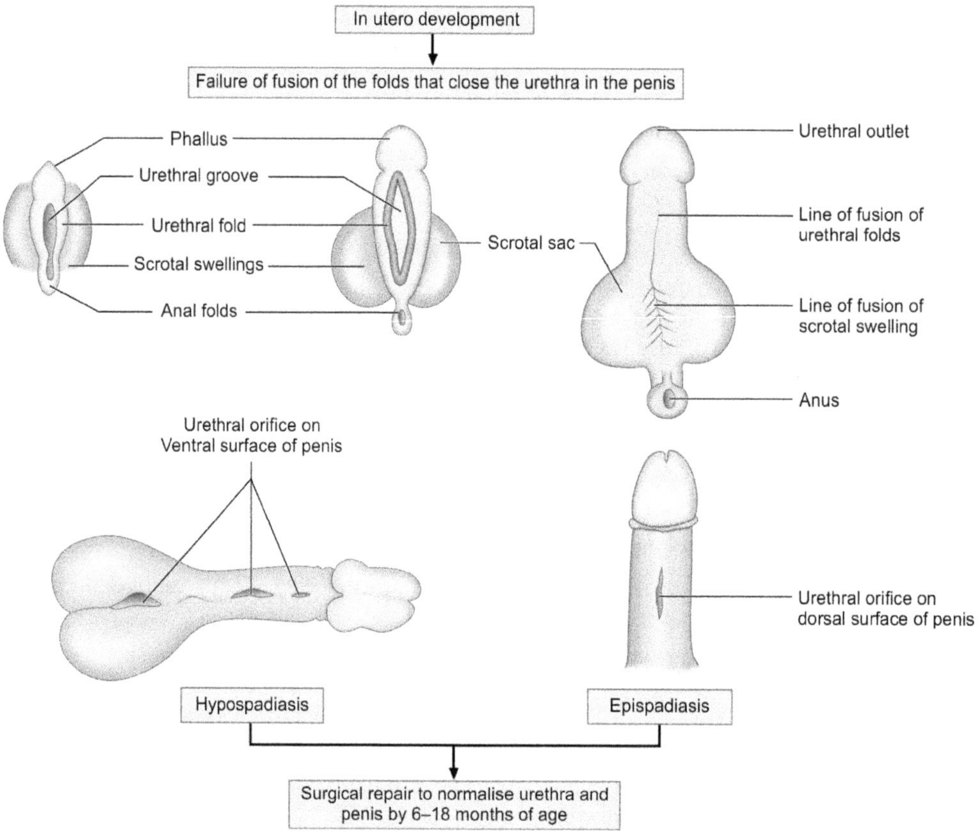

Fig. 15.2: Pathophysiology of hypospadiasis/epispadiasis.

Symptoms of Epispadiasis

Males usually have a short, wide penis with an abnormal curve. The urethra usually opens on the top or side of the penis instead of the tip. However, the urethra may be open along the whole length of the penis.

Females have an abnormal clitoris and labia. The opening is usually between the clitoris and the labia, but it may be in the belly area. They may have trouble controlling urination (urinary incontinence).

Nursing Management

A. Essential Nursing Diagnoses and Nursing Process Associated with this Condition

Nursing diagnosis

High-risk for impaired skin integrity related to external factor of surgical incision.

Assessment: Disruption of skin surface, surgical correction of defect, catheter site irritation.

(Refer Table 12.1 from chapter 12)

Nursing diagnosis

High-risk for fluid volume deficit related to factors influencing fluid needs.

Assessment: NPO preoperatively, temperature elevation with infection, decreased urinary output, inadequate fluid replacement postoperatively.

(Refer Table 14.11 from chapter 14)

Nursing diagnosis

Hyperthermia related to illness (presence of infection).

Assessment: Increase in body temperature above normal range, warm to touch, increased pulse and respiratory rate, evidence of infection at surgical site, evidence of lower urinary tract infection.

(Refer Table 14.18 from chapter 14)

B. Specific Nursing Diagnoses and Nursing Process

Nursing diagnosis

Anxiety of parent(s) related to threat to self-concept, change in health status, change in environment (hospitalization) **(Table 15.9)**.

Assessment: Expressed apprehension and concern about correction of defect by surgery and the imperfect appearance of the penis following surgery, preoperative and postoperative care.

Evaluation
- Verbalizes reduction in anxiety about defect, surgical correction
- Verbalizes positive effects of surgical correction
- Participates in care and support of child and decision making during postoperative experience.

Nursing diagnosis

Pain related to physical injuring agent (surgery) **(Table 15.10)**.

Nursing Process for the Child with Renal Disorder

Table 15.9: Nursing interventions for anxiety of parent(s).

Interventions	Rationales
Assess source and level of anxiety and need for information that will relieve anxiety	Provides information about anxiety level and need to relieve it: source for parent include the type of procedure and appearance of penis after surgery, whether the adequate, possibility that correction may need to be done in stages if child is old enough, sources include fear of castration and change in body image
Allow expression of concerns and time for parent(s) and child to ask questions about condition, procedures, recovery	Provides opportunity to vent feelings and fears and secure environment
Answer questions calmly and honestly; use pictures, drawings, and models for information	Promotes trust and a calm and supportive environment
Allow parent(s) to stay with child during hospitalizations and encourage to assist in care	Allows parent(s) to care for and support child and continue parental role
Give parent(s) as much input into decisions about care and usual routines as possible	Allows for more control over situations and maintains familiar routines for care

Table 15.10: Nursing interventions for pain.

Interventions	Rationales
Assess verbal and nonverbal behavior, type location and severity of pain depending on child's age	Provides information about pain as basis for analgesic therapy
Administer analgesics and sedative	Reduces pain and promotes rest which reduces stimuli and pain
Place in position of comfort and position catheter to avoid tension and kinking	Promotes comfort and prevents pain from pulling on or manipulating catheter
Apply ice pack if ordered	Reduces edema and pain

Assessment: Communication of pain descriptors, crying, irritability, restlessness, withdrawal, increased P, increased R, increased BP.

Evaluation
- Absence of pain and associated responses
- Administers correct medication to prevent and/or control pain
- Controls pain provoking actions when giving care or positioning child.

Nursing diagnosis

High-risk for infection related to inadequate primary defenses (surgical incision); invasive procedure (catheter) **(Table 15.11)**.

Assessment: Redness, swelling, drainage at incisional site; cloudy, foul smelling urine, elevated temperature, positive urine or wound culture.

Nursing Process for the Child with Renal Disorder

Table 15.11: Nursing interventions for high-risk for infection.

Interventions	Rationales
Assess wound for redness, swelling, drainage on dressing, healing	Provides information indicating presence of infection or poor healing
Assess catheter insertion site for redness, irritation, swelling, urine collected in drainage system for cloudiness, foul odor, sediment	Indicates infectious process at catheter site or in urinary bladder
Collect urine specimen for culture and sensitivities	Provides information about specific organism and sensitivity to antibiotic
Administer anti-infective if culture results are 100,000 mL/mm or more as ordered	Treats specific organism causing urinary infection or prevents infection when catheter is in place
Use sterile technique when changing dressings or giving catheter care or emptying drainage bag	Prevents contamination by introducing organisms into sterile wound or cavity
Encourage to increase fluid intake according to age needs	Promotes dilution of urine to prevent urinary infection and after catheter removed will encourage voiding
Maintain catheter and collection bag below level of bladder and a closed drainage system free of kinks in the tubing	Prevent back flow of urine into bladder and stem patency is assured
Immobilize arms and legs with restraints, remove periodically; use a bed cradle following surgery	Prevents accidental removal or disturbance of catheter or contamination of wound, if surgical correction done for a more severe defect
Avoid change of dressing, reinforce as needed, and secure catheter to penis with dressing and taps and to leg or abdomen with taps	Promotes comfort and prevents infection and catheter displacement
Note urinary output of at least 1 mL/kg/h and report if less	Indicates that catheter obstruction may be present with urinary retention which leads to infection

Evaluation
- Absence of urinary tract infection
- Patency and placement of catheter maintained
- Wound healing without infection or complications
- Complies with preventive measures and anti-infective therapy.

Nursing diagnosis

Altered urinary elimination pattern related to mechanical trauma (urethroplasty) **(Table 15.12)**.

Assessment: Dysuria, frequency, urgency, retention, bladder spasms, inadequate output.

Evaluation
- Return of urinary elimination pattern through new or corrected meatus after catheter removed
- Absence of signs and symptoms of urinary retention or dysfunction.

Table 15.12: Nursing interventions for altered urinary elimination pattern.

Interventions	Rationales
Assess 1:0 ratio, voiding stream, color and amount of urine on first voiding and each subsequent voiding	Provides information about voiding pattern after clamping or removal of catheter
Assess for pain, abdominal distention, inability to void for 8 hours after catheter removal	Indicates urinary dysfunction and possible obstruction or continuing edema of meatus
Support child after catheter is removed and provide privacy for voiding	Prevents embarrassment which is common in an older child
Encourage increased fluid intake after catheter removed, offer preferred liquids qlh	Promotes micturition

Nephrotic Syndrome

Nephrotic syndrome is a kidney disease characterized by an increased glomerular capillary wall permeability to protein (albumin) causing proteinuria, hypoproteinemia, hyperlipidemia, and edema. The most common type is minimal change nephritic syndrome (idiopathic nephrosis) which is thought to be caused by some nonspecific illness and affects children between 2-7 years of age. Secondary nephritic syndrome occurs in children during or following a kidney or systemic disease that causes damage to the glomeruli. A congenital type is caused by a recessive gene and presents itself during infancy with early symptoms and death as it does not respond to therapy. Nephritic syndrome requires continuous and close monitoring and care to prevent the complications of hypertension, renal failure or congestive heart failure and relapses associated with prolonged remissions and exacerbations **(Fig. 15.3)**.

Signs and Symptoms of Nephrotic Syndrome

- Pitting edema
- Respiratory tract infection
- Allergy—approximately 30% of children with nephritic syndrome have a history of allergy
- Macrohematuria
- Symptoms of infection—such as fever, lethargy, irritability or abdominal pain due to sepsis or peritonitis
- Hypotension and signs of shock
- Respiratory distress—due to either massive ascites and thoracic compression or frank pulmonary edema, effusions, or both
- Tachypnea
- Seizure
- Anorexia
- Irritability
- Fatigue
- Abdominal discomfort
- Diarrhea
- Hypertension.

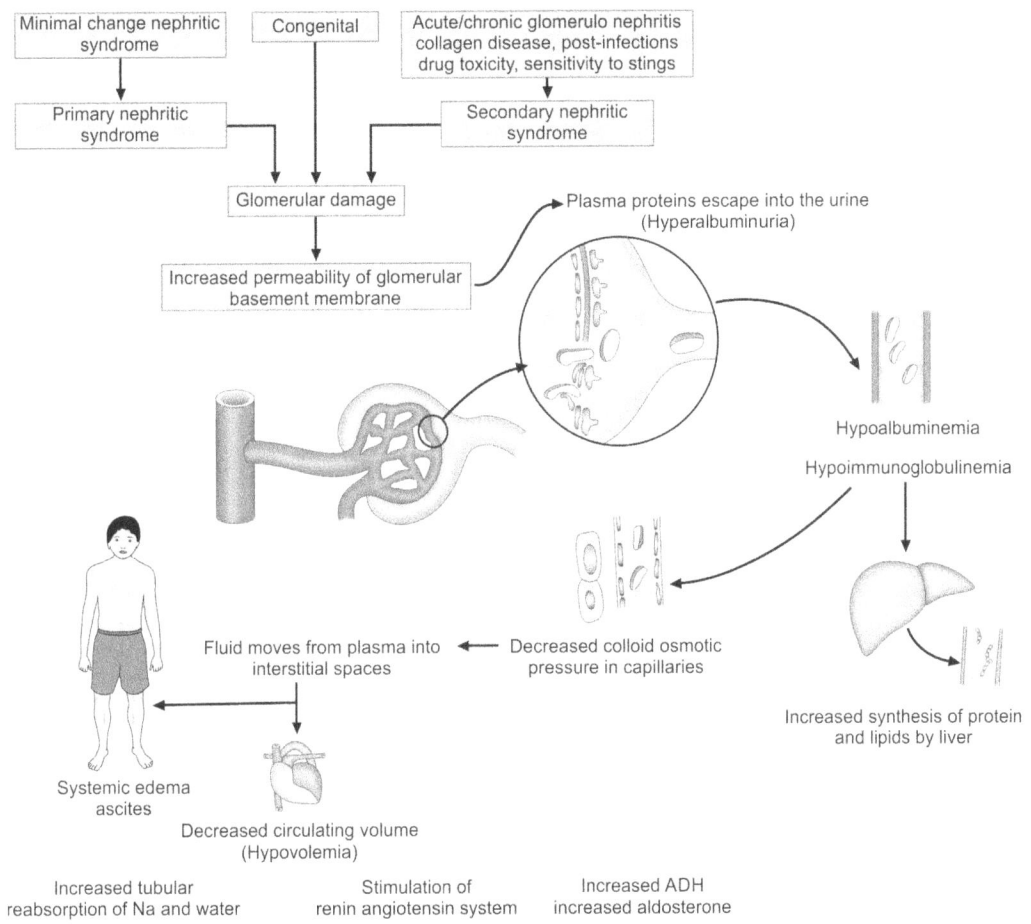

Fig. 15.3: Pathophysiology of nephrotic syndrome.
(ADH: anti-diuretic hormone)

Nursing Management

A. Essential Nursing Diagnoses and Nursing Process Associated with this Condition

Nursing diagnosis

Fluid volume excess related to compromised regulatory mechanism.

Assessment: Edema (pitting), periorbital and facial puffiness in morning and dependent in the evening, abdominal ascites, scrotal or labial edema, edema of mucous membranes of intestines, anasarca, slow weight gain, decreased urine output, altered electrolytes, specific gravity, blood pressure changes, respiratory pattern (dyspnea, tachypnea).

(Refer Table 14.9 from chapter 14)

Nursing diagnosis

Altered nutrition: Less than body requirements related to inability to ingest and digest foods and absorb nutrients.

Nursing Process for the Child with Renal Disorder

Assessment: Anorexia, diarrhea, edema of intestinal tract affecting absorption, weight loss, loss of protein (negative nitrogen balance), rejection of low salt diet.

(Refer Table 14.3 from chapter 14)

Nursing diagnosis

High-risk for impaired skin integrity related to internal factor of edema.

Assessment: Disruption of skin surface, waxy pallor, stretched and shiny appearance, muscle wasting, decreased tissue perfusion, pressure on edematous area, irritation of anal area with diarrhea.

(Refer Table 12.1 from chapter 12)

Nursing diagnosis

Diarrhea related to inflammation, edema, malabsorption of bowel.

Assessment: Increased frequency, loose liquid stools abdominal discomfort.

(Refer Table 13.8 from chapter 13)

Nursing diagnosis

High-risk for fluid volume deficit related to intravascular fluid loss.

Assessment: Diuretic therapy, increased fluid output, urinary frequency, rapid weight loss, hypotension, hypovolemia.

(Refer Table 14.11 from chapter 14)

B. Specific Nursing Diagnoses and Nursing Process

Nursing diagnosis

Fatigue related to states of discomfort **(Table 15.13)**.

Assessment: Extreme edema, lethargy, easily fatigued with any activity.

Table 15.13: Nursing interventions for fatigue.

Interventions	*Rationales*
Assess degree of weakness, fatigue, extent of edema and difficult movement or activity in bed	Provides information about fatigue and tendency of lying in prone position and not moving or changing position
Maintain bed rest during most acute stage	Prevents energy expenditure when edema is severe
Provide selected play activities as tolerated and adjust schedule to allow for rest periods and after activity	Provides stimulation and activity within endurance level as edema is relieved
Plan activities with discretion and observe for behavior changes after activity	Prevents fatigue while improving endurance, inactivity and steroid therapy and disease result in mood swings and irritability in the child
Allow for quiet play followed by unrestricted activity and encourage child to set own limits when feasible	Promotes independence and control of situations

Nursing Process for the Child with Renal Disorder

Table 15.14: Nursing intervention for high-risk for infection.

Interventions	Rationales
Assess temperature elevation, respiratory changes (dyspnea, productive cough with yellow sputum), urinary changes (cloudy, foul smelling urine), skin changes (redness, swelling, pain in an area)	Indicates presence of infectious process resulting from steroid and immunosuppressant therapy given to enhance body defenses and reduce relapse rate
Prevents visits from those with illnesses or infectious processes	Protects child from infected persons that may transmit pathogen to immunosuppressed child
Provide private room or share room with children who are free from infections	Protects child from pathogen transmission
Maintain medical aseptic techniques and handwash when giving care	Promotes measures to prevent infection
Maintain warmth for child. Regulate room environmental temperature and humidly	Prevents chilling and predisposition to upper respiratory infection
Administer antibiotic therapy if ordered	Prevents or treats infection based on culture and sensitivities

Evaluation
- Conserves energy and minimizes fatigue
- Participates in play and activities within capabilities in a progressive fashion
- Balances activity with rest periods.

Nursing diagnosis

High-risk for infection related to inadequate secondary defenses **(Table 15.14)**.

Assessment: Fluid overload, edema, elevated temperature, immunosuppression, suppressed inflammatory response, leukopenia.

Evaluation
- Absence of infections
- Controls transmission of pathogens to child
- Participates in measures to prevent infections.

Nursing diagnosis

Knowledge deficit related to lack of exposure to information about disease **(Table 15.15)**.

Table 15.15: Nursing interventions for knowledge deficit.

Interventions	Rationales
Assess knowledge of disease, signs and symptoms of relapse, dietary and activity aspects of care, medication administration and side effects, monitoring urine and VS	Provides information about teaching needs for follow-up care
Assess level of anxiety and need for support in care of ill child and possible relapse	Anxiety will interfere with learning process

(VS: vital signs)

Assessment: Expressed need for information about disease, medication administration, follow-up care and procedures, anxiety associated with relapse of disease.

Evaluation
- Verbalizes signs and symptoms of disease and importance of immediate reporting
- Complies appropriately with an administration of medications with knowledge of side effects to expect
- Complies with follow-up care requirements in diet and activity
- Collects specimen and tests for albumin
- Monitors for edema, daily weights and, BP
- Minimizes potential for relapse of disease
- Verbalizes comfort with implementation of follow-up care
- Encourages return to school and socialization for child with in limitations imposed by the disease.

Sexually Transmitted Diseases

Sexually transmitted diseases are those disease caused by intimate sexual activities with an individual who is infected with the disease. Among these diseases are gonorrhea, syphilis, herpes, warts, urethritis, and pelvic inflammatory disease. Most occur as a result of social and intellectual immaturity regarding responsible sexual behavior. Each is treated according to identification of the causative agent and response to specific therapy. Important in the prevention and/or treatment is education in early treatment and measures to prevent reinfection or transmission of the infection to others **(Flowchart 15.2)**.

Nursing Management

A. Essential Nursing Diagnoses and Nursing Process Associated with these Conditions

Nursing diagnosis

High-risk for impaired skin integrity related to external factor of excretions and secretions, internal factor of infectious agent invasion.

Assessment: Disruption of skin surface, invasion of body structures, pus from urethra or cervix, vesicles on genitalia, buttocks, thighs, penile or vaginal discharge, chancre lesion on penis or female genitalia, skin rash, papules on skin, blisters and ulcerations on genitalia, itching and burning of lesions or sores.

(Refer Table 12.1 from chapter 12)

Nursing diagnosis

Hyperthermia related to illness (pelvic inflammatory disease).

Assessment: Increase in body temperature above normal range, warm to touch, increased pulse and respiratory rate, evidence of infectious process.

(Refer Table 14.18 from chapter 14)

Flowchart 15.2: Pathophysiology of sexually transmitted diseases.

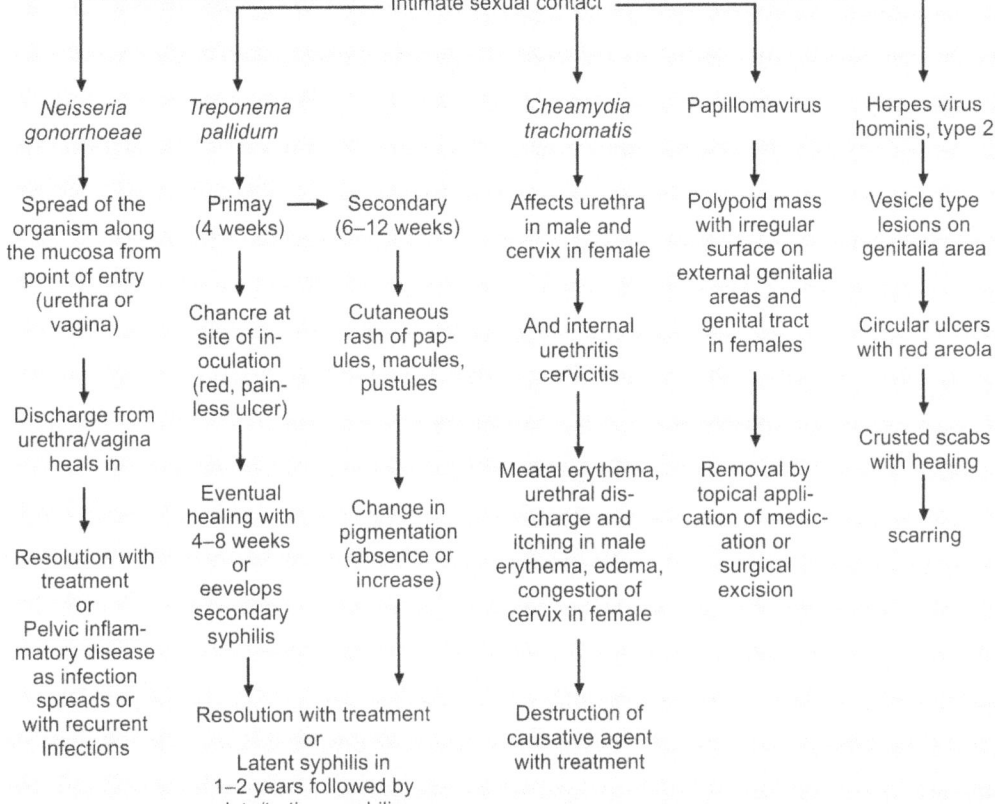

B. Specific Nursing Diagnoses and Nursing Process

Nursing diagnosis

Knowledge deficit related to lack of information about disease **(Table 15.16)**.

Assessment: Expressed need for information about treatment and prevention of recurrence of sexually transmitted disease.

Evaluation
- Verbalizes signs and symptoms specific to disease present
- Administers oral and topical medications correctly with desired effect
- Complies with measures to prevent transmission or recurrence of the disease
- Complies with follow-up treatment
- Absence of signs and symptoms of spread of disease or complications
- Avoids factors that exacerbate disease and maintains nutrition, activity, rest needs for optimal health

Nursing Process for the Child with Renal Disorder

Table 15.16: Nursing interventions for knowledge deficit.

Interventions	Rationales
Assess knowledge of diagnostic and reporting methods, signs and symptoms of specific disease, risk factors in acquiring or transmitting disease and potential complications	Provides information about the disease causes, treatment and preventive measures
Inform of type of culture and blood testing done for diagnosis of disease	Provides information about need to identify specific organisms by culture of discharge from lesions, urethra, vagina, and cervix
Instruct to note pain, tingling, burning, dysuria, frequency, purulent discharge or leucorrhea, itching of genitalia	Indicates active disease caused by lesion, inflammation
Instruct in administration of antibiotics, analgesics, topical agents as ordered; emphasis need to take full course of ordered antibiotic and follow-up exam for syphilis, gonorrhea, pelvic inflammation, chlamydial infection; application of topical chemical agent and removing the drug by washing off in 4–6 hours to remove warts; topical application of topical antiviral to treat herpes	Provides treatment of choice for specific disease and instructions for administration
Inform that disease is contracted and transmitted by sexual contact and to avoid sexual contact with an infected partner and during active phase of the disease; instruct to use male or female condom protection, if sexually active	Prevents spread of the disease to others and recurrence in the infected person
Instruct in hand washing technique to be used following toileting and to avoid touching face with hands	Prevents transmission of infectious agents to genitalia or other body parts
Explain consequences of disease if left untreated or follow-up evaluation avoided specially in gonorrhea and syphilis	Prevents progression or complications of the disease; may lead to infertility or second stage syphilis
Inform that information will be kept confidential according to state laws	Promotes environment conducive to instruction and that is nonjudgmental and accepting
Inform of causes of flare-ups of herpes and to avoid changes in environment extremes, tight clothing, colds, exposure to sun	Prevents recurrence of herpes lesions that commonly occur with illnesses, trauma, or changes that may lower resistance
Inform of importance of reporting the disease and contacts	Promotes control of disease by tracing and treating contacts as well as the infected person

- Verbalizes adequate knowledge about disease, treatment, transmission, prevention and follow-up care
- Participates in sex education classes.

Undescended Testes

Undescended testes (cryptorchidism) is a condition present at birth in which one or both testes fail to descend through the inguinal canal into the scrotal sac. The testes usually descend spontaneously by 1 year of age. If not, child may receive human chorionic gonadotropin therapy or surgery (orchiopexy) performed between 1-2 years of age. Surgery prevents damage to the testes that are affected by exposure to a higher temperature in the abdomen and the risk for tumor formation of the testes. Repair at a younger age also prevents the adverse effect on body image and embarrassment caused by the difference in the appearance of the empty smaller scrotal sac. Undescended testes that are associated with the presence of an inguinal hernia are repaired at the time of herniorrhaphy **(Fig. 15.4)**.

Symptoms of Undescended Testes

There are two types of undescended testes: congenital and acquired.
Congenital—boys who are born with undescended testes.
- In babies born early (premature babies), the testes may not have dropped down yet (usually happens in the eight month of pregnancy).
- Some hormone and genetic disorders can cause undescended testes
- Usually doctors cannot find the cause.

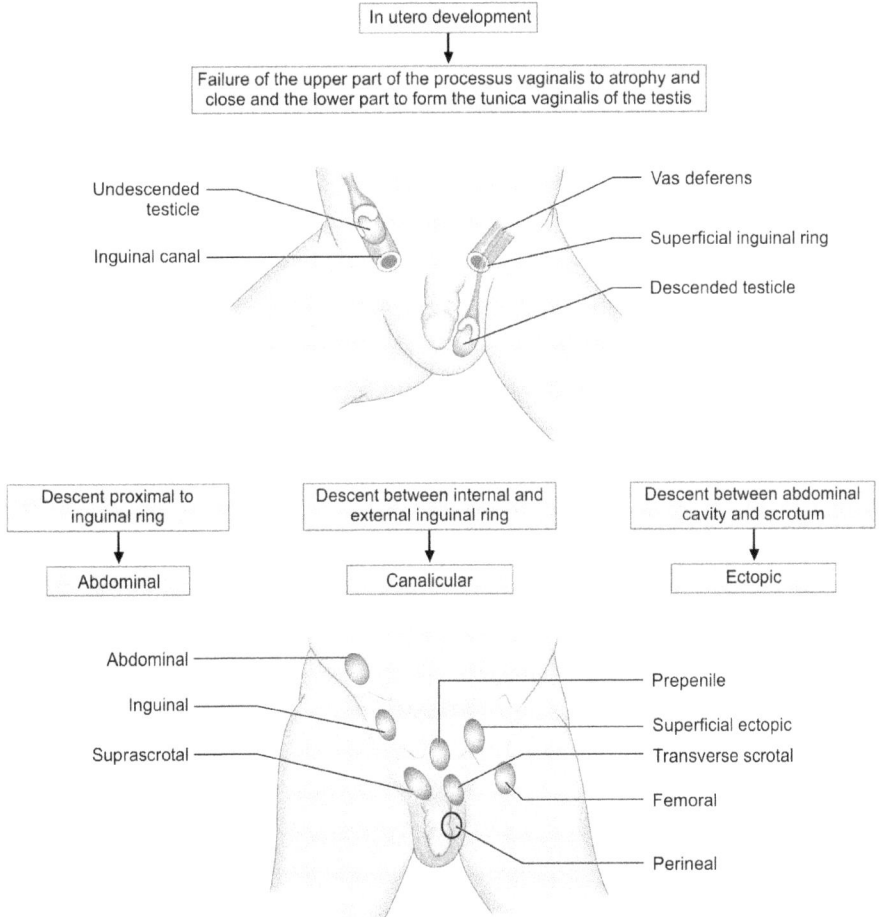

Fig. 15.4: Pathophysiology of undescended testes.

Acquired—boys who develop undescended testes after birth.
- This can happen between 1–10 years of age.
- A boy is born with the testes in the normal place (in the scrotum).
- As the boy grows the cord attached to the testes (spermatic cord), fails to grow at the same rate. It ends up too short and pulls the testes back up into the groin.

Nursing Management

A. Essential Nursing Diagnoses and Nursing Process Associated with this Condition

Nursing diagnosis

High-risk for impaired skin integrity related to external factor of surgical incision.

Assessment: Disruption of skin surface, surgical invasion of body structure(s).

(Refer Table 12.1 from chapter 12)

Nursing diagnosis

Hyperthermia related to illness (presence of infection).

Assessment: Increase in body temperature above normal range, warm to touch, increased pulse and respiratory rate, evidence of infectious process at surgical site.

(Refer Table 14.8 from chapter 14)

B. Specific Nursing Diagnoses and Nursing Process

Nursing diagnosis

Anxiety of parent(s) and child related to threat to self-concept, change in health status of child, hospitalization and surgery of child **(Table 15.17)**.

Assessment: Increased apprehension and expressed concern about future infertility and effect on body image, presence of empty scrotum and smaller size, expressed concern about impending surgery or need for future surgery and procedure performed to correct abnormality.

Evaluation
- Verbalizes reduction in anxiety about abnormality, procedure to correct it, risk of complications
- Verbalizes positive effects of surgical correction
- Participates in decision making and postoperative care
- Complies with activity restrictions, self-examination of testes.

Nursing diagnosis

High-risk for infection related to inadequate primary defenses (broken skin) **(Table 15.18)**.

Assessment: Surgical incision proximity to urine and feces.

Evaluation
- Absence of infection of surgical area
- Maintains clean perineal and wound areas
- Complies with antibiotic regimen as instructed
- Protects surgical area from bathing and urine and/or feces.

Table 15.17: Nursing interventions for anxiety of parent(s) and child.

Interventions	Rationales
Assess source and level of anxiety and how it is manifested; need for information that will relieve anxiety	Provides information about anxiety level and need for interventions to relieve it; source for the parent(s) include fear and uncertainty about treatment and recovery; source for child include embarrassment by different shape and size of scrotum after school age
Allow expression of concerns and opportunity to ask questions about diagnosis, procedures, effect of abnormal placement on testes and future fertility	Provides opportunity to vent feelings and fears and secure information to reduce anxiety
Communicate with parent(s) and child and answer questions calmly and honestly; use pictures, models and drawings as aids where helpful in explanations	Promotes calm and supportive trusting environment
Give parent(s) and child as much input in decisions about care and routines as possible	Allows for more control over situation
Provide as much privacy to the child as possible during assessments	Promotes comfort and prevents embarrassment

Table 15.18: Nursing interventions for high-risk for infection.

Interventions	Rationales
Assess wound for redness, warmth, swelling, discharge	Indicates infection at site
Apply ice to wound postoperatively	Reduces swelling
Carefully cleanse perineal area of any urine or stool as needed	Prevents contamination of wound and risk of infection
Administer antibiotic therapy as ordered	Prevents or treats infection by preventing synthesis of cell wall of microorganisms

Urinary Tract Infection

Urinary tract infection (UTI) is a condition in which an infectious process is present in the upper urinary tract (kidney, ureter) or lower urinary tract (urethra, bladder). It may be caused by the anatomic proximity of the urethra to the anal area and the shortness of this organ in the female; incomplete emptying of the bladder which causes stasis of urine as a result of reflux or anatomic abnormalities or dysfunctional voiding mechanism, catheterization procedure or indwelling catheter placement; alkaline urine and low fluid intake. Ascending spread of the infection via the ureters results in pyelonephritis. Microorganisms responsible for the infection are those found in the perianal and perineal areas. UTI is said to be present when culture results reveal colonization of 100,000/mL or more. The infection is most common in children between 2-6 years of age **(Flowchart 15.3)**.

Flowchart 15.3: Pathophysiology of urinary tract infection.

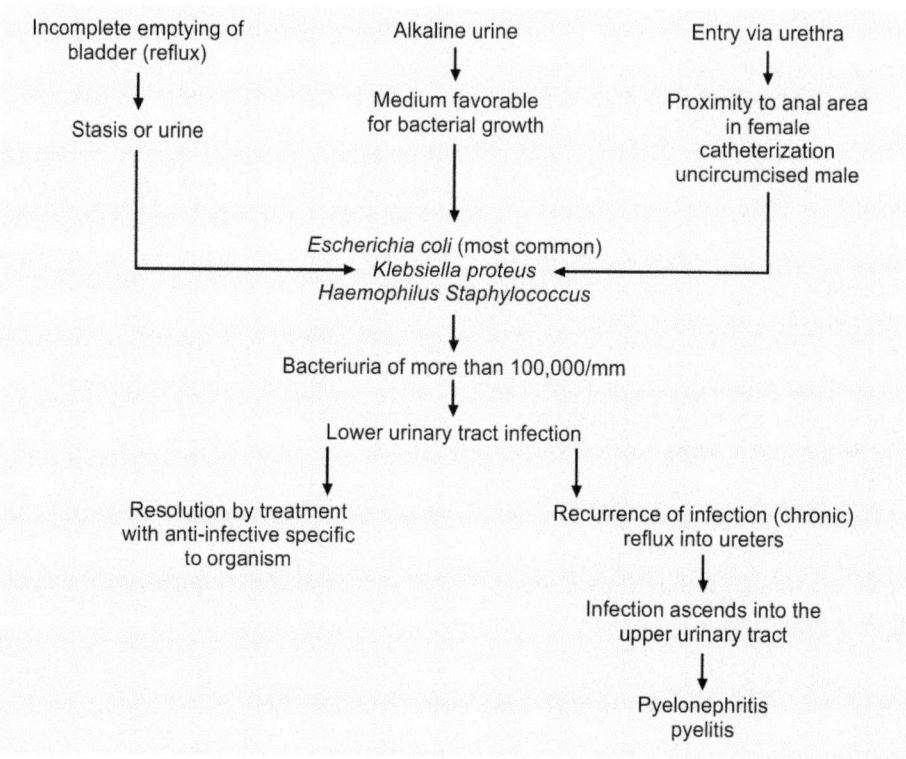

Symptoms of Urinary Tract Infection

Urinary tract infection (UTIs) in children may not cause obvious urinary symptoms.

Symptoms of a UTI in an infant or young child may include:
- Fever: This may be the only symptom in infants
- Irritability
- Lack of appetite
- Failure to gain weight or develop normally
- Foul-smelling urine
- Crying during urination
- Vomiting or diarrhea.

In an older child with a UTI, symptoms are usually easier to recognize and may include:
- Pain or burning when urinating
- Urge to urinate frequently but usually passing only small amounts of urine
- Loss of bladder control, new bedwetting or other changes in urination habits
- Pain in the lower abdomen
- Reddish, pinkish, or cloudy urine
- Foul-smelling urine

- Pain in the flank which is felt just below the rib cage and above the waist on one or both sides of the back.

Nursing Management

A. Essential Nursing Diagnoses and Nursing Process Associated with this Condition

Nursing diagnosis

Hyperthermia related to illness (infection).

Assessment: Increase in body temperature above normal range (low grade), warm to touch, evidence of infection of urinary tract.

(Refer Table 14.18 from chapter 14)

Nursing diagnosis

High-risk for fluid volume deficit related to deviations affecting intake of fluids.

Assessment: Holding back fluid intake to avoid need to void which is frequent, painful, and burns, temperature elevation.

(Refer Table 14.11 from chapter 14)

B. Specific Nursing Diagnoses and Nursing Process

Nursing diagnosis

Knowledge deficit of parent(s) and child related to lack of information about disease (Table 15.19).

Assessment: Expressed need for information about disease, causes, prevention and treatment.

Evaluation
- Verbalizes signs, and symptoms of UTI
- Minimizes recurrent UTI by carrying out preventive measures
- Urinary culture negative for infectious organisms following treatment
- Complies appropriately with administration of anti-infective therapy
- Collects mid-stream urine specimen and takes to laboratory when signs and symptoms of urinary infection are present
- Complies with follow-up care requirements

Table 15.19: Nursing interventions for knowledge deficit of parent(s) and child.

Interventions	Rationales
Assess knowledge of signs and symptoms of urinary tract infection, previous infections, age and gender of child, past treatments for UTI, pressure of anatomic defects affecting renal/urinary system	Provides information needed to develop plan of instruction to ensure compliance of medical regimen; UTI commonly occur in females and are prone to recurrent episodes; vesicoureteral reflux predisposes to UTI

- Prevents spread of infection to upper urinary tract
- Absence of constipation causing bladder neck obstruction and urinary stasis.

Vesicoureteral Reflux

Vesicoureteral reflux is characterized by the retrograde flow of urine into the ureters from the bladder as a result of a congenital defect or infection. The degree of reflux is graded from the effect on the lower ureter to the involvement of the upper urinary tract and ureteral structures causing distention and renal scarring. The disorder is most common in children under 5 years of age before growth changes the shape of the kidney structures and angle of entry into the collecting ducts which prevents reflux into the renal structures. The disorder commonly resolves itself if the degree of reflux is not too severe by vigilant monitoring and treatment of infection; or surgical repair (ureteral reimplantation) if reflux is severe or medical compliance with regimen is not successful **(Flowchart 15.4)**.

Signs and Symptoms of Urinary Reflux

- Urinary reflux does not cause any symptoms in affected babies or children.
- The most common sign of urinary reflux is a UTI (urinary tract infection).
- If child has urinary reflux, it is important to watch out for the signs of a UTI.
- Dilated (widened) urinary tract detected on ultrasound scan; this can sometimes be diagnosed before a baby is born when the mother has an ultrasound scan in pregnancy.

Evaluation: Urinary tract infection

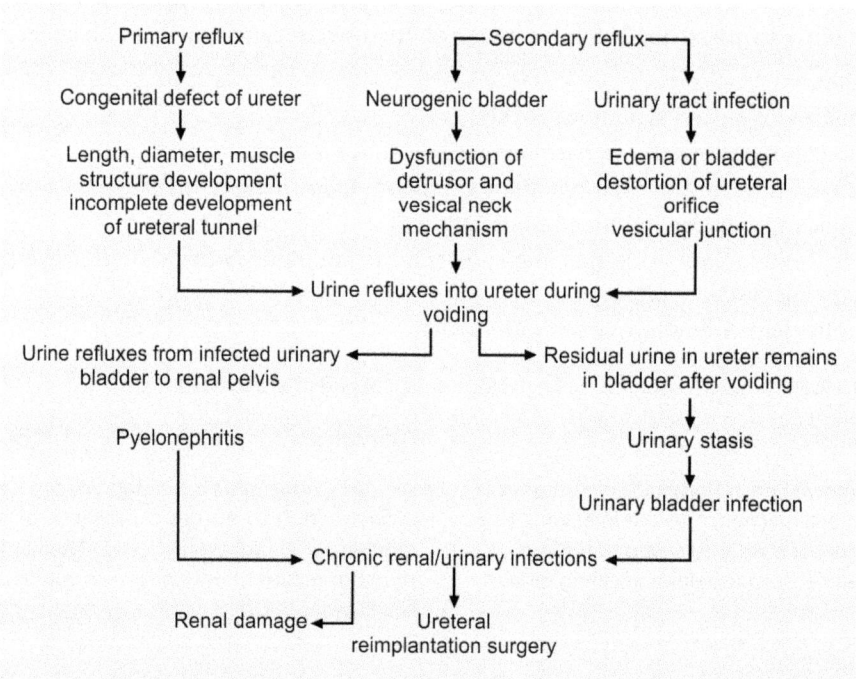

Flowchart 15.4: Pathophysiology of vesicoureteral reflex.

Nursing Management

A. Essential Nursing Diagnoses and Nursing Process Associated with this Condition

Nursing diagnosis

High-risk for fluid volume deficit related to loss of fluid through abnormal routes, deviations affecting intake of fluid.

Assessment: NPO status pre and postoperatively, urinary catheter (Foley or suprapubic), dry skin and mucous membranes, poor skin turgor, decreased urinary output via catheter or stents, temperature elevation.

(Refer Table 14.11 from chapter 14)

Nursing diagnosis

High-risk for impaired skin integrity related to external factor of surgical incision.

Assessment: Disruption of skin surface, catheter site irritation and discomfort.

(Refer Table 12.1 from chapter 12)

Nursing diagnosis

Hyperthermia related to illness (presence of infection).

Assessment: Increase in body temperature above normal range, evidence of infection at surgical or catheter site, or renal/urinary infection.

(Refer Table 14.18 from chapter 14)

B. Specific Nursing Diagnoses and Nursing Process

Nursing diagnosis

Knowledge deficit related to lack of exposure to information about disorder **(Table 15.20)**.

Assessment: Expressed need for information about continuous medical regimen to control renal/bladder infection and measures to prevent infection.

Table 15.20: Nursing interventions for knowledge deficit.

Interventions	Rationales
Instruct parent(s) and child in antibacterial administration including information on action, dose, form, time, frequency, how to take, side effects to report	Promotes compliance with the medication regimen for long-term therapy to prevent recurrent or relapse of urinary infection
Instruct parent(s) and child to develop strategies for administration of medications	Assists to ensure compliance to prescribed regimen
Instruct parent(s) and child to write a contact with an agreement on rules and rewards included for following medical regimen	Promotes compliance and independence and prevent constant reminding by parent to take medication
Inform and instruct parent(s) and child of need to obtain urine cultures by mid-stream and taking to a laboratory or use of dip slide or strip to use at home	Reveals presence of urinary infection and assists to regulate antibacterial therapy

Table 15.21: Nursing interventions for anxiety of parent(s) and child.

Interventions	Rationales
Assess source and level of anxiety and need for information and interventions that will relieve it	Provides information about anxiety level and need to relieve it; source for parent include the procedure and care of child pre and postoperatively source for child includes separation from parent(s), unfamiliar environment, and painful procedures
Allow expression of concerns and time to ask questions about need of surgery, procedure to be done, procedures to prepare for surgery, procedures, care and recovery after surgery	Provides opportunity to vent feelings and fears and to feel secure in the environment
Answer questions calmly and honestly, use pictures, drawings, models and therapeutic play	Promotes trust and a calm and supportive environment
Encourage and allow parent(s) to stay with child and assist in care	Allows parent(s) to care for and support child and continue parental role and increases child's comfort by having a familiar caretaker
Allow as much input into decisions about care and usual routines as possible by parent(s)	Allows for more control over situations and maintains a familiar routine for care
Orient and introduce child to the surgical unit preoperatively	Reduces anxiety caused by fear of the unknown

Evaluation
- Complies with medication regimen
- Complies with urine testing for infectious process
- Absence of recurrent urinary infection.

Nursing diagnosis

Anxiety of parent(s) and child related to change in health status, change in environment (hospitalization for surgery) **(Table 15.21)**.

Assessment: Expressed apprehension and concern about surgery (ureteral reimplantation) and pre and postoperative procedures and care.

Evaluation
- Verbalizes reduction in anxiety about pre and postoperative procedures and care
- Verbalizes positive effects of surgical procedure
- Participates in care and support of child before and after surgery
- Verbalizes what to expect when child returns from surgery.

Nursing diagnosis

Pain related to physical injuring agent (surgery) **(Table 15.22)**.

Assessment: Communication of pain descriptors, crying, irritability, restlessness, withdrawal, flank pain, ureteral edema from surgery, bladder spasms.

Table 15.22: Nursing interventions for pain.

Interventions	Rationales
Assess verbal and nonverbal behavior, type and location and severity of pain depending on age	Provides information about pain as a basis for analgesic therapy
Administer analgesic and possibly sedative based on pain assessment and before pain becomes severe	Reduces pain and promotes rest to reduce stimuli and restlessness
Place in a comfortable position; avoid unnecessary movement or manipulation of suprapubic catheter	Promotes comfort and decreases bladder spasms that cause pain
Administer antispasmodic PO or suppository as ordered	Reduces bladder spasms caused by irritation of suprapubic catheter
Maintain catheter patency by ensuring placement, checking flow and presence of kinks or obstruction	Reduces pain caused by distention as a result of catheter clogging or displacement
Provide distractions and reassurance when spasms occur and stay with child when they occur to inform the child that the pain is temporary	Reduces anxiety which tends to increase pain

Evaluation
- Absence or control of pain
- Administers medications to control pain or factors that predispose to pain
- Controls pain provoking actions when giving care.

Nursing diagnosis
High-risk for infection related to inadequate primary defenses (surgical incision), invasive procedure (catheter) **(Table 15.23)**.

Assessment: Redness, swelling, drainage at incision or catheter site, cloudy, foul smelling urine positive wound culture, temperature elevation.

Evaluation
- Absence of urinary tract infection
- Absence of wound infection with healing in progress
- Complies with preventive measures and anti-infective therapy
- Maintains sterile technique in procedures and catheter patency.

Nursing diagnosis
High-risk for injury related to external physical factor of catheter displacement; internal factor of complications of surgical trauma **(Table 15.24)**.

Assessment: Catheter obstruction, postoperative bleeding catheter dislodgement, bladder distention, reduce urine output, dysuria, frequency, retention following removal of catheter.

Evaluation
- Maintains placement and patency of catheters
- Urinary output of 1 mL/kg/h
- Return of urinary elimination pattern and adequate amount after removal of catheters

Table 15.23: Nursing interventions for high-risk for infection.

Interventions	Rationales
Assess wound for redness, swelling, purulent drainage on dressing, healing	Indicates presence of infectious process or poor healing
Assess catheter site for redness, edema, irritation; urine collected in drainage system for cloudiness and foul odor	Indicates infectious process at catheter site or in urinary bladder
Collect urine for culture and sensitivities	Reveals presence of urinary infection and sensitivity to specific antibacterial agent
Administer antibacterial as ordered	Treats specific microorganism or prevents infection when catheter is in place
Encourage increased fluid intake daily depending on age requirements when PO fluids are allowed	Promotes dilution of urine to prevent infection and encourage voiding after catheter is removed
Use sterile technique when changing dressing, giving catheter care or emptying drainage bag	Prevents contamination of wound or urinary tract by the introduction of pathogens
Maintain catheter and collection bag below level of bladder and maintain a closed, patent system free of kinks or obstructions	Prevents backflow of urine into bladder or retention of urine which predisposes to infection
Provide suprapubic catheter care by cleansing with peroxide solution after removing any meatal crusting, catheter care by washing perineum with mild soap and water, rinsing and applying antiseptic ointment	Promotes comfort and prevent infection at suprapubic or meatal site
Change dressings when soiled or wet 24 hours after surgery	Promotes comfort and allows for wound assessment

(PO: per os or by mouth)

- Prevents and reports risk of complications
- Absence of signs and symptoms of urinary retention or dysfunction.

Wilms Tumor

Wilms tumor is an encapsulated malignant tumor of the kidney. It may be associated with other congenital anomalies of the heart and genitalia/testes. It may be inherited or noninherited. Tumor originates in the renal parenchyma and extends into the surrounding areas with metastasis occurring via the blood stream to the lungs, liver and bone or via the lymphatic system to the retroperitoneal lymph nodes. Staging of the tumor determines prognosis and treatment protocols and is achieved by diagnostic testing, biopsy, or surgical removal and histology. It is most common in children 3 years of age. Histology classifies the tumor into favorable or unfavorable histology with unfavorable associated with a poorer prognosis and more extensive therapy. Clinical stage and histology form the basis for radiation therapy and chemotherapy although postoperative radiotherapy is indicated for those in all stages (except for stage 1) and chemotherapy is indicated for all stages **(Flowchart 15.5)**.

Nursing Process for the Child with Renal Disorder

Table 15.24: Nursing interventions for high-risk for injury related to external physical factor of catheter displacement, internal factor of complications of surgical trauma.

Interventions	Rationales
Assess output via catheter and note characteristics of urine, passage of blood clots, color of urine and return to clear color; and if clots or return to red color occurs after a period of normal characteristics	Provides information about possible complication of bleeding or obstruction
Notify physician immediately, if red color returns	Allows for immediate interventions to treat hemorrhage
Immobilize arms and legs with restraints, remove periodically; use bed cradle following surgery	Prevents accidental dislodgement or removal of catheter.
Secure catheter to abdomen or leg with tape, stents to catheter and avoid placing tension on the catheter when in place by gently holding it when performing care	Prevents movement or manipulation of catheter that may cause displacement
If catheter becomes displaced, notify physician for replacement (have a suprapubic catheter on hand at all times)	Ensures continued drainage of urine
Measure 1:0 qh for an output of 1 mL/kg/h and notify physician if less	Provides information to ensure adequate output via catheters
Note first voiding after catheter removed, time of voiding and amount, difficulty, presence of abdominal distention	Provides information about return of urinary pattern, presence of retention
Support during first voiding (warm water over perineum, sitting or standing position) and privacy	Prevents embarrassment and promotes voiding
Encourage increase in fluid intake according to age requirements	Promotes voiding

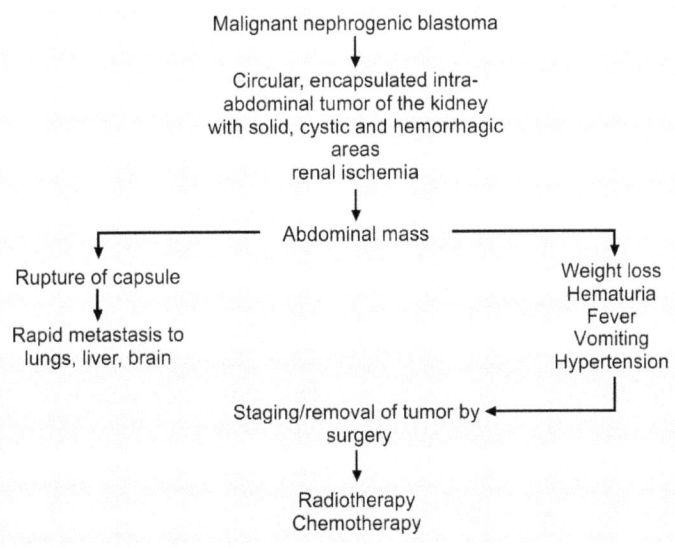

Flowchart 15.5: Pathophysiology of Wilms tumor.

Malignant nephrogenic blastoma
↓
Circular, encapsulated intra-abdominal tumor of the kidney with solid, cystic and hemorrhagic areas
renal ischemia
↓
Abdominal mass

Rupture of capsule
↓
Rapid metastasis to lungs, liver, brain

Weight loss
Hematuria
Fever
Vomiting
Hypertension

Staging/removal of tumor by surgery
↓
Radiotherapy
Chemotherapy

Signs and Symptoms of Wilms Tumor
- Wilms tumors can be hard to find early because they can often grow quite large without causing any symptoms.
- Children may look healthy and play normally.
- Swelling or a hard mass in the abdomen (belly): This is often the first sign of a Wilms tumor.
- It feels firm and is often large enough to be felt on both sides of the belly. It's usually not painful, but it might cause belly pain in some cases.

Other possible symptoms: Some children with Wilms tumor may also have:
- Fever
- Nausea
- Loss of appetite
- Shortness of breath
- Constipation
- Blood in the urine
- Sometimes cause high blood pressure.

Nursing Management

A. Essential Nursing Diagnoses and Nursing Process Associated with this Condition

Nursing diagnosis

Altered nutrition: Less than body requirements related to inability to ingest and digest food.

Assessment: Anorexia, nausea and vomiting from chemotherapy, obstruction postoperatively from chemotherapy causing a dynamic ileus.

(Refer Table 14.3 from chapter 14)

Nursing diagnosis

High-risk for fluid volume deficit related to altered intake, excessive losses through normal routes.

Assessment: Diarrhea, vomiting from radiation, chemotherapy, NPO preoperatively.

(Refer Table 14.11 from chapter 14)

Nursing diagnosis

Diarrhea related to radiation, chemotherapy postoperatively.

Assessment: Increased frequency of bowel sounds and loose, liquid stools.

(Refer Table 13.8 from chapter 13)

Nursing diagnosis

Constipation related to gastrointestinal obstructive lesions postoperatively.

Assessment: Adynamic ileus, decreased bowel sounds, abdominal distention, frequency less than usual pattern.

(Refer Table 12.9 from chapter 12)

Nursing Process for the Child with Renal Disorder

Table 15.25: Nursing intervention for anxiety of parent(s) and child.

Interventions	Rationales
Assess source and level of anxiety and need for information and support that will relieve it	Provides information about degree of anxiety and need for interventions and support; sources for parent(s) may be guilt and uncertainty about surgery, treatments and recovery, possible loss of child; sources for the child may be the multiple procedures of diagnosis and surgery and the effects of postoperative treatments
Allow expression of concerns and inquiries about disease and possible consequences of surgery and prognosis	Provides opportunity to vent feelings, secure information needed to reduce anxiety
Allow parent(s) to stay with the child	Promotes care and support of child by parent(s)
Orient child to the surgical and ICU unit, equipment, noises and staff	Reduces anxiety caused by fear of unknown

(ICU: intensive care unit)

Nursing diagnosis

High-risk for impaired skin integrity related to external factors of radiation. IV chemotherapy, excretions and secretions.

Assessment: Disruption of skin surfaces, destruction of skin layers, redness and excoriation of perianal area from diarrhea, extravasation of chemotherapy (swelling, pain, redness, tissue necrosis).

(Refer Table 12.1 from chapter 12)

B. Specific Nursing Diagnoses and Nursing Process

Nursing diagnosis

Anxiety of parent(s) and child related to change in health status, threat of death, threat to self-concept **(Table 15.25)**.

Assessment: Increased apprehension and fear of diagnosis, expressed concern and worry about preoperative procedures and preparation, postoperative care and effects of therapy, possible metastasis of disease.

Evaluation
- Expresses reduction in anxiety as information and explanation are given
- Participates in care and support of child
- Asks questions, clarifies information about procedures and care before and after surgery
- Reveals concern and vents feelings about seriousness of the disease and postoperative medical regimen and effects
- Expresses positive effects of surgery and major benefits of therapy
- Verbalizes effects of therapy on self-concept and physical well-being.

Nursing diagnosis

High-risk for injury related to internal biochemical factors of regulatory function, abnormal blood profile; internal physical factor of broken skin **(Table 15.26)**.

Nursing Process for the Child with Renal Disorder

Table 15.26: Nursing interventions for anxiety of parent(s) and child.

Interventions	Rationales
Assess blood pressure for increases pre and postoperatively q2h, changes in pulse and respirations	Provides information about vital signs caused by renal function abnormality preoperatively or by nephrectomy postoperatively, postoperative atelectasis
Avoid any palpation of abdominal mass; post sign on bed stating not to palpate preoperatively	Prevents trauma to tumor site and possible metastasis by dissemination of cancer cells
Assess bowel activity postoperatively for elimination pattern, bowel sounds, bowel distention	Provides information about possible adynamic ileus form chemotherapy causing bowel obstruction
Assess incisional site for redness, swelling, drainage, intactness and healing and change dressing when soiled or wet; assess oral and perineal area for stomatitis or skin breakdown or inflammation and provide oral care and anal care after elimination; provide postoperative pulmonary	Indicates infectious process resulting from invasive procedure or inflammation resulting from immunosuppressive therapy
Assess urinary output for presence of cloudy, foul smelling urine; collect specimen for culture analysis and report any change in renal function (hypertension, headache, irritability, weight gain, behavior changes)	Indicates possible renal impairment and/or urinary bladder infection; renal involvement alters rennin excretion which increases BP and immunosuppressive therapy leads to infection

Assessment: Hypertension, leucopenia, thrombocytopenia, decreased Hb, rupture of tumor, reduced urinary output, infectious process of urinary bladder, surgical incision, lungs, oral cavity, intestinal obstruction.

Evaluation
- Absence or resolution of signs and symptoms of pre or postoperative complications; monitors for potential complications
- Maintains safe environment with absence of infection or injury
- Verbalization of type of complications and risks associated with care and treatments preoperatively and radiation/chemotherapy postoperatively.

Nursing diagnosis

Altered oral mucous membrane related to medication (chemotherapy) **(Table 15.27)**.

Assessment: Stomatitis, oral ulcers, hyperemia, oral pain or discomfort, oral plaque.

Evaluation
- Oral mucous membranes intact and reduced inflammation
- Complies with measures to prevent trauma or breakdown of mucosa
- Controls discomfort associated with impaired oral mucosa
- Progressive return to oral mucous membranes baseline following chemotherapy protocol.

Nursing Process for the Child with Renal Disorder

Table 15.27: Nursing intervention for altered mucous membrane.

Interventions	Rationales
Assess oral cavity for pain, ulcers, lesions, gingivitis, mucositis or stomatitis and effect on ability to ingest food and fluids	Provides information about effect of chemotherapy
Provide mouth rinses, cleansing with swabs or soft toothbrush	Provides mouth care without irritating oral mucosa
Administer medication topically (xylocaine) before meals and offer bland, smooth foods that are not hot or spicy	Permits eating with more comfort
Administer an antiseptic mouth rinse (nystatin) 30 minutes before any food or fluid intake	Promotes comfort of oral mucosa and maintains integrity

Table 15.28: Nursing interventions for altered protection.

Interventions	Rationales
Assess for bleeding from any site, WBC, platelet count, HCT, absolute neutrophil, count and febrile episodes	Provides information about frank bleeding or blood profile abnormalities that predispose to bleeding caused by bone marrow suppression and immunosuppression resulting from chemotherapy
Administer blood transfusion as ordered for severe blood loss and monitor patency, vital signs, chills, fever, urticaria, rash, dyspnea, diaphoresis, headache throughout transfusion and terminate if any of these changes occur	Replaces blood loss when symptoms of anemia appear (dizziness, pallor, fatigue, increased pulse and respirations) or when HCT is <20% or platelet count <20,000/cu mm
Pad sides of bed, avoid trauma with use of hard toothbrush or dental floss, apply pressure for 5 minutes after IV administration, discontinue taking rectal temperatures or performing unnecessary invasive procedures	Prevents bleeding caused by trauma during chemotherapy administration which alters platelets and clotting factor
Carry out handwashing technique before giving care, use mask and gown when appropriate, provide a private room, monitor for any signs and symptoms of infection	Prevents transmission of pathogens to a compromised immune system during chemotherapy if the absolute neutrophil count is <1000/cu mm

(HCT: hematocrit; WBC: white blood cell)

Nursing diagnosis

Altered protection related to drug therapy (antineoplastics): abnormal blood profile (leukopenia, thrombocytopenia, anemia, coagulation); treatments (radiation) **(Table 15.28)**.

Assessment: Altered clotting, bone marrow suppression, deficient immunity against infection, hematoma, petechiae, bleeding from nose, gums, hematemesis, blood in stool.

Evaluation
- Absence of excessive bleeding or infection during chemotherapy or radiation
- Complies with measures to prevent bleeding and infection based on blood profile

Nursing Process for the Child with Renal Disorder

- Reports signs and symptoms of complications to physician
- Complies with laboratory blood testing and follow-up visits to physician.

PRACTICE QUESTIONS

1. Write the nursing management of a child with nephritic syndrome.
2. Master Monish 1-year-age admitted in pediatric surgical ward for the corrective surgery of hypospadiasis. Write pre and postoperative management of the child by applying nursing process.

CHAPTER 16

Nursing Process for the Child with a Neoplastic Disorder

LEARNING OBJECTIVES
- To identify the signs and symptoms of a child with neoplastic disorder.
- To frame nursing diagnosis based on the needs of the child.
- To plan nursing interventions and outcome identification.

NURSING PROCESS FOR THE CHILD WITH A NEOPLASTIC DISORDER

1. **Nursing diagnosis:** Risk for infection related to neutropenia and immuno-suppression.
   Goal: Child will be free from infection.
   Interventions: Preventing infection.
   - Assess for fever, pain, cough, tachypnea, adventitious breath sounds, skin ulceration, stomatitis and perirectal fissures to identify potential infection
   - Administer antibiotics for temperature >38.4°C to decrease like-hood of over-whelming sepsis
   - Maintain meticulous hand washing procedures (include family, visitors, staff) to minimize spread of infectious organisms
   - Maintain isolation as prescribed to minimize exposure to infectious organisms
   - Avoid rectal temperatures and examinations, intramuscular injections, and urinary catheterization when child is neutropenic to decrease possibility of introducing microorganisms
   - Educate family and visitors that child should be restricted from contact with known infectious exposures (in hospital and at home) to encourage cooperation with infection control
   - Strictly observe medical asepsis to avoid unintentional introduction of microorganisms
   - Promote nutrition and appropriate rest to maximize body's potential to heal
   - Inform family to contact provider if child has known exposure to chickenpox or measles, so that preventive measures can be taken
   - Administer vaccines as prescribed to prevent common childhood communicable diseases
   - Teach family to monitor for fever at home and report temperature elevations to oncologist immediately, so that antibiotic therapy may be instituted as soon as possible.

   Evaluation: Child not experienced over-whelming infection or able to recover if becomes infected.

2. **Nursing diagnosis:** Pain related to invasive diagnostic testing, surgical procedure, neuropathy, disease progression or adverse effects of treatment as evidenced by verbalization of pain, elevated pain scale ratings, guarding, withdrawal from play or refusal to participate in activities of daily living or physiologic indicators such as elevated heart rate, diaphoresis, muscle tension or rigidity.

Goal: Child will be able to demonstrate pain relief.
Intervention: Promoting comfort.
- Determine level of pain using child interview, pain scale and assessment of physiologic variables to determine baseline
- Document location, intensity, description of pain to determine baseline
- Discuss with the child and parent techniques that have helped alleviate pain in the past to incorporate successful interventions into the plan of care
- Administer acetaminophen for mild pain (avoid salicylate and non-steroidal anti-inflammatory drugs due to increased risk for bleeding)
- Administer medications as ordered using the least invasive method possible to avoid pain (intramuscular, subcutaneous and rectal route should be avoided in the child with thrombocytopenia)
- Monitor frequently for adverse effects (particularly respiratory effects) of opioid analgesics, as opioids reduce responsiveness of carbon dioxide receptors in the brain's respiratory center
- Use nonpharmacologic measures such as play therapy, games, TV, guided breathing, imagery, hypnosis, or meditation as appropriate (distracts child's attention from the pain)
- Use massage, positioning, or heat to relieve pain in a particular area
- Use EMLA before needle sticks and conscious sedation with lumbar puncture and bone marrow aspiration to reduce recurrent acute painful episodes associated with frequent blood draws and diagnostic/treatment procedures
- Have the child lie flat for 30 minutes after a lumbar puncture and increase fluid intake for 24 hours after the procedure to decrease incidence of head ache.

Evaluation: Child participates in play, activities of daily living or therapeutic interventions.

3. **Nursing diagnosis:** Impaired oral mucous membranes related to chemotherapy, radiation therapy, immune-compromise, decreased platelet count, malnutrition or dehydration as evidenced by oral lesions, ulcers, plaques, hyperemia or bleeding, difficulty eating or swallowing or complaint of oral discomfort.
Goal: Child will be able to maintain intact, moist mucosa.
Interventions: Restoring healthy oral mucosa.
- Frequently assess oral cavity for redness, lesions, ulcers, plaques or bleeding to provide baseline for comparison and identify alterations early
- Offer ice chips frequently while nil per orals (NPO) to maintain hydration of mucosa
- Use only a soft toothbrush or toothette for dental care, avoiding excessive pressure with brushing, to decrease incidence of bleeding with mouth care
- Keep lips lubricated with petroleum jelly or fragrance free lip balm to maintain moist, hydrated lips
- Rinse with salt solution or mouth wash every 1-2 hours to keep oral cavity clean and moist
- Administer glutamine and/or carotene supplements, which have been shown to decrease the incidence and severity of mucositis
- Have child swish and spit 1:1 Benadryl/Maalox solution to decrease pain
- Administer antifungal solution to prevent or treat oral candidiasis
- Avoid spicy, acidic or very hot or very cold foods to decrease pain
- Administer pain medication (usually acetaminophen or codeine) as ordered to decrease pain.

Evaluation: Child is free from redness, ulceration or debris.

4. **Nursing diagnosis:** Nausea related to adverse effects of chemotherapy or radiation therapy as evidenced by verbalization of nausea, increased salivation, swallowing movements or vomiting.
   Goal: Child will be able to experience decreased nausea.
   Interventions: Alleviating nausea and vomiting.
   - Administer antiemetics prior to chemotherapy and as needed thereafter to decrease frequency of nausea
   - Assess frequency of vomiting and level of hydration to provide baseline data and recognize alterations early
   - Offer frequent, smaller meals or snacks; smaller amounts are less likely to be vomited
   - Avoid spicy foods to avoid stomach upset
   - Allow bubbles to dissipate from carbonated beverages before they are ingested (carbonation may contribute to nausea)
   - Remove cover from meal tray before entering child's room (this will allow the food odor to dissipate outside of the room; food odors may trigger nausea and vomiting).

   Evaluation: Child verbalizes symptom relief and free from vomiting.

5. **Nursing diagnosis: Imbalanced nutrition:** Less than body requirements related to anorexia, nausea, vomiting or mucosal irritation associated with chemotherapy or radiation as evidenced by decreased oral intake and weight, length/height, and/or BMI below average for age or individual child's usual measures.
   Goal: Child will be able to improve nutritional intake.
   Interventions: Promoting adequate nutrition.
   - Determine body weight and length/height normal for age or find out what the child's pretreatment measurements were to determine goal to work toward
   - Determine child's food preferences and provide favorite foods as able to increase the likelihood that the child will consume adequate amounts of foods
   - Administer antiemetics as ordered to increase the likelihood that the child will retain the food he or she ingests
   - Weigh child daily or weekly (according to physician order or institutional standard) and measure length/height weekly to monitor for growth
   - Offer highest-calorie meals at the time of day when the child's appetite is the greatest (to increase likelihood of increased caloric intake)
   - Provide increased-calorie shakes or puddings within diet restriction (high-calorie foods increase weight gain)
   - Administer vitamin and mineral supplements as prescribed to attain/maintain vitamin and mineral balance in the body
   - Administer total parenteral nutrition and intravenous lipids as ordered to provide adequate nutrition for healing.

   Evaluation: Child improved weight steadily.

6. **Nursing diagnosis:** Constipation related to effects of vinca alkaloids, opioid use, decreased activity and dietary changes as evidenced by hard stool or stool, i.e., difficult to pass.
   Goal: Child's bowel function will return to usual pattern.
   Interventions: Preventing or managing constipation
   - Ensure that child increases fluid intake to provide enough water in the intestines for soft stool formation

- Increase fiber in the diet to provide bulk for stool formation
- Administer stool softeners such as mineral oil, docusate sodium; these help soften the stool, aiding in passage
- Provide motivator laxatives such as magnesium hydroxide, lactulose or sorbitol to stimulate stool passage
- Use stimulant laxatives such as senna or bisacodyl only intermittently rather than on a daily basis to avoid dependency and diarrhea.

Evaluation: Child will pass a formed, soft stool every day.

7. **Nursing diagnosis:** Diarrhea related to effects of radiation therapy as evidenced by loose or watery stools, possibly frequent.
Goal: Child's bowel function will return to usual pattern.
Interventions: Managing diarrhea.
- Assess frequency of diarrhea and level of hydration to provide data about severity
- Obtain weight daily on same scale to determine extent of fluid loss
- Maintain accurate intake and output records to determine extent of fluid loss
- Administer oral rehydration solutions or intravenous fluids as ordered to maintain or restore adequate hydration
- Restrict roughage and residue in diet to decrease likelihood of diarrhea
- Avoid milk products during acute diarrheal phase (lactose often worsens diarrhea)
- Provide an elemental diet to relieve symptoms (absorbed in the upper small bowel)
- Provide meticulous perineal care to avoid skin breakdown related to frequent of loose stools
- Administer antidiarrheal medications if ordered to decrease frequency of stools
- If severe and related to radiation therapy, may require a 3-4 days rest period from radiation to begin recovery of normal absorptive capabilities of bowel.

Evaluation: Child passed a formed, soft stool daily (or modify this criterion according to child's usual pattern).

8. **Nursing diagnosis:** Risk for impaired skin integrity related to radiation therapy.
Goal: Child's skin will be able to remain intact.
Interventions: Promoting skin integrity.
- Assess skin frequently for erythema, erosions, ulcers, or blisters to provide baseline data and intervene early if skin is impaired
- Use a mild soap for cleansing and pat dry rather than rubbing to avoid skin irritation
- Use Aloe vera lotion to moisturize the skin
- Avoid perfumed lotions, soaps, heat, cold or sun, as these will further irritate the skin in the irradiated area
- Do not scrub ink from marked radiation field, and avoid adhesive tape in that area, to avoid further skin irritation
- Administer diphenhydramine or apply hydrocortisone 1% cream to reduce itching and urge to scratch
- For areas of desquamation related to radiation, apply Silvadene cream once or twice a day to hasten skin repair

Evaluation: Areas of redness in radiation fields will not progress to desquamation.

9. **Nursing diagnosis:** Activity intolerance related to treatment adverse effects, anemia or generalized weakness as evidenced by verbalization of weakness or fatigue, elevation of

heart rate, respiratory rate or blood pressure with activity, complaint of shortness of breath with play or activity.
Goal: Child will be able to display increased activity tolerance.
Interventions: Promoting skin integrity.
- Encourage activity or ambulation per physician's orders; early mobilization results in better outcomes
- Observe child for symptoms of activity intolerance such as pallor, nausea, light headedness or dizziness, or changes in vital signs to determine level of tolerance
- If child is on bed rest, perform range-of-motion exercises and frequent position changes: negative changes to the musculoskeletal system occur quickly with inactivity and immobility
- Cluster nursing care activities and plan for periods of rest before and after exertion to decrease oxygen need and consumption
- Refer the child to physical therapy for exercise prescription to increase skeletal muscle strength.

Evaluation: Child desires to play without developing symptoms of exertion.

10. **Nursing diagnosis:** Disturbed body image related to hair loss as evidenced by verbalization of dissatisfaction with appearance.
    Goal: Child or adolescent will be able to display appropriate body image.
    Interventions: Promoting body image.
    - Acknowledge child's feelings of anger over body changes and illness; venting feedings is associated with less body image disturbance
    - Encourage the child or teen to choose a wig or hats and scarves to involve the child in making decisions about appearance
    - Support the child's or teen's choices of comfortable, fashionable clothing to disguise weight loss or scarring while promoting self-esteem
    - Involve the child in the decision-making process, as a sense of control will improve body image
    - Encourage the child to spend time with peers who have experienced hair, limb, or weight loss, as peers' opinions are often better accepted than those of persons in authority, such as parents or healthcare professionals.

    Evaluation: Child looks at self in mirror and participates in social activities.

11. **Nursing diagnosis:** Risk for situational low self-esteem related to loss of control and inability to progress with quest for independence (adolescents).
    Goal: Adolescent will be able to maintain or increase self-esteem.
    Interventions: Promoting self-esteem.
    - Identify the adolescent's positive abilities to promote self-esteem
    - Give genuine and honest positive feedback, as the child or adolescent desires honesty
    - Explore strengths and weaknesses with the adolescent: helps the teen to see similarities and differences with healthy peers of the same age
    - Encourage the teen to perform self-care as possible to promote independence
    - Offer emotional support (reduces psychological distress and increases coping abilities)
    - Encourage participation in a support group to allow teens to discuss body changes and the reactions they perceive in others

- When the adolescent is physically able, encourage attendance at camp or an adventure/wilderness event (these programs have been shown to improve mental health and coping skills).

Evaluation: Adolescent will display increased coping responses and verbalize control as appropriate as well as discuss plans for future.

12. **Nursing diagnosis:** Compromised family coping related to potentially life-threatening illness and stressors involved with cancer treatment.

    Goal: Child and/or family will be able to demonstrate adequate coping skills.

    Interventions: Promoting child and family coping.
    - Provide emotional support to child and family (improves coping abilities)
    - Actively listen to the child's and family concerns (validates their feelings, establishes trust)
    - Provide open communication with the child and sibling; children appreciate honesty about their illness and coping is improved
    - Refer families to community resources such as parent support groups and grief counseling (such support improves coping abilities)
    - Give terminally ill children the permission to discuss their feelings about their illness, allowing them to conquer fears and express love for their family and friends
    - Encourage families to be honest with siblings about the treatment and prognosis of the child with cancer (children often sense what is going on and cope better when they are prepared and are given an honest explanation of events)
    - Prepare siblings for the death of the child with cancer, using the child life specialist and chaplain as necessary: the bereavement period is eased when siblings are prepared.

    Evaluation: Child and family verbalize feeling supported and demonstrate healthy family interactions.

13. **Nursing diagnosis:** Anticipatory grieving (family) related to diagnosis of cancer in a child and impending loss of child as evidenced by crying, disbelief of diagnosis and expressions of grief.

    Goal: Family will be able to express feelings of grief.

    Interventions: Supporting the grieving family.
    - Use therapeutic communication with open-ended questions to encourage an open and trusting relationship for better communication
    - Actively listen to family's expression of grief; just being present and listening conveys support
    - Encourage the family to cry and express feelings away from the child to work through feelings while not upsetting the child
    - Assess for spiritual distress and refer the family to the hospital chaplain or clergy of choice for support
    - Educate the family about the child's condition honestly: knowing what is going on, what is to be expected, and what the treatment plan is gives the family a sense of control
    - Support the family through discussions with the child about anticipated death when the illness is deemed terminal.

    Evaluation: Family seeking help in dealing with feelings.

PRACTICE QUESTIONS

1. Write nursing care plan for a child diagnosed with leukemia by applying nursing process.
2. A 3-year toddler got admitted in the pediatric ICU for bone marrow transplantation. Draw a nursing care plan for the child by applying nursing process.

CHAPTER 17

Nursing Process for the Child with Communicable Diseases

LEARNING OBJECTIVES
- To identify the signs and symptoms of a child with communicable diseases.
- To frame nursing diagnosis based on the needs of the child.
- To plan nursing interventions and outcome identification.

NURSING PROCESS FOR THE CHILD WITH COMMUNICABLE DISEASES

1. **Nursing diagnosis: Altered body temperature:** Fever related to infectious disease process as evidenced by rectal temperature more than 38°C or 100.4°F.
   Goal: Child will be able to maintain temperature with adaptive levels and will be comfortable and remain hydrated.
   Interventions: Managing fever.
   - Assess temperature at least every 4–6 hours, 30–60 minutes after antipyretic is given and with any change in condition; recognizing the pattern of fever may help identify source
   - Use same site and device for temperature measurement to reflect a more accurate trend in temperature, since different sites can result in significant difference in temperature reading
   - Administer antipyretics per physician order when the child is experiencing discomfort or cannot keep up with the metabolic demands of the fever. Fever is a protective response of the body to fight infection. Antipyretics provide symptomatic relief but do not change the course of the infection. The major benefits to decreasing fever are increasing comfort in the child and decreasing fluid requirements, helping to prevent dehydration.
   - Notify physician of temperature per institution or specific order guidelines; increases in temperature may indicate worsening infection and relevant changes in condition.
   - Assess fluid intake and encourage oral intake or administer intravenous fluids per physician order; increased metabolic rate and diaphoresis related to fever can cause fluid loss and lead to fluid volume deficit.
   - Keep linens and clothing clean and dry; diaphoresis can leave clothing and linen soaked and increases discomfort for the child.
   - Use of nonpharmacologic measures such as tepid bath and removal of clothing and blankets is controversial. If used, discontinue if shivering begins.
   Evaluation: Child verbalizes or exhibits signs of comfort during febrile episode; child demonstrates adequate signs of hydration.
2. **Nursing diagnosis:** Impaired comfort related to infectious and/or inflammatory process as evidenced by hyperthermia, pruritis, rash or skin lesions, sore throat or joint pain.
   Goal: Pain or discomfort will be reduced to level acceptable to child.
   Interventions: Improving comfort.

- Assess pain and response to interventions frequently with use of pain scales or other pain measurement tools; provides baseline of pain and allows for evaluation of effectiveness of interventions
- Administer analgesics and antipruritics as ordered to relieve pain via interruption of CNS pathways and to decrease discomfort related to itching
- Apply cold compresses to areas of pruritus or provide a cool bath to decrease inflammation and soothe pruritus
- Keep child's fingernails short (use mitts, gloves or socks over hands if necessary); short fingernails can help prevent injury to the skin, which leads to increased pain
- Encourage child to press on rather than scratch the area of pruritus; pressing on the area that itches can help soothe the itching and prevent scratching, which can lead to injury to the skin
- Provide frequent fluids and offer warm fluids such as soup or cold foods such as popsicles to help ease the discomfort of a sore throat
- Provide cool mist humidification to help ease the discomfort of a sore throat
- Dress the child in light clothing; restrictive clothing and diaphoresis can lead to increased pruritus
- Use diversional activities and distraction appropriate to developmental level: distraction from pain can reduce the need for pharmacologic agents and distraction for pruritus can minimize scratching.

Evaluation: Child verbalizes absence or decrease of pain using a pain scale such as FLACC (Face, Legs, Activity, Cry, Consolability scale) or linear pain scale will verbalize decrease in uncomfortable sensation such as itching and aches; infants will exhibit decreased crying and ability to rest quietly.

3. **Nursing diagnosis:** Impaired skin integrity related to mechanical trauma secondary to infectious disease process as evidenced by rash, pruritus and scratching.
   Goal: Child will maintain or regain skin integrity.
   Interventions: Promoting skin integrity.
   - Monitor skin for color changes, temperature, redness, swelling, warmth, pain or signs of infection, changes in rash lesions, distribution or size to help identify problems early and allow for prevention of infection; can also provide information regarding the course of the illness
   - Encourage fluid intake and proper nutrition to promote wound healing
   - Keep child's fingernails short (use mitts, gloves, or socks over hands if necessary); short fingernails can help prevent injury to the skin, which leads to increased pain
   - Encourage child to press on rather than scratch the area of pruritus; pressing on the area that itches can help soothe the itching and prevent scratching, which can lead to injury to the skin
   - Use antipruritics and topical ointments or creams as ordered to minimize scratching to prevent injury to skin; can aid in healing.

   Evaluation: Child did not demonstrate increased skin breakdown. Child or parent able to or demonstrate measures to protect and heal skin and proper care for any lesions.

4. **Nursing diagnosis:** Risk for infection related to insufficient knowledge regarding measures to avoid exposure to pathogens, increased environmental exposure to pathogens, transmission toothers secondary to contagious organism or presence of infectious organisms.

Goal: Child will be able to exhibit signs or symptoms of local or systemic infection. Child will not spread infection to others.
Interventions: Preventing and controlling infection.
- Monitor vital signs; elevation in temperature may indicate infection
- Monitor skin lesions for signs of local infection: redness, warmth, drainage, swelling, and pain at lesions can indicate infection
- Maintain aseptic technique and practice good hand washing to prevent introduction of further infectious agents and prevent transmission to others
- Administer antibiotics as prescribed to prevent or treat bacterial infection
- Encourage nutritious diet and proper hydration according to child's preferences and ability to feed orally to assist body's natural defenses against infection
- Isolate child as required based on transmission-based precautions to prevent nosocomial spread of infection
- Teach child and family preventive measures such as good hand washing, covering mouth and nose with cough or sneeze and adequate disposal of used tissues to prevent nosocomial or community spread of infection.

Evaluation: Symptoms of infection decreased over time; others remain free of infection. Child and family will demonstrate appropriate hygiene measures using proper technique, such as hand washing to prevent the spread of infection.

5. **Nursing diagnosis:** Fluid volume deficit, risk, related to increased metabolic demands and insensible loss due to fever, vomiting, poor feeding or intake.
   Goal: Fluid volume will be maintained and balance.
   Interventions: Promoting adequate fluid balance.
   - Administer IV fluids if ordered to maintain adequate hydration in children who are NPO, unable to tolerate oral intake or unable to keep up with fluid losses
   - When oral intake is allowed and tolerated, encourage oral fluids to promote intake and maintain hydration
   - Assess for signs of adequate hydration such as pink and moist oral mucosa, elastic skin turgor, adequate urine output; discrepancies may identify fluid imbalance
   - Monitor intake and output to identify fluid imbalance
   - Assess urine specific gravity, urine and serum electrolytes, blood urea nitrogen, creatinine, and osmolality, and daily weights; these are reliable indicators of fluid status.

   Evaluation: Oral mucosa remains moist and pink. Skin turgor is elastic; urine output is at least 1–2 mL/kg/h.

6. **Nursing diagnosis:** Social isolation related to required isolation from peers secondary to transmission-based precautions, as evidenced by disruption in usual play secondary to inability to leave hospital room, activity intolerance and fatigue.
   Goal: Child will be able to participate in stimulating activities.
   Interventions: Preventing social isolation.
   - Explain reasons for transmission-based precautions and length of time; this helps increase understanding and decrease anxiety about isolation. Children sometimes mistake isolation as punishment. Explaining length of time gives child an end point he or she can work toward

Nursing Process for the Child with Communicable Diseases

- Visit child frequently, at least every hour, and try to spend some uninterrupted time to play and allow child time to verbalize feelings about separation from others; helps establish a therapeutic relationship and demonstrates caring
- Let child see caregiver's face before applying mask if appropriate to help child identify and relate to those caring for him or her and minimize anxiety about strangers and the unknown
- Consult child life specialist to arrange for stimulating activities child enjoy; can help child to better understand reasons for isolation
- Contact volunteers to spend time with child, if appropriate: gives child attention and support, which will assist child with coping and decrease stress.

Evaluation: Child verbalizes reason for isolation and length of isolation (if developmentally appropriate); child verbalizes interest in activities.

7. **Nursing diagnosis:** Knowledge deficit related to lack of information regarding medical condition, prognosis and medical needs as evidenced by verbalization, questions or actions demonstrating lack of understanding regarding child's condition or care.
   Goal: Child and family will be able to verbalize accurate information and understanding about condition, prognosis and medical needs.
   Interventions: Provide patient and family teaching.
   - Assess child's and family's willingness to learn: child and family must be willing to learn in order to teaching to be effective
   - Provide family with time to adjust to diagnosis to help facilitate adjustment and ability to learn and participate in child's care
   - Repeat information—allows family and child time to learn and understand
   - Teach in short sessions—many short sessions are found to be more helpful than one long session
   - Gear teaching to level of understanding of the child and family (depends on age of child, physical condition, memory) to ensure understanding
   - Provide reinforcement and rewards to facilitate the teaching/learning process
   - Use multiple modes of learning involving many senses (provide written, verbal, demonstration and videos) when possible; the child and family are more likely to retain information when it is presented in different ways using many senses.

   Evaluation: Child and family demonstrate knowledge of condition, prognosis and medical needs, including possible causes, contributing factors and treatment measures.

PRACTICE QUESTIONS

1. Write a nursing care plan for a 7-year child diagnosed with tuberculosis by applying nursing process.
2. Baby Renuka 5-year child diagnosed with HIV/AIDS. Draw nursing care plan for the child by applying nursing process.

CHAPTER 18

Nursing Process for the Child with Hematologic Disorder

LEARNING OBJECTIVES
- To identify the signs and symptoms of a child with hematological disorder.
- To frame nursing diagnosis based on the needs of the child.
- To plan nursing interventions and outcome identification.

INTRODUCTION

The hematologic system includes the blood (plasma and cells) and the blood-forming tissues/organs (red bone marrow, lymph, lymph nodes, spleen, thymus, and tonsils). The cellular portion of the blood contains the erythrocytes (RBC), leukocytes (WBC), and thrombocytes (platelets). The plasms portion contains water and solutes, which include albumin, electrolytes, and proteins (clotting factors, fibrinogen, globulins, and antibodies). The system provides the body with cells that have certain functions in the transport of oxygen, nutrients, and substances to all the tissues; assists in clotting to prevent blood loss; regulates heat to maintain body temperature; and provides protection to the body from infectious agents (immunologic function).

Changes in the hematologic system occur adult parameters are reached. These changes make the child more vulnerable to disorders common to the system such as anemia, immunologic disorders, hemostatic problems, and malignancies involving the lymphatic system and blood cell production. Further disturbances in the function of any cellular or transport activities in children cause a multiple number of disorders and pathologies that affect all organ systems of the body.

NURSING PROCESS FOR THE CHILD WITH HEMATOLOGIC DISORDER (IN GENERAL)

1. **Nursing diagnosis:** Fatigue related to decreased oxygen supply in the body as evidenced by lack of energy, increased sleep requirements or decreased interest in play activities.
   Goal: Child will be able to display increased endurance.
   Intervention: Decreasing fatigue.
   - Cluster nursing care activities and plan for periods of rest before and after exertional activities to decrease oxygen need and consumption
   - Encourage activity or ambulation per physician's orders: early mobilization results in better outcomes

- Observe child for symptoms of activity intolerance such as pallor, nausea, light headedness or dizziness, or changes in vital signs to determine level of tolerance
- If child is on bed rest, perform range-of-motion exercises and frequent position changes, as negative changes to the musculoskeletal system occur quickly with inactivity and immobility
- Refer the child to physical therapy for exercise prescription to increase skeletal muscle strength.

Evaluation: Child desires to play without developing symptoms of exertion.

2. **Nursing diagnosis:** Impaired physical mobility related to pain from sickle cell crises or acute bleeds or imposed activity restrictions as evidenced by guarding of painful extremity, resistance to activity.
   Goal: Child will be able to engage in activities within age parameter and limits of disease.
   Intervention: Promoting physical mobility.
   - Encourage gross and fine motor activities as able as within limits of mobility
   - Collaborate with physical therapy to strengthen muscles and promote optimal mobility to facilitate motor development
   - Use passive and active range-of-motion exercises and teach child and family how to perform them: these exercises prevent contractures and facilitate joint mobility and muscle development (active ROM) to help increase mobility
   - Praise accomplishments and emphasize child's abilities to improve self-esteem and encourage feelings of confidence and competence.

   Evaluation: Child able to move extremities moves about environment and participates in exercise programs within limits of age and disease.

3. **Nursing diagnosis:** Ineffective health maintenance related to knowledge and skill acquisition regarding nutritional and medical treatment of anemia, prevention of infection, home administration of intravenous clotting factors or protection from injury as evidenced by new diagnosis and inability to verbalize appropriate treatment regimen or demonstrate medication administration skills.
   Goal: Child's health will be maintained.
   Intervention: Educating parents about effective health maintenance.
   - Educate the family about iron-rich foods to be promoted in the child with iron deficiency anemia and limited in the child with thalassemia
   - Limit cow's milk intake in the child with iron deficiency anemia to decrease risk of microscopic GI bleeding and increase appetite for other foods
   - Provide ongoing evaluation of nutritional intake to ensure that appropriate dietary restrictions are followed
   - Ensure that parents can verbalize understanding of home medication regimen; iron or folic acid supplementation for anemia, prophylactic antibiotics for sickle cell anemia, and chelation for Thalassemia and factor replacement for hemophilia
   - Have parents provide return demonstration of subcutaneous infusion of deferoxamine or intravenous factor as appropriate to ensure accuracy and independence in the home environment
   - Educate families about when to call or visit medical provider to ensure timely intervention when signs and symptoms develop.

Evaluation: Child received supplements, medications as prescribed and taken appropriate diet.

4. **Nursing diagnosis:** Anxiety related to diagnostic testing as evidenced by parent verbalization, child resistance or crying with procedures.
   Goal: Child's anxiety will be minimized.
   Intervention: Relieving anxiety.
   - Use topical anesthetic creams or agents for nonemergency laboratory draws to decrease stress related to needle sticks or venipunctures
   - Maintain a quiet and calm environment to reduce the child's stress
   - Educate the child as appropriate, and the family regarding the need for obtaining any laboratory specimens: knowledge helps to alleviate anxiety related to the unknown
   - Identify the need for the specific test and explain the procedure before obtaining the specimen to decrease the anxiety and time required for the procedure
   - Provide developmentally appropriate activities for the child (activities can reduce stress and also provide stimulus for children; the use of safe and developmentally appropriate acts as a role model for the family).

   Evaluation: Child verbalizes less fear, experience less pain with procedures.

5. **Nursing diagnosis:** Ineffective family coping related to hospitalization of child or chronic, possibly life-threatening genetic disorder as evidenced by excessive fearfulness or denial statements, withdrawal or verbalization of inadequate coping skills.
   Goal: Child and/or family will be able to demonstrate adequate coping skills.
   Intervention: Promoting effective family coping.
   - Provide emotional support to the child and family to improve coping abilities
   - Actively listen to the child's and family's concerns to validate the child's and family's feelings and establish trust
   - Encourage parents to talk about their child and the illness; verbalization brings feelings out in the open
   - Validate feelings of guilt, shock, frustration, resentment, or depression to promote trusting communication and begin avenue for appropriate coping
   - Provide open communication with the child and siblings: children appreciate honesty about their illness, and coping is improved
   - Refer families to community resources such as parent support groups, grief counseling (involvement with emotional and instrumental support improve scoping abilities)
   - Encourage role-playing and play activities to identify the child's fears and provide a method for working through feelings.

   Evaluation: Child verbalizes feelings and demonstrates healthy family interactions.

6. **Nursing diagnosis:** Risk for injury related to alteration in peripheral sensory perception, decreased platelet count, deficient coagulation factor, or excessive iron load.
   Goal: Child will be free from hemorrhage.
   Intervention: Preventing injury.
   - Assess petechiae, purpura, bruising or bleeding (provides baseline data for comparison; if present, may warrant intervention).
   - Encourage quiet activities or play to avoid trauma with active play
   - Avoid rectal temperatures and examinations. Post sign at head of bed "no rectal temperatures or medications" to avoid rectal mucosa damage resulting in bleeding

- Avoid intramuscular injections and lumbar puncture if possible to decrease risk of bleeding from a puncture site
- If bone marrow aspiration must be performed, apply pressure dressing to site to prevent bleeding
- Teach families about preferred physical activities for the child with idiopathic thrombocytopenic purpura (ITP) or hemophilia to provide safe physical activity and decrease risk for injury.

Evaluation: Experience decreased bruising or episodes of prolonged bleeding.

NURSING PROCESS FOR SPECIFIC HEMATOLOGICAL DISORDERS

Acquired Immunodeficiency Syndrome

Acquired immunodeficiency syndrome (AIDS) is a disorder of the immune system believed to be caused by a retrovirus. AIDS is identified as the human T-cell lymphotropic virus type III (HTLV-III), which is presently termed human immunodeficiency virus (HIV) type 1. It is known to be found in the blood and body fluids and is transmitted to infants or children through in utero exposure from an infected mother or through blood products received to treat hemophilia. Older children may become infected when involved in high-risk behaviors such as sexual contact and/or intravenous drug use. AIDS is not known to be transmitted by casual contact. Diagnosis of the disease in children includes the presence of opportunistic infections (viral, bacterial, fungal, protozoal) and cancer; confirmed HIV in blood or tissues; or presence of the HIV antibody. Treatment is focused on prevention and management of opportunistic infections and control of disease progression. Most children with the disease are under 2 years of age and have a poor prognosis. No cure is available at this time **(Fig. 18.1)**.

Symptoms of Acquired Immunodeficiency Syndrome

The symptoms vary depending on the age of the child. The following are the most common symptoms of HIV infection. However, each infant, child, or adolescent may experience symptoms differently. Symptoms may include:

Infants

At birth, infants born to an HIV-infected mother may test negative for the virus and have no symptoms. This does not mean that the infant does not have the virus. Blood tests will be done at various stages after birth up to and past 6 months of age to determine an infant's HIV status.

Symptoms may include the following:

- Failure to thrive-delayed physical and developmental growth as evidenced by poor weight gain and bone growth
- Swollen abdomen (due to swelling of the liver and spleen)
- Swollen lymph nodes
- Intermittent diarrhea (diarrhea that may come and go)
- Pneumonia
- Oral thrush—a fungal infection in the mouth that is characterized by white patches on the cheeks and tongue. These lesions may be painful to the infant.

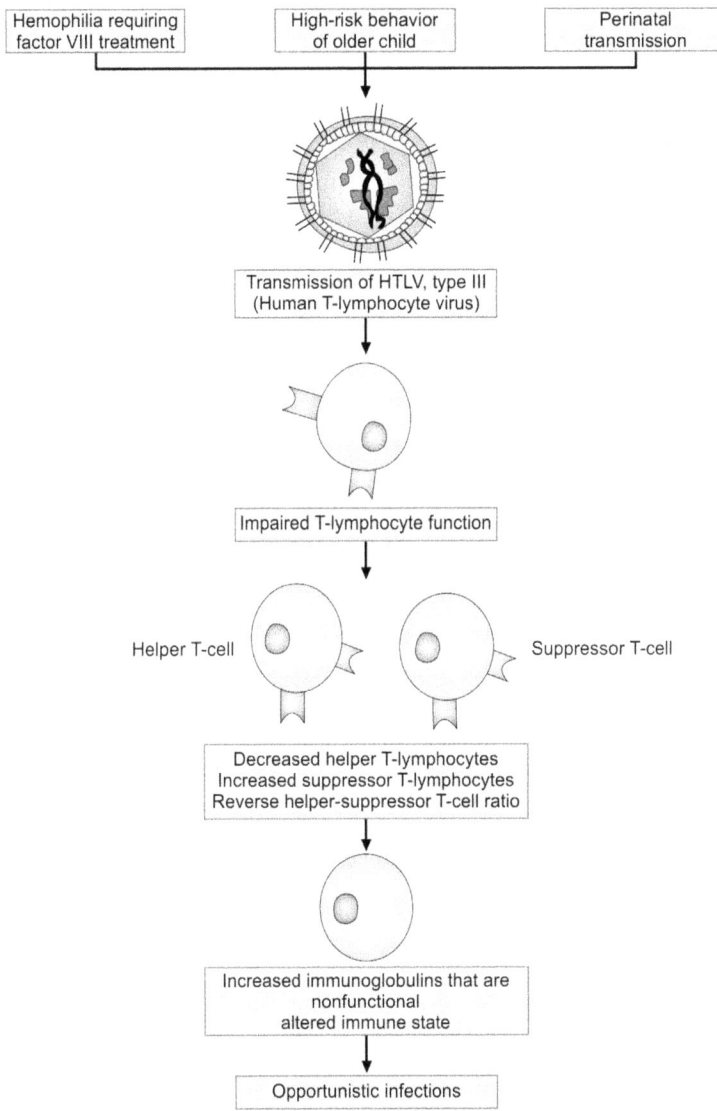

Fig. 18.1: Pathophysiology of acquired immunodeficiency syndrome.

Children

Symptoms seen in children older than 1 year of age can be divided into three different categories, from mild to severe. They may include the above symptoms, but may also include the following:

Mild
- Swollen lymph nodes
- Swelling of the parotid gland (salivary glands located in front of the ear)
- Constant or recurring sinus infections
- Constant or recurring ear infections

- Dermatitis—an itchy, rash on the skin
- Abdominal swelling from increased live and spleen size.

Moderate

- Pneumonitis—swelling of lung tissue
- Oral thrush that lasts for more than 2 months (a fungal infection in the mouth that is characterized by white patches on the cheeks and tongue). These lesions may be painful to the child.
- Constant or recurring diarrhea
- A fever that persists for more than one month
- Hepatitis—an inflammation of the liver that is often caused by an infection
- Complicated chickenpox.

Severe

- Two serious bacterial infections in a 2 year period (meningitis, blood infection, or pneumonia)
- A yeast infection that occurs in the digestive track or lungs
- Encephalopathy—a deterioration of the brain
- Tumors or malignant lesions
- PCP or *Pneumocystis* carinii pneumonia (the type of pneumonia most commonly seen with HIV)
- Kidney disease.

Adolescents

Symptoms of HIV in teens may be the same as in children, and may also be more similar to the symptoms commonly seen in adults with HIV. Some teens and adults may develop a flu-like illness within a month or two after exposure to the HIV virus, although, many people do not develop any symptoms at all when they first become infected. In addition, the symptoms that do appear, which usually disappear within a week to a month, are often mistaken for those of another viral infection.

Symptoms may include:

- Fever
- Headache
- Malaise (not feeling well)
- Enlarged lymph nodes.

Persistent or severe symptoms may not surface for 10 years or more, after HIV infection first enters the body in teens and adults. This asymptomatic period of the infection is highly variable from person to person. But, during the asymptomatic period, HIV is actively infecting and killing cells of the immune system. Its most obvious effect is a decline in the blood levels of CD4+ cells (also called T4 cells)—the immune system's key infection fighters. The virus initially disables or destroys these cells without causing symptoms.

An HIV-infected child is usually diagnosed with AIDS when the immune system becomes severely damaged or other types of infections occur. As the immune system deteriorates, complications begin to develop. The following are some common complications, or symptoms, of AIDS. However, each child may experience symptoms differently.

Symptoms may include:
- Lymph nodes that remain enlarged for more than 3 months
- Lack of energy
- Weight loss
- Frequent fevers and sweats
- Persistent or frequent yeast infection (oral or vaginal)
- Persistent skin rashes or flaky skin
- Pelvic inflammatory disease that does not respond to treatment
- Short-term memory loss

Some people develop frequent and severe herpes infections that cause mouth, genital, or anal sores, or a reactivation of chickenpox known as shingles.

Nursing Management

A. Essential Nursing Diagnosis and Nursing Process Associated with this Condition

Nursing diagnosis

Ineffective airway clearance related to obstruction, secretions, decreased energy, and fatigue.

Assessment: Abnormal breath sounds, changes in rate, ease, and depth of respirations, tachypnea, fever, weakness, cough infective with or without sputum.

(Refer Table 11.1 from chapter 11)

Nursing diagnosis

Ineffective breathing pattern related to illness (infection).

Assessment: Increase in body temperature above normal ranged, increased respiratory rate, tachycardia.

(Refer Table 14.2 from chapter 14)

Nursing diagnosis

Diarrhea related to irritation of bowel.

Assessment: Chronic, increased frequency of loose, liquid stools; cramping, abdominal pain.

(Refer Table 13.8 from chapter 13)

Nursing diagnosis

Altered nutrition: Less than body requirement related to inability to ingest, digest, or absorb nutrients.

Assessment: Anorexia, weight loss, lack of interest in feeding, failure to thrive.

(Refer Table 14.3 from chapter 14)

Nursing diagnosis

Altered thought processes related to physiological changes (brain infection).

Nursing Process for the Child with Hematologic Disorder

Table 18.1: Nursing interventions for anxiety of parent(s) and child.

Interventions	Rationales
Assess level of anxiety of parent(s) and child and how it is manifested; and need for information that will relieve anxiety	Provides information about source and level of anxiety and need for interventions to relieve it; sources for the child may be procedures, fear of mutilation or death, unfamiliar environment of hospital, and may be manifested by restlessness and inability to play, sleep or eat
Assess possible need for special counseling or social services for child	Reduces anxiety, supports child's dealing with illness, and promotes adjustment to lifestyle changes
Allow open expression of concerns about illness, procedures, treatments, and prognosis	Provides opportunity to vent feelings and fears to reduce anxiety
Communicate with child at appropriate age level and answer questions calmly and honestly; use pictures, models, and drawings for explanations	Promotes understanding and trust
Allow child as much input in decisions about care and routines as possible	Allows child more control and independence in situations
Allow parent(s) to stay with child	Promotes parental care and support

Assessment: Cognitive dissonance; changes in consciousness, with disorientation, irritability, confusion.
(Refer Table 12.14 from chapter 12)

B. Specific Nursing Diagnoses and Nursing Process

Nursing Diagnosis

Anxiety of parent(s) and child related to change in health status, threat of death, threat to self-concept, fear of interpersonal transmission and contagion **(Table 18.1)**.

Assessment: Increased apprehension and fear of diagnosis; expressed concern and worry about early death, effect of lifestyle changes on physical and emotional status, possible opportunistic infections.

Evaluation
- Expresses reduction in anxiety as information and explanations are given
- States concerns and reason for anxiety and behavior
- Verbalizes knowledge of and participates in decision making regarding care
- Explores and notes anger and sorrow about diagnosis, prognosis, and proposed changes in lifestyle
- Utilizes existing and new support systems.

Nursing Diagnosis

Anticipatory grieving related to perceived potential loss of infant/child by parent(s), perceived loss of physiopsychosocial well-being by child **(Table 18.2)**.

Nursing Process for the Child with Hematologic Disorder

Table 18.2: Nursing interventions for anticipatory grieving.

Interventions	Rationales
Assess stage of grief process, problems encountered, feelings regarding long-term illness and potential loss	Provides information about stage of grieving as time to work through the process varies with individuals as they move toward acceptance
Provide emotional and spiritual comfort in an accepting environment and avoid conversations that will cause guilt or anger	Provides for emotional needs of parent(s) and child as appropriate, and helps them to cope with illness, and its implications without adding stressors that are difficult to resolve
Allow for parent(s) and child's responses and expressions of concern, fear, anxiety, or guilt	Promotes ventilation of feelings
Assist in identifying and using effective coping mechanisms and in understanding situations over which they have no control	Promotes constructive use of coping skills
Allow for discussion of likelihood of child's death with parent(s) and child if appropriate, and encourage them to discuss this with family members, friends	Presents realistic view of probable outcome of illness

Assessment: Expression of distress at potential loss, fatal prognosis of the disease, premature death of child.

Evaluation
- Verbalizes understanding of grief process and responses
- Shares feelings with professionals, family members, friends
- Secures assistance from support groups and individuals
- Identifies and uses coping skills with a positive effect
- Discusses death and dying with appropriate professionals and friends.

Nursing diagnosis

High-risk for infection related to inadequate secondary defenses (immunosuppression), insufficient knowledge to avoid exposure to pathogens **(Table 18.3)**.

Assessment: Presence of infective organism, opportunistic infectious process and malignancy, expressed need for information about transmission prevention.

Evaluation
- Absence or control of opportunistic infections
- Prevents transmission of the virus to others
- Provides precautions to prevent infection in child
- Follows Center for Disease Control Guidelines and Universal Precaution in care of child to prevent infection transmission of disease to others
- Administers medications correctly to prevent progression of disease and treat infections if present

Nursing Process for the Child with Hematologic Disorder

Table 18.3: Nursing interventions for high-risk for infection.

Interventions	Rationales
Assess for fever, malaise, fatigue, night sweats, weight loss, chronic diarrhea, oral infection or lesions, pain in joints and muscles, lymphadenopathy, upper and lower respiratory infections	Provides information about signs and symptoms of infection during the prodromal stage of AIDS with responses that are age-dependent at onset of AIDS in infants/children; long-term opportunistic infections including *Pneumocystis carinii* pneumonia, Kaposi's sarcoma, and lymphoma
Provides protective isolation for immunosuppressed child; use gloves, mask, and gown for visitors and during care, proper handwashing when needed	Protects child from contact with infectious process in others
Wear gloves for all care, especially when in contact with body fluids (changing diapers, handling any secretions or excretions); avoid recapping needles; clean all spills and disinfect articles or areas; use bleach solution in home; wash, disinfect, or dispose of all contaminated articles used; double bag all illness and specimens with proper precautionary labeling	Prevents transmission of virus to personnel or caretaker; follows guidelines published by the Centers for Disease Control
Use medical or surgical asepsis for all procedures and care as appropriate	Prevents transmission of pathogens to child
Administer medications as ordered to control disease progression or treat any infection as ordered	Prevents or treats infectious process, compensates for immunosuppression by improving functioning of immune system
Restrict contact with persons with infections or illness, allow child to share room with another child who does not have an infection	Prevents transmission of infection to child

- Verbalizes risk factors in acquiring or transmitting disease
- Attends school within limitations imposed by the disease
- Verbalizes precaution to prevent disease by sexual contact or IV drug use
- Provides immunizations for child.

Nursing Diagnosis

Social isolation related to altered state of wellness, unaccepted social behavior **(Table 18.4)**.

Assessment: Protective isolation; absence of support by family, friends, others; seeks to be alone; expresses feelings of rejection, indifference of others, aloneness; withdrawal; displays behavior unaccepted by dominant culture; evidence of altered state of wellness.

Table 18.4: Nursing interventions for social isolation.

Interventions	Rationales
Assess child and family for feelings about stigma associated with the disease, rejection by others	Provides information about extent of isolation felt by the family and child
Provide accepting, warm environment for child and parent(s) to express their feelings	Promotes trust and comfort to enhance adaptation to presence of positive testing or actual symptoms of the disease
Encourage child to interact with peers, attend school and activities	Promotes feelings of belonging, and provides growth and development needs
Inform peers, and personnel about AIDS and safe activities for child and other children	Provides information and education about AIDS
Discuss with child and parent(s) misconceptions that the public has and ways to correct the situation by providing information about causes and mode of transmission and by answering questions and concerns	Promotes correct information dissemination and dispels myths about the disease, thereby reducing fear and rejection by others
Inform parent(s) and child that confidentiality will be maintained at school and elsewhere if needed	Protects child from stigma associated with the disease

(AIDS: acquired immune deficiency syndrome)

Evaluation
- Participates in family and peer activities, including school
- Exhibits a positive, secure feeling in child
- Verbalizes feeling of acceptance.

Anemias

Anemia, the most common hematologic disease of childhood is a disorder of the red blood cell (RBC), characterized by the alteration in the function or production of the cells. Anemia is the result of an underlying disease. The types included in this nursing process are iron deficiency anemia which is caused by an inadequate supply of iron, aplastic anemia, which is caused by decreased production from bone marrow depression, and sickle cell anemia, which is caused by an inherited trait that causes sickling of the RBC when oxygen tension and pH are lowered. Iron deficiency anemia usually occurs in infants between 6 and 9 months of age if the milk and food intake is not iron fortified and in the older infant and young child between 1 and 1½ years of age. It is treated by iron administration. Aplastic anemia usually occurs between 3 and 5 years of age and is treated with medication to inhibit the autoimmune process and administration of blood transfusions. Sickle cell anemia occurs primarily in blacks late in infancy because of the presence of fetal hemogbulin with sickling usually apparent by 4 months of age and is treated with blood transfusions and symptomatic support as needed to prevent crisis situations **(Flowchart 18.1)**.

Nursing Process for the Child with Hematologic Disorder

Flowchart 18.1: Pathophysiology of anemias.

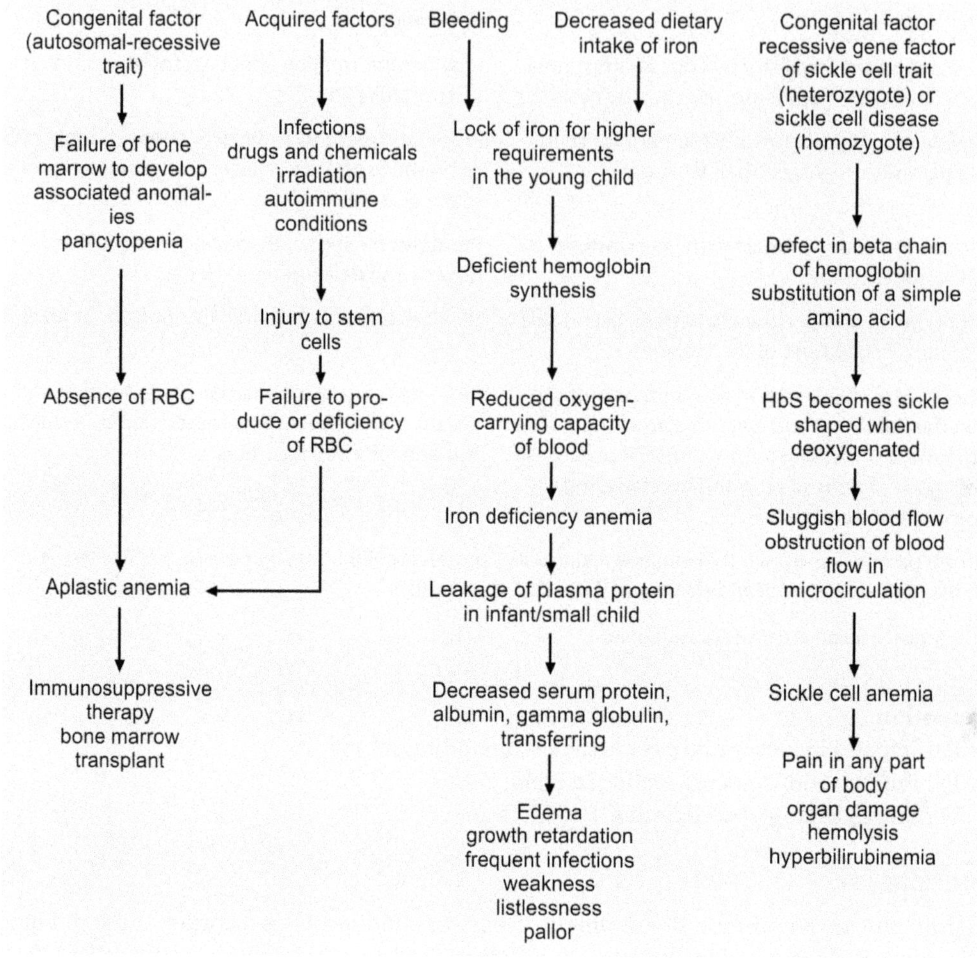

```
Congenital factor        Acquired factors      Bleeding        Decreased dietary      Congenital factor
(autosomal-recessive                                            intake of iron         recessive gene factor
    trait)                                                                             of sickle cell trait
      ↓                        ↓                  ↓                    ↓               (heterozygote) or
  Failure of bone          Infections       Lock of iron for higher                    sickle cell disease
  marrow to develop    drugs and chemicals     requirements                            (homozygote)
  associated anomal-       irradiation        in the young child                              ↓
      ies                  autoimmune                 ↓                                Defect in beta chain
  pancytopenia             conditions         Deficient hemoglobin                     of hemoglobin
      ↓                        ↓                  synthesis                            substitution of a simple
                         Injury to stem             ↓                                  amino acid
                            cells                                                            ↓
      ↓                        ↓                    ↓                                  HbS becomes sickle
  Absence of RBC        Failure to pro-      Reduced oxygen-                           shaped when
                        duce or deficiency   carrying capacity                         deoxygenated
                        of RBC               of blood                                         ↓
                                                    ↓                                  Sluggish blood flow
                                             Iron deficiency anemia                    obstruction of blood
                                                    ↓                                  flow in
      ↓                                                                                microcirculation
  Aplastic anemia  ←                         Leakage of plasma protein                        ↓
      ↓                                      in infant/small child
  Immunosuppressive                                 ↓                                  Sickle cell anemia
     therapy                                 Decreased serum protein,                         ↓
  bone marrow                                albumin, gamma globulin,
  transplant                                 transferring                              Pain in any part
                                                    ↓                                  of body
                                                  Edema                                organ damage
                                             growth retardation                        hemolysis
                                             frequent infections                       hyperbilirubinemia
                                             weakness
                                             listlessness
                                             pallor
```

Nursing Management

A. Essential Nursing Diagnoses and Nursing Process Associated with these Conditions

Nursing diagnosis

Altered tissue perfusion related to interruption of arterial or venous flow, hypovolemia.

Assessment: Cyanosis, dyspnea, cool extremities, tissue anoxia, delayed capillary filling, changes in BP in extremities, thick and brittle nails, pallor, fatigue, bleeding from mucous membranes, leg ulcers, tachycardia.

(Refer Table 14.12 from chapter 14)

Nursing diagnosis

High-risk for fluid volume deficit related to failure of regulatory mechanisms (renal function).

Assessment: Dilute urine, increased urinary output, altered intake, dehydration, hemoconcentration.

(Refer Table 14.11 from chapter 14)

Nursing diagnosis

Altered nutrition: Less than body requirements related to inadequate ingestion of iron in food/feeding.

Assessment: Reported inadequate intake of iron rich foods, weakness, anorexia, malnutrition, poor weight gain, pallor, decreased Hb level.

(Refer Table 14.3 from chapter 14)

Nursing diagnosis

High-risk for impaired skin integrity related to internal factor of medication (horse serum).

Assessment: Allergic response to ATG administration, itching, rash, urticaria, face and lymph node swelling.

(Refer Table 12.1 from chapter 12)

B. Specific Nursing Diagnoses and Nursing Process

Nursing diagnosis

Pain related to biological injuring agents (tissue anoxia) **(Table 18.5)**.

Assessment: Communication of pain descriptors, guarding and protective behavior of area, soft tissue swelling, warmth over painful area, crying, clinging behavior.

Table 18.5: Nursing interventions for pain.

Interventions	Rationales
Assess for location, severity, and duration of pain	Provides information about pain caused by vaso-occlusive resulting from RBC sickling that leads to occlusion, ischemia, and necrosis in soft tissue, joints, abdomen, back, or wherever occlusion occurs
Administer analgesic as ordered; administer intermittently over 24 hours period before pain becomes severe rather than wait for request or compliant from child	Controls pain and promotes comfort
Provide rest periods, refrain from disturbing child unless necessary	Decreases stimuli that increase pain and promotes rest, decreases oxygen expenditure
Apply dry heat to area and note response of pain decrease	Promotes vasodilatation and circulation to area to reduce pain
Maintain position of comfort, handle painful areas gently and support with pillows	Promotes comfort and prevents pain from movement

(RBC: red blood corpuscle)

Nursing Process for the Child with Hematologic Disorder

Table 18.6: Nursing interventions for activity intolerance.

Interventions	Rationales
Assess temperature, respirations, and pulse: change in behavior (irritability, lightheadedness, short attention span), if easily fatigued, unable to sleep, or weak, ability to tolerate any activity or ADL	Provides information about VS changes caused by hypoxia and about behavior changes caused by reduced oxygenation of the brain
Assist with activities that require exertion and are beyond tolerance and ability	Minimizes physical exertion, which increases oxygen to tissues
Provides rest periods, plan care and activities around rest/sleep	Decreases oxygen expenditure to enhance tissue oxygenation
Provide appropriate quite play and activities, and allow interaction with child of same age, if possible	Promotes diversional activity and prevents with drawl
Administer oxygen therapy as ordered	Provides supplemental oxygen, if needed, to treat hypoxia
Administer transfusion of blood, packed RBC, platelets as ordered	Replaces blood or blood components depending on type of anemia and need

(RBC: red blood corpuscle; ADL: activities of daily living; VS: vegetative state)

Evaluation
- Controls or manages pain effectively
- Maintains comfort and rest with measures that prevent sickling and pain
- Administers analgesic with effective results
- Avoids pain-provoking situations.

Nursing diagnosis

Activity intolerance related to generalized weakness, imbalance between oxygen supply and demand **(Table 18.6)**.

Assessment: Reduced oxygen delivery to tissues from reduced RBC or RBC sickling, fatigue, verbalization of weakness, changes in respiratory rate, depth, and ease, irritability, low tolerance to activity, increased pulse.

Evaluation
- Minimizes oxygen expenditure and hypoxia
- Reduces activity, intolerance, fatigue, weakness
- Promotes restful environment
- Provides oxygen, transfusion, other treatments and procedures without incident
- Provides play and diversional activities with minimal exertion.

Nursing diagnosis

High-risk for infection related to inadequate secondary defenses (decreased Hgb, leucopenia, immunosuppressive therapy), pharmaceutical agents (ATG, steroid therapy) **(Table 18.7)**.

Nursing Process for the Child with Hematologic Disorder

Table 18.7: Nursing interventions for high-risk for infection.

Interventions	Rationales
Assess for signs, symptoms, and laboratory tests indicating infectious process irritability and malaise, swelling in soft tissue or lymph nodes	Provides information about infection in a child made susceptible by steroid and globulin therapy, particularly in aplastic anemia, or pneumococcal and *Salmonella* infections in child with sickle cell anemia
If an infection is present, administer antibiotics as ordered	Prevents and/or treats infection; children with sickle cell anemia are prone to infections, which precipitate a crisis episode
Provide protective isolation if neutrophil count is <200/cu mm; use mask and gown and good handwashing when caring for child	Prevents transmission of pathogens to a susceptible child
Obtain culture of body fluid for examination	Identifies pathogens and sensitivity to antibiotic therapy if an infection is present

Assessment: Temperature elevation; positive throat, urine or blood culture; changes in respirations and sputum characteristics; cloudy, foul-smelling urine.

Evaluation
- Absence of infection in any area
- Protects child from exposure to infectious agents
- Administers antibiotic therapy properly and correctly
- Reports signs and symptoms of infectious process.

Nursing diagnosis

High-risk for injury related to internal factor of abnormal blood profile (thrombocytopenia) reaction to transfusion or ATG administration **(Table 18.8)**.

Assessment: Fever, restlessness, chills, shortness of breath, chest pain, tachycardia, hypotension, headache, thrombocytopenia at 20,000/cu mm level, bruising, petechiae, bleeding from mucous membranes, blood in urine, sputum, stool, nosebleed, blood in vomitus, stomatitis.

Evaluation
- Bleeding absent or controlled
- Absence of allergic reactions or complications to transfusion or medication
- Complies with correct administration of medications
- Provides protective measures to prevent trauma, bleeding, or allergic reaction
- Assesses test, and reports bleeding from any site.

Nursing diagnosis

Knowledge deficit of parent(s) and child related to lack of information about anemia **(Table 18.9)**.

Assessment: Request of information about pathophysiology of anemia, changes that occur, preventive measures and treatments.

Table 18.8: Nursing interventions for high-risk for injury related to internal factor of abnormal blood profile (thrombocytopenia) reaction to transfusion or ATG administration.

Interventions	Rationales
Assess for signs of bleeding from any site as manifested in skin changes; also, blood from nose, oral cavity, urinary or gastrointestinal tract, and factors that precipitate or increase bleeding	Provides information indicating blood loss as tendency increases with therapy for aplastic anemia
Assess blood in urine with dipsticks and hematests	Identifies occult blood in urine or stool
Protect child from trauma by padding bed and toys, using soft toothbrush and towels or swabs for cleaning mouth, avoiding rectal temperature and injections	Prevents bleeding in skin layers, deeper tissues, or mucous membranes
Discontinue transfusion if allergic reaction occurs, notify physician	Prevents irreversible reaction to blood or blood products
If ordered, perform skin test for ATG before dose, administer steroid daily 30 minutes before ATG, which is given in normal saline IV	Alerts to possible sensitivity to horse serum and protects from allergic reaction to ATG
Inform parent(s) and child of activities to avoid while on therapy, such as contact sports or activities that cause falls	Prevents trauma, which causes bleeding when tendency is present
Advise parent(s) to avoid aspirin and aspirin products	Encourages bleeding by its effect on platelet aggregation
Instruct parent(s) to report any bleeding from any site, nosebleed that would not stop, blood in urine or stool	Provides for early interventions to control bleeding

(ATG: antithymocyte globulin; IV: intravenous)

Evaluation
- Verbalizations of knowledge of disease, cause, implications and interventions for compliance of medical regimen
- Applies knowledge to care and measures to prevent complications
- Seeks out counseling (genetic) information and support form groups and agencies
- Complies with correct medication/replacement administration.

Hemophilia A

Hemophilia A is a sex-linked, recessive, inherited disorder affecting male children but passed to the child by the mother. It is characterized by a defect in the action of factor VIII necessary in the clotting process. Other types, hemophilia B (factor IX deficiency) and hemophilia C (factor XI deficiency) also exist, but they are not as common as hemophilia A. The result of the disorder is a prolonged bleeding caused by trauma anywhere in the body a spontaneous bleeding into any tissue of the body. Hemophilia A forms can range from mild to severe, determined by the tendency and degree of bleeding. Treatment is concerned with administration of the deficient factor, prevention of bleeding episodes, and control and support of bleeding episodes if they occur **(Fig. 18.2)**.

Table 18.9: Nursing interventions for knowledge deficit of parent(s) and child.

Interventions	Rationales
Assess for knowledge level of type of anemia, cause, treatment, prevention	Provides information needed for appropriate teaching content for parent(s) and child
Inform of RBC physiology and the changes that occur in each of the anemias as pertain to the child	Promotes understanding of RBC function to provide a rationale for signs, symptoms, and treatments
Inform parent(s) of importance of genetic counseling for sickle cell anemia	Provide information about risk of offspring having the disease
Inform parent(s) and child of bone marrow transplant treatment if appropriate	Provides information of this therapy if child has aplastic anemia
Instruct child to carry or wear identification information, including condition, treatments, and physician's name and number	Provides information in the event of an emergency
Instruct parent(s) and child in dietary intake of iron, including foods such as iron-rich formula for infant, meats, whole grains, green leafy vegetables, dried fruits	Provides iron intake or replacement in iron-deficiency anemia
Administer oral iron replacement and instruct to take with orange juice to promote absorption; give iron preparation between meals, avoid administering with milk, use straw or dropper and have child rinse mouth after ingestion	Provides iron replacement therapy
Inform parent(s) of importance of child attending school and participating in family activities	Treats child as member of family and integrates him or her into social, mental, and physical activities, which will enhance growth and development needs
Reinforce risks to avoid, including signs and symptoms of infection, bleeding, hypoxia, malnutrition, immunizations, high altitudes, side effects of steroid therapy, emotional and physical stress	Prevents complications of disease

(RBC: red blood cell)

Symptoms of Hemophilia

- Frequent bruising
- Frequent bleeding from the nose or gums
- Pain and swelling in joints or muscles
- Bleeding that lasts a long time
- Bowel movements that are black
- Urine that is pink or red.

Nursing Management

A. Essential Nursing Diagnoses and Nursing Process Associated with this Condition

Nursing Diagnosis

Impaired physical mobility related to pain and discomfort, musculoskeletal impairment.

Nursing Process for the Child with Hematologic Disorder

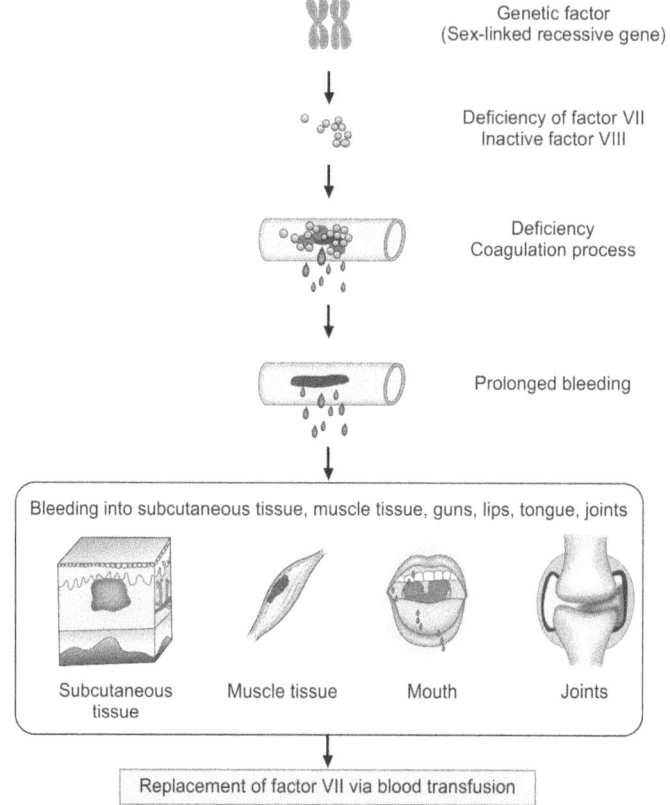

Fig. 18.2: Pathophysiology of hemophilia.

Assessment: Reluctance to attempt movement, arthropathy, muscle contracture, imposed restriction in movement during bleeding into joints, pain in joints.

(Refer Table 14.19 from chapter 14)

Nursing diagnosis

High-risk for impaired skin integrity related to altered circulation (bleeding tendency).

Assessment: Breaks in skin with IV therapy, bleeding into tissue caused by trauma, bleeding from mucous membrane, soft tissue hemorrhages.

(Refer Table 12.1 from chapter 12)

B. Specific Nursing Diagnoses and Nursing Process

Nursing diagnosis

Pain related to biological injuring agent **(Table 18.10)**.

Assessment: Hemarthroses, verbal descriptors of pain, guarding and protective behavior of painful area, irritability, refusal to move or change position, crying, restlessness.

Nursing Process for the Child with Hematologic Disorder

Table 18.10: Nursing interventions for pain.

Interventions	Rationales
Assess for joint pain, swelling, and limited ROM	Provides information about pain level caused by bleeding into the joints during acute episodes
Administer analgesics PO and avoid aspirin or aspirin-combination products	Relieves pain; aspirin avoided as it prolongs bleeding time
Immobilize and support extremities with pillow or sand bag; apply ice to painful area and avoid any heat applications	Relieves pain; heat promotes vasodilation and circulation, which would increase bleeding in the area
Provide bed cradle over painful extremity	Prevents pressure of linens on painful area
Avoid handling or movement of extremity during acute pain; apply splint or sling if prescribed	Prevents increase of pain caused by movement and increased bleeding

(ROM: range of motion; PO, per os or by mouth)

Evaluation
- Verbalizes that pain is reduced or absent
- Administers correct analgesic for pain control
- Maintains continuous comfort level.

Nursing Diagnosis

Altered protection related to abnormal blood profile **(Table 18.11)**

Assessment: Altered clotting (deficient factor VIII), fatigue, weakness, soft tissue hemorrhage, hematomas, ecchymoses, bleeding from mucous membranes.

Table 18.11: Nursing interventions for altered protection.

Interventions	Rationales
Assess signs and symptoms of bleeding, hemarthroses, traumatized areas, bleeding gums, continued oozing of blood from breaks in skin	Provides information about active bleeding; common sites are joints, muscles, and any area that has been traumatized
Provide soft toys, soft toothbrush or toothettes, padded sides on bed; avoid rectal temperatures, performing unnecessary invasive procedures	Prevents bleeding caused by trauma as a result of in factor VIII deficiency
Administer deficient factor IV, fibrin, or Gelfoam to open bleeding sites; after IV administration, apply pressure to puncture site for 5 minutes and rotate sites; when possible, perform finger stick for blood specimen instead of venipuncture	Controls bleeding to prevent complications by immediate treatment of bleeding or prevention of bleeding; cryoprecipitate or other concentrates may be used
Note vital signs and laboratory values for coagulation factors	Reflects changes in hemodynamic status, indicating blood loss and blood clotting capability
Elevate, immobilize bleeding site after bleeding episode and apply ice to the area	Decreases blood flow to the area and prevents possible emboli
Provide environment free of hazards, including clear pathways, and supervise child during ambulation and play without being overprotective	Prevents trauma caused by falls; infants and toddlers frequently fall or sustain injuries

Evaluation
- Absence of excessive bleeding
- Complies with measures to prevent trauma, which results in bleeding
- Reports signs and symptoms of bleeding to physician
- Complies with protocol in administration of concentrates and measures to control bleeding
- Prevents joint degeneration from prolonged bleeding and repeated hemarthrosis
- Participates in acceptable activities and physical therapy to prevent trauma and joint damage.

Nursing Diagnosis

Ineffective family coping: compromised related to inadequate or incorrect information or understanding, prolonged disease or disability progression that exhausts the physical and emotional supportive capacity of caretakers **(Table 18.12)**

Assessment: Expression and/or confirmation of concern and inadequate knowledge about long-term care needs, problems and complications, anxiety and guilt, overprotection of child.

Evaluation
- Verbalizes and clarifies child's and family's knowledge about long-term needs and care
- Develops and uses coping skills and problem-solving techniques effectively
- Family members supports and cares for child while meeting own needs
- Preserves family relationships, minimizes family stressors, resolves differences
- Family progressively adapts and accepts hemophilia condition and therapy by family

Table 18.12: Nursing interventions for ineffective family coping compromised.

Interventions	Rationales
Assess family's coping methods and their effectiveness; family interactions and expectations related to long-term care, developmental level of family; response of siblings; knowledge and use of support systems and resources; presence of guilt and anxiety; overprotection and/or overindulgent behavior	Identifies coping methods that work and the need to develop new coping skills and behaviors, family attitudes; child with special long-term needs may strengthen or strain family relationships and an undue degree of overprotection may be detrimental to child's growth and development (disallowing school attendance or peer activities, avoiding discipline of child, and disallowing child to assume responsibility for ADL)
Encourage family members to express problem areas and explore solutions responsibly	Reduces anxiety and enhances understanding; provides family an opportunity to identify problems and develop problem-solving strategies
Help family establish short- and long-term goals for child and integrate child into family activities, include participation of all family members in care routines	Promotes involvement and control over situations and maintains role of family members and parent(s)
Provide assistance of social worker, counselor, or other as needed	Gives support to the family faced with long-term care of child with a serious illness
Allow family members to express feelings, such as how they deal with the chronic needs of family member and coping patterns that help or hinder adjustment to the problems	Allows for venting of feelings, which relieves guilt and anxiety and helps determine need for information and support

(ADL: activities of daily living)

- Implements preventive measures of follow-up-care to ensure optimal function and heart of child.

Idiopathic Thrombocytopenic Purpura

Idiopathic thrombocytopenia purpura (ITP) is a condition characterized by a decrease in platelets as a result of destruction of or the inadequate formation or function of the cells. The reduction of platelets (thrombocytopenia) leads to hemorrhaging in the form of petechiae, ecchymoses, hematomas, and bleeding from mucous membranes anywhere in the body. The disease may be acute, chronic, or recurrent with a favorable prognosis. Treatment is symptomatic and supportive except in those children who do not response to therapy or who experience severe hemorrhaging, in which case a splenectomy is performed. The disorder most commonly affects children between 2 and 6 years of age, and most have experienced a viral infection before the disease onset **(Fig. 18.3)**.

Symptoms of Idiopathic Thrombocytopenic Purpura

Normal platelet count is in the range of 150,000 to 450,000. With ITP, the platelet count is <100,000. By the time significant bleeding occurs, the child may have a platelet count of <10,000. The lower the platelet count, the greater the risk of bleeding.

Because platelets help stop bleeding, the symptoms of ITP are related to increased bleeding. However, each child may experience symptoms differently.

Symptoms may include:
- Purpura
- Petechiae
- Nosebleeds
- Bleeding in the mouth and/or in and around the gums
- Blood in the vomit, urine, or stool
- Bleeding in the head

Nursing Management

A. Essential Nursing Diagnoses and Nursing Process Associated with this Condition

Nursing Diagnosis

High-risk for impaired skin integrity related to altered circulation (bleeding tendency) **(Table 18.13)**.

Assessment: Petechiae, ecchymoses, hematomas, damage from trauma.

(Refer Table 12.1 from chapter 12)

Nursing Diagnosis

Hyperthermia related to illness.

Assessment: Infectious process, increase in body temperature above normal range.

(Refer Table 14.8 from chapter 14)

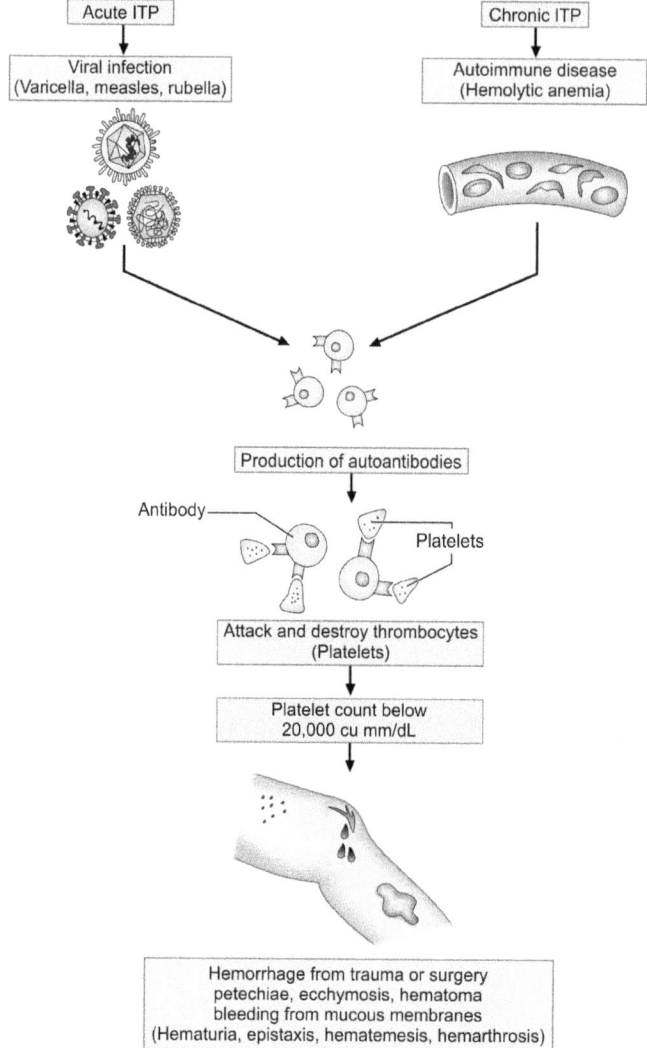

Fig. 18.3: Pathophysiology of idiopathic thrombocytopenic purpura.

B. Specific Nursing Diagnoses and Nursing Process

Nursing Diagnosis

Altered protection related to abnormal blood profile (thrombocytopenia) **(Table 18.13)**.

Assessment: Platelet count below 20,000 cu mm/dL, petechiae, ecchymoses, bleeding from any mucous membrane area, hematomas on legs.

Evaluation
- Absence of bleeding from any area
- Complies with measures to prevent bleeding or infection
- Reports signs and symptoms of bleeding to physician.

Table 18.13: Nursing interventions for altered protection.

Interventions	Rationales
Assess for bleeding from gums, hematemesis, hematuria, hemarthrosis, hematomas, epistaxis or evidence of easy bruising, petechial rash	Provides information and data indicating low platelet level and increased tendency for bleeding
Avoid trauma to tissues by avoiding use of hard toothbrush or dental floss, taking rectal temperatures, performing unnecessary invasive procedures, and if administering an IM injection, applying pressure for 5 minutes to site	Prevents bleeding caused by trauma to sensitive areas
Administer anti-inflammatories PO, gamma globulin IV as ordered	Administered to children who are at highest risk for excessive bleeding
Administer transfusion of platelets, whole blood as ordered and monitor for responses, expected and adverse reactions	Administered to replace blood loss or increase platelets
Provide support in a warm, accepting environment for parent(s) and child	Promotes trust and comfort during periods of stress

(IM: intramuscular; PO: per os or by mouth; IV: intravenous)

Leukemia/Lymphoma

Leukemia is a malignant disease of the bone marrow and lymphatics characterized by an unrestricted proliferation of immature white blood cells in the blood-forming tissues. The nonfunctional cells invade the organs of the body, with the spleen and liver the most highly susceptible. Bone marrow depression decreases the production of blood components, causing anemia (erythrocytes), infection (neutrophils), and bleeding (platelets). These effects on the bone marrow result in the common signs and symptoms of this disease, which include fatigue, anorexia, fever, pallor, bone pain, and petechiae. All organs (brain, kidneys, testes, ovaries, lungs, gastrointestinal tract, liver, and spleen) eventually become involved. The most common types of leukemia affecting children are acute lymphoid (ALL) contracted by children between 2 and 5 years of age, and acute nonlymphoid or myelogenous (ANLL) in adolescents. Prognosis is based on age, sex, initial WBC, histologic type, and morphology. Lymphoma may be Hodgkin's disease or non-Hodgkin's, with the non-Hodgkin's (lymphosarcoma) more common in children under 15 years of age. It primarily involves the lymphoid system and lymph nodes, although diffuse in its involvement and invasion of other organs, especially the mediastinum and meninges. It typically spreads rapidly, by metastasis, to the bone marrow and central nervous system. Prognosis is based on lymph node involvement limited to one or two adjacent regions, presence of an extranodal site, and gastrointestinal involvement.

Treatment of these malignancies includes chemotherapy protocols, radiation therapy, and bone marrow transplantation (**Fig. 18.4**).

Symptoms of Leukemia

Acute lymphoblastic leukemias (ALLs) signs and symptoms are common to other, less serious illnesses.
- Aches in the arms, legs of back
- Black-and-blue marks (bruises) for no clear reason

Nursing Process for the Child with Hematologic Disorder

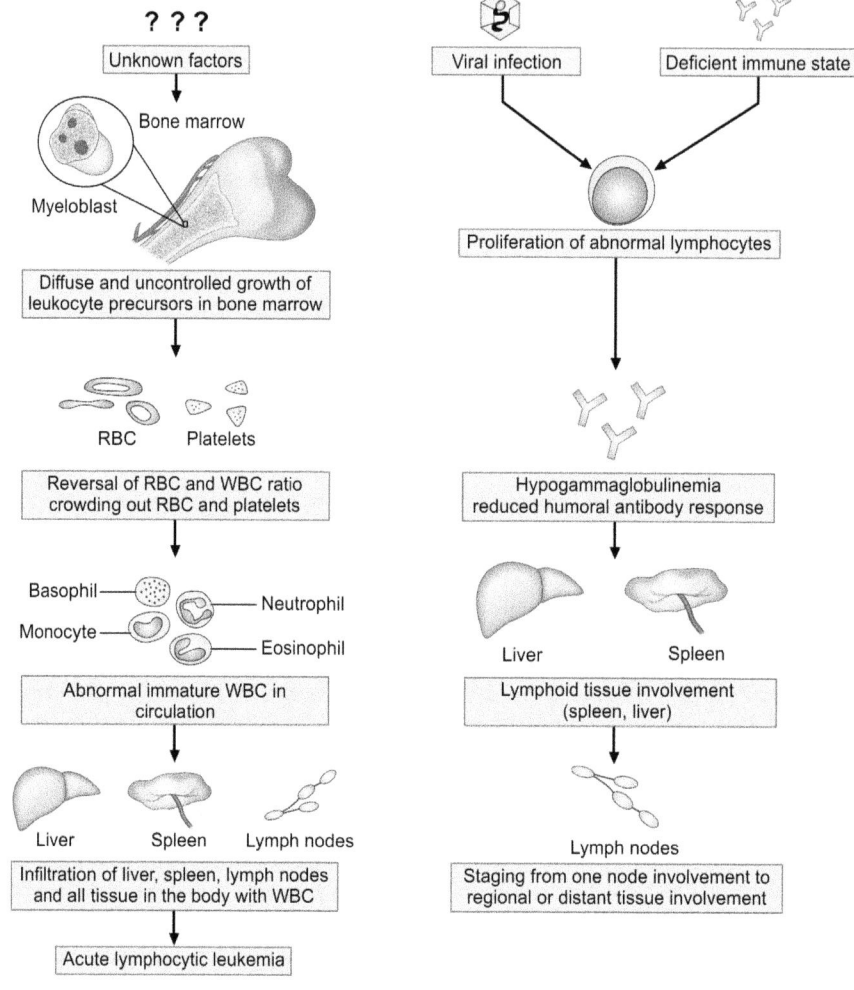

Fig. 18.4: Pathophysiology of leukemia/lymphoma.
(RBC: red blood corpuscle; WBC: white blood cell)

- Enlarged lymph nodes
- Fever without an obvious cause of a lasting, low-grade fever
- Headaches
- Pale skin
- Pinhead-size red spots under the skin (called petechiae)
- Prolonged bleeding from minor cuts
- Shortness of breath during normal physical activity
- Tiredness or no energy
- Vomiting
- Unexplained weight loss.

Symptoms of Lymphoma
- The most common symptom of lymphoma is one or more enlarged lymph nodes in the neck, underarm, or groin, which are usually painless.
- Enlarged lymph nodes in children with lymphoma may resemble the swollen glands of children who have a throat infection involving the lymph nodes.

Other frequent symptoms of lymphoma can include:
- Unexplained fever
- Night sweats
- Loss of appetite or weight loss
- Coughing or difficulty breathing
- Abdominal swelling (lymphomas in the chest or abdomen can grow to a very large size before symptoms appear).

Nursing Management

A. Essential Nursing Diagnoses and Nursing Process Associated with these Conditions

Nursing diagnosis

Altered nutrition: Less than body requirements related to inability to ingest and digest food, chemotherapy and radiation therapy.

Assessment: Anorexia, nausea, vomiting, anxiety, grieving, weight loss, mucositis, gustatory changes, abdominal cramps.

(Refer Table 14.3 from chapter 14)

Nursing diagnosis

High-risk for fluid volume deficit related to altered intake; excessive losses through normal routes.

Assessment: Diarrhea, vomiting from chemotherapy.

(Refer Table 14.11 from chapter 14)

Nursing diagnosis

Diarrhea related to chemotherapy and/or radiation therapy.

Assessment: Increased frequency of bowel sounds and lose, liquid stools.

(Refer Table 13.8 from chapter 13)

Nursing diagnosis

High-risk for impaired skin integrity related to external factor of radiation therapy, IV chemotherapy, excretions and secretions.

Assessment: Disruption of skin surfaces, destruction of skin layers, redness and excoriation of perianal area, extravasation from chemotherapy (swelling, phlebitis, pain, redness, tissue necrosis) impaired wound healing, hyperpigmentation, hirsutism, alopecia, rash, pruritis.

(Refer Table 12.1 from chapter 12)

Table 18.14: Nursing interventions for anxiety of parent(s) and child.

Interventions	Rationales
Assess level of anxiety of parent(s) and child and how it is manifested, and the need for information that will relieve anxiety	Provides information about sources and level of anxiety and need for interventions to relieve it; sources for the child may be procedures, fear of mutilation or death, unfamiliar environment of hospital, and may be manifested by restlessness or inability to play, sleep, or eat
Assess possible need for special counseling services for child	Reduces anxiety and supports child dealing with illness; promotes adjustment to lifestyle changes
Allow open expression of concern about illness, procedures, treatments and prognosis	Provides opportunity to vent feelings and fears in order to reduce anxiety
Communicate with child at appropriate age level and answer questions calmly and honestly; use pictures, models, and drawings for explanations	Promotes understanding and trust
Allow parent(s) to stay with child or have open visitation; provide a telephone number to call for information	Promotes care and support by parent(s)

Nursing Diagnosis

Hyperthermia related to illness (infection).

Assessment: Increase in body temperature above normal range, flushed skin, warm to touch, increased pulse and respiration rates.

(Refer Table 14.18 from chapter 14)

B. Specific Nursing Diagnoses and Nursing Process

Nursing Diagnosis

Anxiety of parent(s) and child related to change in health status, threat of death, threat to self-concept **(Table 18.14)**.

Assessment: Increased apprehension and fear of diagnosis, expressed concern and worry about diagnostic procedures and preparation, early death, effects of therapy on physical and emotional status, possible metastasis of disease.

Evaluation
- Expresses reduction in anxiety as information and explanations are given
- States concerns and reason for anxiety and behavior
- Verbalizes knowledge of and participates in decision making regarding care
- Explores and notes anger about diagnosis and proposed changes in body structure and function
- Utilizes existing and new support systems.

Nursing Diagnosis

Pain related to biological injuring agent **(Table 18.15)**.

Table 18.15: Nursing interventions for pain.

Interventions	Rationales
Assess verbal and nonverbal behavior; type, location (bone, joint, abdomen), and severity of pain depending on age using a pain scale: presence of crying, whining, irritability, and restlessness	Provides information about pain that varies with age, developmental level, and is unique to a particular child's learned emotional response; degree of pain and fatigue influence ability of child to perceive and identify discomfort
Administer analgesic and sedative PO, IV as indicated or ordered and monitor side effects	Relieves pain and promotes comfort and rest when administered according to severity
Promote rest and avoid disturbing child unnecessarily	Decreases stimuli that increase pain, and promotes rest to conserve energy
Maintain body alignment and support, and immobilize limbs with pillows and sand bags	Promotes comfort and prevents contractures
Apply heat (moist or dry) to painful areas	Relieves pain by promoting circulation to the area
Provide toys and activities for quiet play appropriate for age; use music, relaxation technique; remain with child when pain is most acute	Provides diversion and distraction from pain

(PO: per os or by mouth; IV: intravenous)

Assessment: Verbal descriptors of pain, guarding and protective behavior of painful area, irritability, refusal to move or change position, crying, clinging behavior.

Evaluation
- Verbalizes that pain is reduced or absent
- Participates in pain-reducing techniques
- Maintains continuous comfort level.

Nursing diagnosis

Altered oral mucous membrane related to medication (chemotherapy), radiation therapy **(Table 18.16)**.

Assessment: Stomatitis, oral ulcers, hyperemia, oral pain or discomfort, oral plaque.

Evaluation
- Oral mucous membranes intact and reduced inflammation present
- Complies with measures to prevent trauma or breakdown of mucosa
- Controls discomfort associated with impaired oral mucosa
- Progressive return to oral mucous membrane baseline following chemotherapy protocol/radiation therapy.

Nursing diagnosis

Altered protection related to drug therapy (chemotherapy): treatments (radiation therapy); abnormal blood profile (leucopenia, thrombocytopenia, anemia, coagulation) **(Table 18.17)**.

Nursing Process for the Child with Hematologic Disorder

Table 18.16: Nursing interventions for altered mucous membrane.

Interventions	Rationales
Assess oral cavity for pain, ulcers, lesions, gingivitis, mucositis, or stomatitis, and effect on ability to ingest food and fluids	Provides information about effect of chemotherapy and/or radiation therapy
Provide mouth rinses, cleansing with swabs or soft toothbrush	Provides mouth care without irritating oral mucosa
Administer medication topically (Xylocaine) before meals and offer bland, smooth foods	Permits eating with more comfort
Administer an antiseptic mouth rinse (nystatin) 30 minutes before any food or fluid intake	Promotes comfort of oral mucosa and maintains integrity
Encourage child to select allowable foods that they prefer	Allows for independence and control over situation to reduce helplessness and increase nutrition

Assessment: Altered clotting, bone marrow suppression, deficient immunity against infection, hematoma, petechiae, bleeding from nose, gums, hematemesis, blood in stool, fatigue.

Evaluation
- Absence of excessive bleeding or infection during chemotherapy
- Complies with measures based on blood profile that prevent excessive bleeding or infection
- Reports signs and symptoms of complications to physician
- Complies with laboratory blood testing and follow-up visits to physician.

Nursing diagnosis

Body image disturbance related to biophysical and psychosocial factors **(Table 18.18)**.

Table 18.17: Nursing interventions for altered protection.

Interventions	Rationales
Assess for bleeding from any site, WBC, platelet count, HCT, absolute neutrophil count, and febrile episodes	Provides information about frank bleeding or blood profile abnormalities that predispose to bleeding caused by bone marrow suppression and immunosuppression resulting from chemotherapy or radiation therapy
Avoid trauma by not using hard toothbrush or dental floss, not taking rectal temperatures, not performing unnecessary invasive procedures	Prevents bleeding during chemotherapy regimen which alters platelet level and clotting factors
Carry out handwashing technique before giving care, use mask and gown when appropriate, provide a private room, monitor for any signs and symptoms of infection, especially pulmonary	Prevents transmission of pathogens to a compromised immune system during chemotherapy if neutrophil count is <1,000 cu mm

(WBC: white blood cell; HCT: hematocrit)

Table 18.18: Nursing interventions for body image disturbance.

Interventions	Rationales
Assess child for feelings about multiple restrictions in lifestyle, chronic illness, difficulty in school and social situations, inability to keep up with peers and participate in activities	Provides information about status of self-concept and body image, which may require special attention
Encourage expression of feelings and concerns and support communication with parent(s), teachers and peers	Provides opportunity to vent feelings and reduce negative feelings about changes in appearance
Avoid negative comments and stress positive activities and accomplishments	Enhances body image and confidence
Note withdrawal behavior and signs of depression	Reveals responses to body image changes and possible poor adjustment to changes
Show support and acceptance of changes in appearance of child; provide privacy as needed	Promotes trust and demonstrates respect for child

Assessment: Verbal and nonverbal responses to change in body appearance (alopecia, weight loss), weakness, negative feelings about body, multiple stressors, and change in daily living limitations and social relationships.

Evaluation
- Verbalizes improved body image and sense of well-being
- Participates in family, school, and social activities as appropriate
- Verbalizes feelings about special long-term needs in positive terms
- Supports positive body image and promotes adjustment to illness
- Identifies need and seeks out social services and psychological counseling as appropriate.

Nursing diagnosis

Ineffective family coping: Compromised related to inadequate or incorrect information or understanding; prolonged disease or disability progression that exhausts the physical and emotional supportive capacity of caretakers **(Table 18.19)**.

Assessment: Expression and/or confirmation of concern and inadequate knowledge about long-term care needs, problems and complications, anxiety and guilt, overprotection of child.

Evaluation
- Verbalizes and clarifies knowledge about child long-term need and care
- Develops and use coping skill and problem solving techniques effectively
- Family members support and care for child while meeting own needs
- Family relationships preserves family relationships and family stressor, minimize with differences resolved
- Progressive adaptation and acceptance of condition and therapy by family
- Implement preventive measures of follow-up care to ensure optimal function and health of child.

Nursing Process for the Child with Hematologic Disorder

Table 18.19: Nursing interventions for ineffective family coping.

Interventions	Rationales
Assess effectiveness of family coping methods; family interactions and expectations related to long-term, developmental level of family; response of siblings; knowledge and use of support systems and resources; presence of guilt, anxiety, overprotective and/or overindulgent behavior	Provides information identifying successful coping methods or the need to develop new coping skills, behaviors, and family attitudes; child with overprotection (e.g., not allowing child to attend school, participate in activities with peers, or assume responsibilities for ADL; avoiding disciplining of child) may be detrimental to child's growth and development
Encourage family members to express problem areas and explore solutions responsibly	Reduces anxiety and enhances understanding; allows family to identify problems and develop problem-solving strategies
Assist family in establishing short- and long-term goals for child and in integrating child into family activities; include participation of all family members in care routines	Promotes involvement and control over situations, and maintains role of family members and parent(s)
Provide assistance of social worker, counselor, clergy, or other as needed	Provides support to the family faced with long-term care of child with a serious, life-threatening illness
Allow family members to express feelings on how they deal with the chronic needs of family member and on coping patterns that help or hinder adjustment to the problems	Allows for venting of feelings to determine need for information and support, and relieves guilt and anxiety

PRACTICE QUESTIONS

1. Master Ram admitted in pediatric oncology ward with the diagnosis of leukemia. Draw a nursing care plan for master Ram based on 3 priority problems.
2. Draw a nursing care plan of the child with hemophilia by applying nursing process.

CHAPTER 19

Nursing Process for the Child with Endocrine Disorders

LEARNING OBJECTIVES
- To identify the signs and symptoms of a child with endocrine disorder.
- To frame nursing diagnosis based on the needs of the child.
- To plan nursing interventions and outcome identification.

INTRODUCTION

The endocrine system includes the cells of certain glands that produce hormones; the organ or tissue sites that receive the hormone; and the transport system of the blood, lymph, and extracellular fluids that move the hormones from the point utilization. Hormones may regulate general cell physiologic activities or may affect specific cells of the body. Glands included in this system are the pituitary, thyroid, parathyroid, adrenal, isles of Langerhans, ovaries, and testes. With the neurologic system; the system regulates and integrates functions with the neurologic system that assist the body to adjust behavior, growth, development, and sexual reproduction, in children, abnormal conditions involving these glands are caused by over secretion or under secretion of hormones or by a problem in the response to these hormones by the receiving organ or tissue. These abnormalities may result from congenital or acquired factors. They are usually treated by partial or complete surgical removal of the gland and/or drug therapy to replace deficiencies.

NURSING PROCESS FOR THE CHILD WITH ENDOCRINE DISORDERS (IN GENERAL)

1. **Nursing diagnosis:** Delayed growth and development related to hypo- or hyper-function of gland/hormone as evidenced by weight and/or height less than expected for age, failure to meet expected age-appropriate developmental milestones.
   Goal: Nutritional status will be maximized and development will be enhanced.
   Interventions: Enhancing growth and development.
   - Monitor growth parameters using standard growth charts
   - Encourage favorite foods (within prescribed diet restrictions if present) to maximize oral intake
   - Consult dietitian for appropriate diet supplementation recommendations
   - Encourage compliance with hormone supplementation to enhance ability to achieve appropriate growth
   - Provide care related to any complications of dysfunction such as correcting fluid and electrolyte imbalances or diarrhea
   - Screen for developmental capabilities to determine child's current level of functioning
   - Offer age-appropriate toys, play and activities (including gross motor) to encourage further development

- Provide support to families of children with developmental delay (progress in achieving developmental milestones in the child to maintain motivation.

For the child with diabetes mellitus:
- Provide a calorie-appropriate, no restricted, well-balanced diet to maintain appropriate growth
- Encourage three meals with two or three snacks with consistent carbohydrates to maintain appropriate blood glucose levels and promote growth.

Evaluation: Child maintains or gained weight appropriately and attained progress toward expected developmental milestones.

2. **Nursing diagnosis:** Disturbed body image related to abnormal growth and development/changes in physical appearance due to hormone dysfunction as evidenced by verbalization of dissatisfaction with the child's or adolescent's looks.
   Goal: Child will be able to develop self-esteem in relation to body image.
   Interventions: Promoting healthy body image.
   - Provide opportunities for child to explore feelings related to appearance; venting feelings is associated with less body image disturbance
   - Relate to child on age level, not appearance level: 'babying' a child who looks younger due to his or her small size reduces self-image
   - Involve the child and especially the teen in the decision-making process: a sense of control will improve body image
   - Encourage the child to spend time with peers who have similar endocrine disorders: peer's opinions are often better accepted than those of persons in authority, such as parents or healthcare professionals
   - Refer to counseling or support groups to further support the child.

   Evaluation: Expresses positive feelings about self and participates in social activities.

3. **Nursing diagnosis:** Deficient knowledge related to therapeutic regimen as evidenced by questions about endocrine disorder and self-management.
   Goal: Child and family will be able to understand and develop skills for self-management.
   Interventions: Promoting knowledge required for self-management.
   - Assess child's developmental level and family's ability to absorb instruction to determine how to approach teaching sessions
   - Establish teaching plan with child and family to gain cooperation and involvement
   - Teach and give printed instructions on disorder, complications, home care, and follow-up requirements, so family has source to refer to at home
   - Evaluate teaching with return demonstrations to determine whether child/family is skilled enough for home management of the disorder

   For the child with diabetes mellitus:
   - First teach 'survival skills' (e.g., glucose and urine testing, administering insulin, record-keeping, food guidelines, when to call physician) to provide initial base of knowledge for self-management
   - Implement second-phase home management program with more extensive instruction: providing additional teaching over time is necessary for management of a significant chronic illness

- Monitor outcomes of teaching with every contact to ensure progress with patient/family education.

    Evaluation: Child and family verbalize about disorder, complications/adverse effects, home care regimen and long-term needs, and provide return demonstrations of medication administration or other procedures.

4. **Nursing diagnosis:** Interrupted family processes or adjustment issues related to lifestyle changes required to manage chronic illness and possible lifestyle changes as evidenced by family's presence in the hospital, missed work, demonstration of inadequate coping.

    Goal: Family will be able to maintain functional system of support; demonstrate adequate coping, adaptation of roles and functions, and decreased anxiety.

    Intervention: Encouraging healthy family processes.
    - Encourage parents and family members to verbalize concerns related to child's illness, diagnosis and prognosis; allows the nurse to identify concerns and areas where further education may be needed
    - Explain treatments, medications, procedures, child's behaviors, and plan of care to parents; understanding of the child's current status and plan of care helps decrease anxiety
    - Identify support system for family and child: helps nurse identify needs and resources available for coping
    - Provide family with information about support groups, financial resources and special clinics in the area for the particular type of disorder to provide family with wide base of support
    - Encourage parents to become involved in care; allows parents to feel needed and valued and gives them a sense of control over their child's health
    - Evaluate coping processes on follow-up visits to determine restoration of family processes.

    Evaluation: Parents are involved in child's care, ask appropriate questions, express tears and concerns, identify needs, seek appropriate resources and support, can discuss child's care and condition calmly.

5. **Nursing diagnosis: Imbalanced nutrition:** Less than or more than body requirements related to pathophysiology of dysfunction as evidenced by growth parameters significantly less or more than expected for age.

    Goal: Child will be able to maintain balanced nutritional status.

    Interventions: Maintaining adequate nutrition.
    - Determine body weight and length/height normal for age or what the child's pretreatment measurements were to determine goal to work toward
    - Weigh daily or weekly (according to physician order or institutional standard) and measure length/height weekly to monitor for appropriate growth
    - Determine child's food preferences and provide favorite foods as able to increase the likelihood that the child will consume appropriate amounts of foods
    - Instruct child and family about nutritional requirements, so that they are involved and are prepared for home care

    For the child who needs to gain weight: Consult dietician

- Offer highest-calorie meals at the time of day when the child's appetite is the greatest to increase likelihood of increased caloric intake
- Provide increased-calorie shakes or puddings within dietary restrictions (high-calorie foods increase weight gain)
- Administer vitamin and mineral supplements as prescribed to attain/maintain vitamin and mineral balance in the body.

Evaluation: Child demonstrates adequate growth (weight and height) pattern within normal range for age and gender or, in the child who has difficulty in growing, a progressive increase over time.

6. **Nursing diagnosis:** Deficient or excess fluid volume related to pathophysiology of endocrine dysfunction as evidenced by signs and symptoms of dehydration (deficient fluid volume) or edema and excessive urine output (excess fluid volume).
   Goal: Child will be able to maintain adequate fluid volume.
   Interventions: Maintaining adequate fluid volume.
   - Assess hydration status (skin turgor, oral mucosa, presence of tears) every 4–8 hours to evaluate maintenance of adequate fluid volume
   - Assess adequacy of urine output to evaluate end-organ perfusion
   - Maintain strict intake and output record to evaluate effectiveness of rehydration
   - Weigh child daily: accurate weight is one of the best indicators of fluid volume status in children
   - Administer specific hormone, fluid and electrolyte requirements as ordered to aid in fluid balance.
   - Maintain IV line and administer IV fluid as ordered to maintain fluid volume.
   - Maintain fluid restriction as ordered to restore homeostasis.

   Evaluation: Improved skin turgor; absence of edema; moist, pink oral mucosa; presence of tears; urine output 1 mL/kg/h or more; vital signs within normal range for age; and normal electrolyte/hormone serum levels.

7. **Nursing diagnosis:** Non-compliance related to long-term/complex management of some disorders as evidenced by failure to keep appointments, development of complications or exacerbation of symptoms, or child/family verbalization of inability to maintain treatment plan.
   Goal: Child and family will be able to comply with treatment regimen.
   Interventions: Encouraging compliance.
   - Listen non-judgmental while child/family describe reasons for non-compliance; assessment of problem should begin with non-threatening discussion
   - Help child/family develop a schedule for medication administration and other home regimens that works best for them; involving child and family in planning care will increase compliance by making them feel respected and valued
   - Work with the child and family to develop a written treatment plan or schedule that best suits their needs to provide support for maintenance of treatment plan
   - Establish follow-up visits to fit family's situation to promote compliance
   - Encourage monitoring with pediatric endocrinologist and specialists: multidisciplinary involvement has been shown to increase compliance
   - Recognize that behavioral change comes slowly; allows time for child and family to adjust to chronic nature of illness.

Evaluation: Child and family verbalize treatment expectations and agree to follow through them.

NURSING PROCESS FOR SPECIFIC ENDOCRINE DISORDERS

Diabetes Mellitus (Insulin Dependent) Type 1

Diabetes mellitus, type 1 (insulin dependent or juvenile onset diabetes) is a metabolic disorder caused by a deficiency of insulin. The deficiency is thought to occur in those individuals who are genetically predisposed to the disease and who have experienced a viral infection causing an autoimmune condition affecting the beta cells of the pancreas. It is treated by injection of insulin and regulation of diet and activity that maintain body functions. Complications that occur from improper coordination of these include hypoglycemia and hyperglycemia which, if untreated, lead to insulin shock or ketoacidosis. Long-term effects of the disease include neuropathy, nephropathy, retinopathy, atherosclerosis, and microangiopathy **(Fig. 19.1)**.

Symptoms of Diabetes Mellitus-Insulin Dependent Type

The signs and symptoms of type 1 diabetes in children usually develop quickly, over a period of weeks
- Increased thirst and frequent urination
- Extreme hunger
- Weight loss
- Fatigue
- Irritability or unusual behavior
- Blurred vision
- Yeast infection.

Nursing Management

A. Essential Nursing Diagnoses and Nursing Process Associated with this Condition

Nursing diagnosis

Altered nutrition: Less than body requirements related to inability to ingest, digest food.

Assessment: Loss of weight with adequate food intake, lack of interest in food, inadequate intake, insufficient insulin, too much insulin.

(Refer Table 14.3 from chapter 14)

Nursing diagnosis

High-risk for impaired skin integrity related to external factor of SC injections, internal factor of altered metabolic state, sensation, nutritional state.

Assessment: Disruption of skin surfaces with daily injections (lipodystrophy), failure to rotate sites, weight loss, poor wound healing, dry skin.

(Refer Table 12.1 from chapter 12)

Nursing Process for the Child with Endocrine Disorders

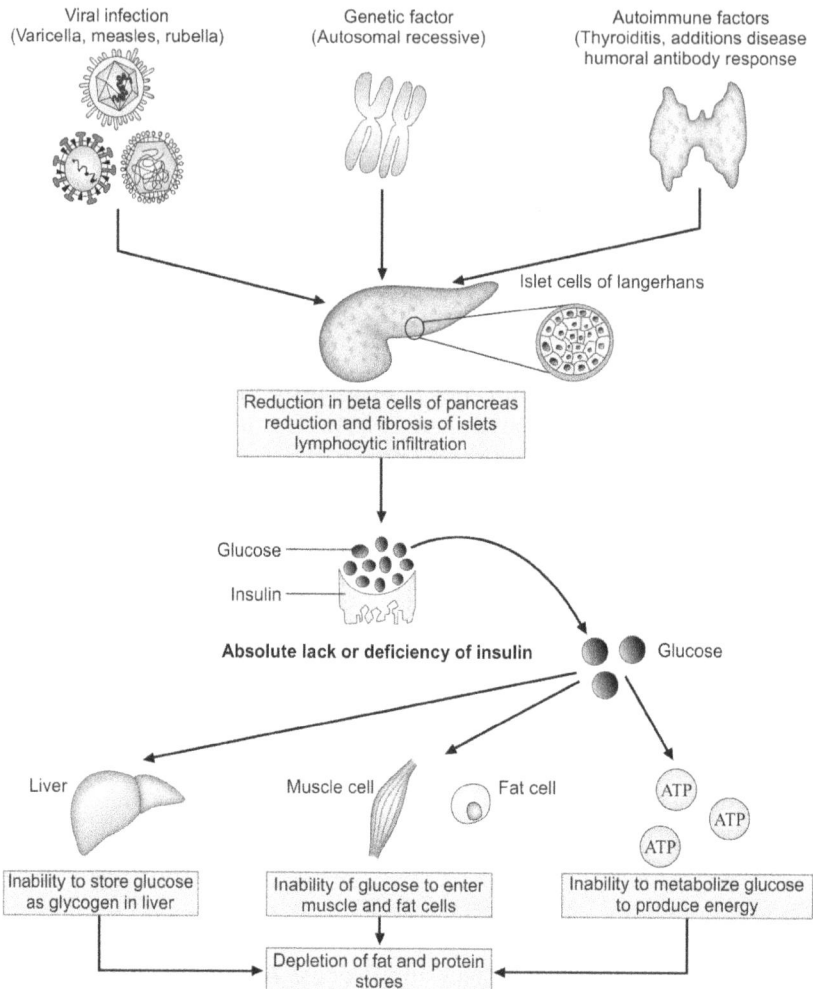

Fig. 19.1: Pathophysiology of diabetes mellitus (Insulin dependent type).

Nursing diagnosis

High-risk for fluid volume deficit related to active loss (osmotic diuresis).

Assessment: Output greater than intake, decreased urine output, dry skin and mucous membranes, poor skin turgor, dehydration with electrolyte depletion (K, Na, Cl, Mg, PO_4) with ketoacidosis, polyuria, polydipsia.

(Refer Table 14.11 from chapter 14)

B. Specific Nursing Diagnoses and Nursing Process

Nursing diagnosis

High-risk for injury related to internal biochemical factors of hyperglycemia or hypoglycemia **(Table 19.1)**.

Table 19.1: Nursing interventions for high-risk for injury related to internal biochemical factors of hyperglycemia or hypoglycemia.

Interventions	Rationales
Assess for signs and symptoms of hyperglycemia, blood glucose and ketones, pH and electrolyte levels	Provides information about complication caused by increased glucose levels resulting from improper diet, an illness, or omission of insulin administration; glucose is unable to enter the cells, and protein is broken down and converted to glucose by the liver, causing the hyperglycemia; fat and protein stores are depleted to provide energy for the body when carbohydrates are not able to be used for energy
Administer insulin SC as ordered, rotate sites, increase dosage as indicated by glucose levels; decrease food intake during an infection or illness and adjust dosage during an illness	Provides insulin replacement to maintain normal blood glucose levels without causing hypoglycemia; two or more injections may be given daily SC with a portable syringe pump or by intermittent bolus injections with a syringe and needle
Provide diet with calories that balances expenditure for energy and corresponds to type and action of insulin, and snacks between meals and at bedtime as appropriate	Provides child's nutritional needs for proper growth and development by consulting dietician
Promote exercise program consistent with dietary and insulin regimen; increase carbohydrate intake before vigorous activities	Aids in the utilization of dietary intake, regular activity may reduce amount of insulin required; a decrease in insulin and increased carbohydrate intake before vigorous exercise or activity may prevent hypoglycemia
Assess for signs and symptoms of hypoglycemia, blood glucose level	Provides information about episodes of hypoglycemia resulting from increased activity without additional food intake or omission or incomplete ingestion of meals, incorrect insulin administration, illness

(SC: subcutaneous)

Assessment: Hyperglycemia-fatigue, irritability, headache, abdominal discomfort, weight loss, polyuria, polydipsia, polyphagia, dehydration, blurred vision.

Hypoglycemia-nervousness, sweating, hunger, palpitations, weakness, dizziness, pallor, behavior changes, uncoordinated gait.

Evaluation
- Maintains blood glucose level of less than 120 mg/dL or more than 60 mg/dL
- Absence of blood ketones and urine acetone
- Absence of signs and symptoms of hyperglycemia or hypoglycemia
- Provides and complies with medical regimen to maintain growth and development and to control severe blood glucose fluctuations
- Verbalizes causes and measures to take to prevent complications.

Nursing Process for the Child with Endocrine Disorders

Nursing diagnosis

Knowledge deficit of parent(s) and child related to lack of information about disease (Table 19.2).

Assessment: New diagnosis of diabetes mellitus, type 1; request for information about pathology, insulin therapy, dietary requirements, activity/exercise needs, blood and urine testing, personal hygiene and health promotion.

Table 19.2: Nursing interventions for knowledge deficit of parent(s) and child.

Interventions	Rationales
Assess parent(s) and child for knowledge of disease and reliability in performing procedures and care, for educational level and learning capacity, and for developmental level	Provides information needs to plan teaching program; children over the age of 10 may be able to take responsibility for some of the care
Inform of cause of disease, disease process and pathology; use pamphlets and other aids appropriate for age of child and level of comprehension of parent(s)	Provides basic information that may be used as a rationale for treatment and care and allows for different teaching strategies
Provide a quiet, comfortable environment; allow time for teaching small amounts at a time and for reinforcement, demonstrations and return demonstrations; start teaching 3–4 days following diagnosis and limit sessions to 15–20 minutes	Prevents distractions and facilitates learning
Include as many family members in teaching sessions as possible	Promotes understanding and support of family and feeling of security for child
Instruct parent(s) and child in insulin administration including storing insulin, drawing up insulin into syringe, rotating vial instead of shaking, drawing clear insulin first if mixing 2 types in same syringe, injecting SC, rotating sites, adjusting dosages, reusing syringe and needle, and disposing of them	Promotes accurate administration of insulin, which prevents complications
Instruct in use of syringe-loaded injector	Provides temporary method of insulin administration if child is afraid to puncture skin
Instruct parent(s) and child in operation and use of a portable insulin pump to adjust insulin delivery	Provides continuous subcutaneous insulin infusion
Instruct parent(s) and child in collection and testing of blood for glucose with a lancet and blood-testing meter or a reagent strip compared to a color chart; collection and testing of urine with ketostix or Clinitest	Monitors glucose and ketone levels in blood and urine
Instruct parent(s) and child in dietary planning with emphasis on proper meal times and adequate caloric intake according to age; offer food lists, and assist in preparing sample menus; inform that food intake depends on activity, and describe methods to judge amounts of foods	Provides information about an important aspect of total care of the child

Contd...

Contd...

Interventions	Rationales
Inform parent(s) and child of role of exercise and alterations needed in food and insulin intake with increased or decreased activity	Provides information about usual activity pattern and effect on dietary intake and insulin needs
Inform parent(s) and child of skin problems associated with diabetes, need for regular dental examinations, foot care, protection of and proper care of nails, prevention of infections and exposure to infections, eye examinations, immunizations	Provides information about common problems resulting from long-term effects of the disease
Instruct parent(s) and child of record keeping for insulin, test results, responses to diet and exercise, noncompliance in medical regimen and effects	Provides a method to enhance self-care and demonstrates the need to notify physician for treatment evaluation and possible change
Inform parent(s) and child to wear or carry identification and information about the disease, treatment, and physician	Provides information in event of emergency

(SC: subcutaneous)

Evaluation
- Complies with medical regimen to control diabetes
- Prevents complications of diabetes
- Demonstrates correct insulin, dietary, and exercise procedures and interventions
- Promotes personal hygiene and health
- Verbalized understanding of information and instructions to manage total care
- Facilitate self-care by maintaining accurate daily record
- Recognizes importance of compliance with medical regimen
- Maintains identification information at all times.

Nursing diagnosis

Ineffective family coping: Compromised related to inadequate or incorrect information or understanding, prolonged disease or disability progression that exhausts the physical and emotional supportive capacity of caretakers **(Table 19.3)**.

Assessment: Expression and/or confirmation of concern and inadequate knowledge about long-term care needs, problems and complications, anxiety and guilty, overprotection of child.

Evaluation
- Verbalizes and clarifies child's and family's knowledge about long-term needs and care
- Develops and uses coping skills and problem-solving techniques effectively
- Family members provide support and care for child while meeting own needs
- Family relationships preserved and family stressors minimized; with differences resolved
- Progressive adaptation and acceptance by family of chronic condition and therapy
- Implements preventive measures of follow-up care to ensure optimal function and health of child.

Nursing Process for the Child with Endocrine Disorders

Table 19.3: Nursing interventions for ineffective family coping.

Interventions	Rationales
Assess family coping methods and effectiveness, family interactions and expectations related to long-term care, developmental level of family, response of siblings, knowledge and use of support systems and resources, presence of guilt and anxiety, overprotection and/or overindulgent behaviors	Identifies coping methods that work and the need to develop new coping skills and behaviors, family attitudes; child with special long-term needs may strengthen or strain family relationships, and overprotection may be detrimental to child's growth and development (e.g., not allowing child to attend school or participate in peer activities; avoiding discipline of child; and not allowing child to assume responsibilities for care)
Encourage family members and child to express problem areas, anxiety and explore solutions responsibly	Reduces anxiety and enhances understanding; provides family an opportunity to identify problems and develop problem-solving strategies
Assist family to establish short- and long-term goals for child and to integrate child into family activities include participation of all family members in care routines	Promotes involvement in and control over situations and maintains role of family members and parent(s)
Provide assistance of social worker, counselor, clergy, or other as needed	Provides support to the family faced with long-term care of child with a chronic illness
Allow family members to express feelings, to tell how they deal with the chronic needs of family member, and to describe coping patterns that help or hinder adjustment to the problems	Allows for venting of feelings to determines need for information and support and to relieve guilt and anxiety

Hypothyroidism

Hypothyroidism is the result of thyroid hormone production which is inadequate to maintain body processes. It may be the result of congenital thyroid abnormality and therefore present in infancy or it may become notable during the first two years of life. It appears later when production is inadequate to maintain body processes as rapid growth increases the need for hormones. Acquired causes of the condition may be thyrotoxicosis, thyroidectomy, irradiation, infections, and dietary deficiency of iodine. Secretions of the thyroid gland include thyroid hormone (thyroxine T4 and triiodothyronine, T3) and thyrocalcitonin, which are bound to proteins in the blood thyroxine-binding globulin (TBG) and thyrocalcitonin (maintains calcium levels in blood). The hormones are controlled by the thyroid-stimulating hormone (TSH) which is secreted by the anterior pituitary gland. Treatment of the deficiency is thyroid hormone replacement, which involves prompt intervention in the infant and gradual by increasing amounts of hormone administration in the child. Treatment is maintained throughout life to ensure restoration of thyroid deficiency. Hypothyroidism in infants accounts for one-third of diagnosed cases and, in children, accounts for two-thirds of cases **(Fig. 19.2)**.

Symptoms of Hypothyroidism

Hypothyroidism is common condition which can go understand if symptoms are mild. Symptoms of hypothyroidism are usually very suitable and gradual and may include:

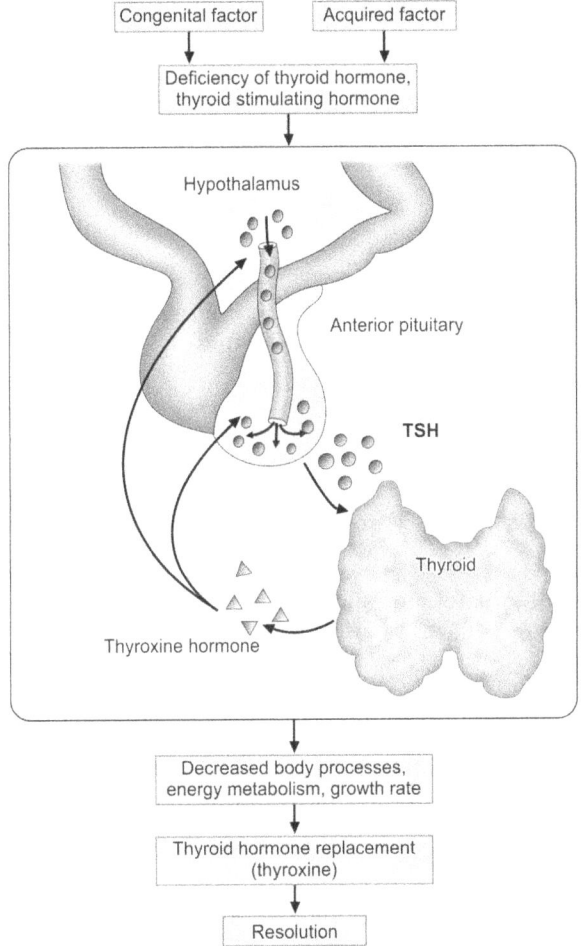

Fig. 19.2: Pathophysiology of hypothyroidism.
(TSH: thyroid stimulating hormone)

- Fatigue and/or exercise intolerance
- Slower reaction time (an important issue for drivers)
- Weight gain
- Constipation
- Sparse, coarse and dry hair
- Coarse, dry and thickened skin
- Slow pulse
- Cold intolerance
- Muscle cramps
- Sides of eyebrows thin or fall out
- Dull facial expression
- Hoarse voice

- Slow speech
- Droopy eyelids
- Puffy and swollen face
- Increased menstrual flow and cramping in girl and women.

Nursing Management

A. Essential Nursing Diagnosis and Nursing Process Associated with this Condition

Nursing diagnosis

High-risk for impaired skin integrity related to internal factor of altered metabolic state (hypothyroidism).

Assessment: Skin pale, cool, dry, and scaly.

(Refer Table 12.1 from chapter 12)

Nursing diagnosis

Altered nutrition: Less than body requirements related to inability to ingest or digest food; decreased body processes.

Assessment: Poor feeding, choking, thick tongue in infant; lethargy, reduced metabolic process, anorexia in child.

(Refer Table 14.3 from chapter 14)

Nursing diagnosis

Constipation related to less than adequate physical activity, decreased body process.

Assessment: Lethargy, decreased peristalsis, fatigue, reduced activity level.

(Refer Table 12.9 from chapter 12)

B. Specific Nursing Diagnoses and Nursing Process

Nursing diagnosis

Knowledge deficit of parent(s) and child related to lack of information about disorder (Table 19.4).

Table 19.4: Nursing interventions for knowledge deficit of parent(s) and child.

Interventions	Rationales
Assess knowledge of disorder, signs and symptoms for infant or child as appropriate, replacement therapy	Provides information needed to develop plan of instruction to ensure compliance with medical regimen
Inform parent(s) and child of cause of thyroid deficiency and need for prompt treatment in infants and for gradual increases in thyroxine in children to achieve euthyroidism	Provides thyroid replacement over 4–8 weeks in the child without causing hyperthyroidism

Contd...

Contd...

Interventions	Rationales
Instruct parent(s) and child in thyroid replacement including administering daily for life without missing doses, crushing and mixing with food, giving at breakfast time	Ensures compliance with correct administration of thyroid via oral route
Inform parent(s) and child to report nervousness, irritability, tachycardia, tremors, diarrhea	Indicates an excess of thyroid hormone and need for and adjustment in dosage
Inform parent(s) and child that improvement will be gradual as hormone levels are achieved and sleep, elimination, appetite, growth, and activity levels will improve	Promotes comfort and reduces anxiety caused by physical and mental changes brought about by the disorder; maintains realistic expectations from the treatment
Inform parent(s) that periodic laboratory tests are needed to monitor	Informs physician of thyroid levels maintained at a therapeutic level

Assessment: Request for information about cause and treatment of the disorder, thyroid replacement.

Evaluation
- Euthyroidism achieved
- Absence of signs and symptoms of hyperthyroidism
- Complies with daily thyroid replacement regimen
- Complies with periodic monitoring and follow-up care.

PRACTICE QUESTIONS

1. Baby Chandana 7-years child is diagnosed with juvenile diabetes. Draw a nursing care plan for baby Chandana by applying nursing process.
2. Write pre and postoperative management of a child undergone thyroidectomy.

CHAPTER 20

Nursing Process for the Child with Disorder of Eyes, Ears, Nose and Throat

LEARNING OBJECTIVES
- To identify the signs and symptoms of a child with eye, ear, nose and throat disorder.
- To frame nursing diagnosis based on the needs of the child.
- To plan nursing interventions and outcome identification.

INTRODUCTION

The eye, ear, nose and throat is a group affecting special organs that include eye (vision), ear (hearing), nose and throat, common disorders of these organs in children include chronic infections and the surgical procedures to correct them. Other conditions affecting these organs are included in the neurologic system.

NURSING PROCESS FOR THE CHILD WITH DISORDER OF EYES, EARS, NOSE AND THROAT

1. **Nursing diagnosis:** Sensory perception, disturbed (visual) related to visual impairment or blindness as evidenced by lack of reaction to visual stimuli, squinting and holding items close.
   Goal: Child will be able to reach maximal vision potential.
   Interventions: Improving vision.
   - Encourage corrective lens use for enhancement of vision
   - For the severely impaired or blind child, identify yourself via voice and name items in environment for the child, so that the child is aware of his or her surroundings
   - Support the family's efforts at vision therapy and other habilitation programs to promote vision enhancement
   - Engage the parents in bedside care giving because the parents' voice and presence are reassuring to the child.
   Evaluation: Child uses corrective lenses appropriately and is able to participate in play and schoolwork.
2. **Nursing diagnosis:** Sensory perception, disturbed (auditory) related to hearing loss as evidenced by lack of reaction to verbal stimuli, delayed attainment of language milestones.
   Goal: Child will reach maximal hearing and speech potential.
   Interventions: Improving hearing.
   - Assess hearing ability frequently because early detection of hearing loss allows for earlier intervention and correction
   - Assess language development at each visit to allow for early detection of hearing loss (earlier intervention and correction)
   - Encourage hearing aid use for amplification of sound

- Teach about hearing aid battery safety to avoid aspiration of battery
- Assist child with focusing on sounds in the environment to encourage listening skills
- Refer for and encourage attendance at communication habilitation program to maximize communication potential.

Evaluation: Child uses aids appropriately and communication effectively.

3. **Nursing diagnosis:** Risk for infection related to presence of infectious organisms as evidenced by fever, presence of virus or bacteria on laboratory screening.
   Goal: Child will be able to exhibit no signs of secondary infection and will not spread infection toothers.
   Interventions: Reducing infection risk.
   - Maintain aseptic technique and practice good handwashing to prevent introduction of further infectious agents
   - Limit number of visitors, screening for recent illness, to prevent further infection
   - Administer antibiotics if prescribed to prevent or treat bacterial infection
   - Encourage nutritious diet according to child's preferences to assist body's natural infection-fighting mechanisms
   - Isolate the child as required to prevent nosocomial spread of infection
   - Teach child and family preventive measures such as good handwashing, covering mouth and nose when coughing or sneezing, adequate disposal of used tissues to prevent nosocomial or community spread of infection.

   Evaluation: Symptoms of infection decrease over time, and others remain free from infection.

4. **Nursing diagnosis:** Growth and development delay, related to sensory impairment as evidenced by delay in attainment of developmental milestones.
   Goal: Child will be able to achieve optimum independence for age.
   Interventions: Encouraging growth and development.
   - Encourage attainment of development milestones with use of assistive devices as needed for timely developmental achievements
   - Foster independence in activities of daily livings (ADLs) to promote sense of accomplishment
   - Encourage participation in play with another child or within a group to promote socialization
   - Assist family to set limits and apply discipline because structure and routine provide a secure environment in which the developing child can grow
   - Encourage friendships with other children with a sensory impairment to promote socialization and let the child know that he or she is not the only one with these challenges.

   Evaluation: Child participates in age appropriate developmental activities.

5. **Nursing diagnosis:** Impaired verbal communication related to hearing loss as evidenced by lack of or inarticulate speech, lack of alternate communication channel.
   Goal: The child will be able to communicate effectively with the method chosen by the family.
   Interventions: Improving communication.
   - Encourage choice of and attendance at communication habilitation program to promote continued learning

- Provide consistency between home and hospital in regard to communication style/devices to promote continued learning
- Support the child's efforts at correct speech to promote speech development through reinforcement and praise
- Encourage family to use spoken language and read books at home to continue to promote appropriate language development.

Evaluation: Uses sign language, oral/deaf speech, cued speech or augmentative alternative communication device as per the preferences of family.

6. **Nursing diagnosis:** Deficient knowledge related to sensory impairment (vision or hearing) as evidenced by new diagnosis and parents' questions.
   Goal: Parents will able to express understanding of diagnosis and care of child.
   Interventions: Educating the family.
   - Review diagnosis and plan of care with the parents to promote understanding of the disease process
   - Refer family to resources available for sensory impaired children to provide further education and support to the parents
   - Demonstrate medical treatments prescribed or use of assistive devices, requiring a return demonstration, which shows the parents' ability to provide the prescribed care for the child
   - Encourage exploration of different communication and learning modes available for the sensory impaired child to allow the child and family to find the right educational and communication style fit.

   Evaluation: Parents verbalize understanding, demonstrate use of assistive devices or independently perform medical treatments.

7. **Nursing diagnosis:** Family processes, interrupted, related to child's sensory impairment as evidenced by parent verbalization, non-verbal language altered coping.
   Goal: Parents will be able to demonstrate adequate coping and decreased anxiety.
   Interventions: Encouraging appropriate family interactions.
   - Encourage parents verbalization of grief if child is hearing or vision impaired, parents must deal with their own feelings of loss to successfully care for the child with an impairment
   - Encourage parent's verbalization of concerns related to child's illness; this allows for identification of concerns and demonstrates to the family that the nurse also cares about them, not just the child
   - Explain therapy, procedures, and child's behavior to parents; developing an understanding of the child's current status helps decrease anxiety
   - Encourage parental involvement in care, so that parents may continue to feel needed and valued.

   Evaluation: Parents are involved in child's care, ask appropriate questions, and are able to discuss child's care and condition calmly.

8. **Nursing diagnosis:** Risk for injury related to vision loss as evidenced by difficulty navigating surroundings.
   Goal: The infant or child will be able to remain free from injury.

Interventions: Preventing injury.
- Orient the child to hospital surroundings because awareness is the first step to preventing injury
- Encourage parent to be at bedside, so that the child feels more comfortable
- Encourage use of assistive devise to promote safety.

Evaluation: The infant or child remains free from injury.

NURSING PROCESS FOR SPECIFIC EYE, EAR, NOSE AND THROAT DISORDERS

Allergic Rhinitis

Allergic rhinitis is an episodic or perennial upper respiratory tract condition characterized by sneezing, itching nose and eyes, and discharge from the nose and throat. Chronic nasal stuffiness and obstruction to air flow cause mouth breathing, otitis media, and Eustachian tube abnormalities. Allergic rhinitis may manifest itself at any age in childhood (**Fig. 20.1**).

Symptoms of Allergic Rhinitis

- Itchy nose, mouth, eyes, throat, skin, or any area
- Problems with smell
- Runny nose
- Sneezing
- Watery eyes.

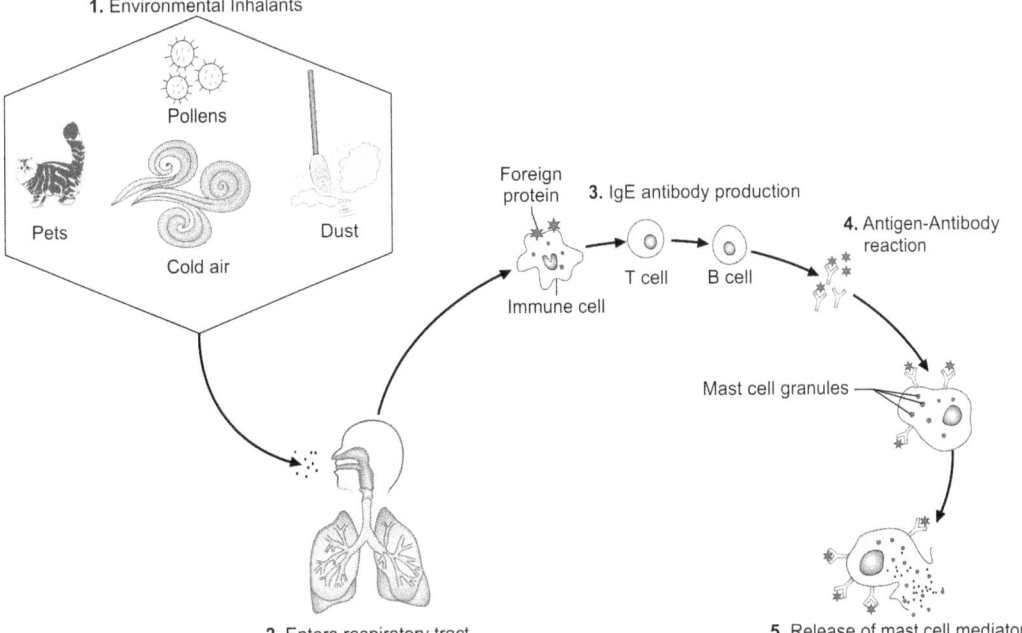

Fig. 20.1: Pathophysiology of allergic rhinitis.

Symptoms that may develop later include:
- Stuffy nose (nasal congestion)
- Coughing
- Clogged ears and decreased sense of smell
- Sore throat
- Dark circles under the eyes
- Puffiness under the eye
- Fatigue and irritability
- Headache.

Nursing Management

A. Essential Nursing Diagnoses and Nursing Process Associated with this Condition

Nursing diagnosis

Ineffective breathing pattern related to inflammatory process, obstruction.

Assessment: Nose stuffiness and obstruction, mouth breathing, mucus secretion and drainage, respiratory changes, breathing difficulty.

(Refer Table 14.2 from chapter 14)

Nursing diagnosis

Sleep pattern disturbance related to internal factors of illness.

Assessment: Interrupted sleep, irritability, restlessness, inability to breath through nose.

(Refer Table 14.10 from chapter 14)

B. Specific Nursing Diagnoses and Nursing Process

Nursing diagnosis

High-risk for infection related to chronic disease (allergy), insufficient knowledge to avoid exposure to pathogens **(Table 20.1)**.

Assessment: Nasal discharge, red, itchy conjunctiva, purulent discharge from nose or eyes, allergic shiners, frequent colds, otitis media with pain and temperature elevation, pharyngitis.

Evaluation
- Demonstrates proper disposal of materials contaminated with respiratory secretions
- Demonstrates proper handwashing technique
- Protects from exposure to upper respiratory infections
- Correctly administers full course of antibiotic
- Complies with desensitization schedule
- Maintains an allergen-free environment
- Reports signs and symptoms of impending or existing infectious process
- Relieves allergic rhinitis symptoms with prescribed antihistamines, decongestants, steroid administration by oral, spray or inhalation route.

Table 20.1: Nursing interventions for high-risk for infection.

Interventions	Rationales
Assess for rubbing of nose, nasal discharge and its characteristics (clear, amount, purulent, (dark areas around eye, nose itching and pushing hand up and back of nose, frequent sneezing, red and itchy eyes with drainage or watering	Provides information about physical and behavioral effects of allergic rhinitis; chronic nasal obstruction causes edema and discoloration of the eyes and mouth breathing, wrinkling of face is caused by attempt to avoid rubbing or scratching of nose
Inspect nasal passages and throat with penlight for redness, swelling, and presence of mucus and/or exudates; check skin around nares for redness, irritation	Reveals inflammation and risk of infection spread
Assess for knowledge and use of preventive measures needed to avoid spread of microorganisms	Provides basis for information needed for health maintenance
Assess for frequency of upper respiratory infections among family members; attendance at school, day-care, nursery school	Persistent reinfection usually the result of repeated exposures to microorganisms
Assess use of over-the-counter medications and type used	Combination products are not particularly useful; symptomatic treatment more effective in controlling upper respiratory responses
Provide vaporizer or humidifier if nasal and oral mucous membranes	Maintains moist mucous membranes to prevent breaks and soreness
Administer antihistamines and immunotherapy if ordered alone or in combination with decongestants	Provides control of the symptoms when exposed to allergens

Otitis Media/Myringotomy and Insertion of Tube

Otitis media, the most common disease of childhood, is a viral or bacterial infection of the middle ear. It often results from an upper respiratory infection. Otitis media may be acute or chronic, with recurrent episodes in infants and young children. Acute otitis media is most frequently caused by *Streptococcus pneumoniae* or *Haemophilus influenzae*, while chronic otitis media is caused by *Staphylococcus aureus* or *Haemophilus influenzae*. The most serious complication of the disorder is hearing impairment from prolonged middle ear disorders. It may be a functional impairment with hearing loss that is conductive and not severe. It may also be a structural impairment in which the tympanic membrane retracts as negative pressure with in the ear causes the membrane to be drawn inward. This results in impaired sound transmission.

Myringotomy is a surgical procedure performed to equalize middle ear pressure by inserting tubes into the tympanic membrane to facilitate drainage. The tympanostomy tubes remain in place about 6 months, at which time they spontaneously fall out. The procedure prevents fluid retention in the middle ear, promotes healing of the membrane, and prevent scarring of the membrane **(Fig. 20.2)**.

Symptoms of Otitis Media

Adolescents and older children:
- Ear aching or pain and temporary hearing loss. These symptoms usually come on suddenly.

Nursing Process for the Child with Disorder of Eyes, Ears, Nose and Throat

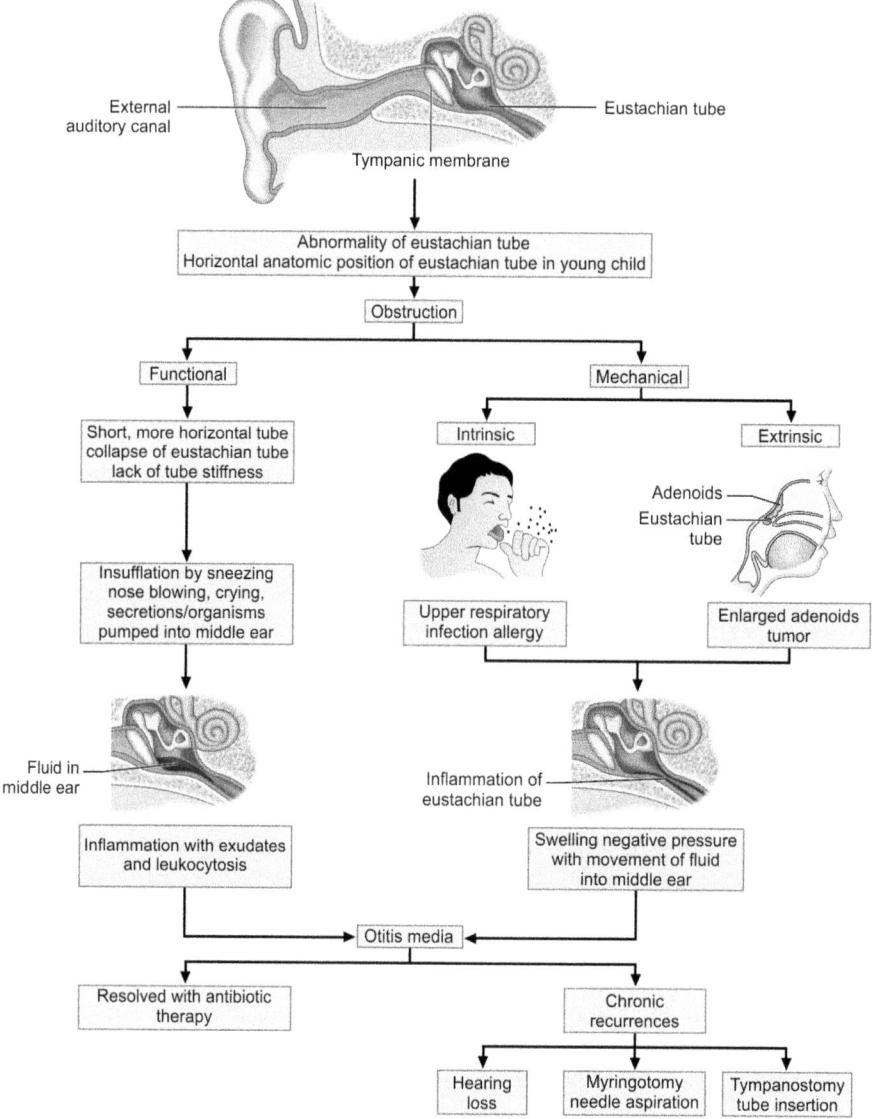

Fig. 20.2: Pathophysiology of otitis media/myringotomy and insertion of tube.

Infants and young children:
- Fever (temperature higher than 100.4°F or 38°C)
- Pulling on the ear
- Fussiness or irritability
- Decreased activity
- Lack of appetite or difficulty eating
- Vomiting or diarrhea

Myringotomy (Tympanostomy; Tympanotomy; Ear Tubes Surgery)

Definition

A myringotomy is a procedure to put a hole in the ear drum. This is done so that fluid trapped in the middle ear can drain out. The fluid may be blood, pus, and/or water. In many cases, a small tube is inserted into the hole in the ear drum. The tube helps to maintain drainage.

Possible Complications

Problems from the procedure are rare, but all procedures have some risk.
- Bleeding
- Infection
- Chronic scarring
- Failure of the myringotomy incision in the ear drum to heal as expected, which may result in frequent drainage
- Hearing loss
- Injury to ear structures other than the ear drum
- Need for repeat surgery.

Nursing Management

A. Essential Nursing Diagnoses and Nursing Process Associated with the Conditions

Nursing diagnosis

Hyperthermia related to illness (inflammation).

Assessment: Increase in body temperature above normal range; flushed skin, warm to touch; increased pulse and respiration rate.

(Refer Table 14.18 from chapter 14)

Nursing diagnosis

Altered nutrition: Less than body requirements related to ingest food.

Assessment: Anorexia, vomiting.

(Refer Table 14.3 from chapter 14)

Nursing diagnosis

High-risk for fluid volume deficit related to excessive losses through normal routes.

Assessment: Vomiting, diarrhea, diaphoresis, elevated temperature, altered intake.

(Refer Table 14.11 from chapter 14)

B. Specific Nursing Diagnoses and Nursing Process

Nursing diagnosis

Pain related to biological injuring agents (infection) **(Table 20.2)**.

Assessment: Communication of pain descriptors, red tympanic membrane, irritability, pulling on ear, earache, tilting of the head, cough, drainage from ear.

Nursing Process for the Child with Disorder of Eyes, Ears, Nose and Throat

Table 20.2: Nursing interventions for pain.

Interventions	Rationales
Assess verbal and non-verbal behavior, type and location and severity. Using a pain scale and include irritability; fever; pulling at ear; red, bulging tympanic membrane, in the infant, anorexia and earache, fever, cough, congestion, drainage from ear, temporary change in auditory acuity, red, bulging tympanic membrane	Provides information about pain and manifestations that vary with age
Administer analgesic, antipyretic, and antibiotic as ordered	Reduces pain and fever; destroys cell and wall of bacterial agents to decrease infectious process; usually given for 10 days
Promote rest and avoid disturbing unnecessarily	Promotes rest and reduces stimuli that decrease pain
Apply dry heat or cold to affected ear based on pain relief and comfort achievement	Facilitates drainage if heat is applied; reduces edema and pressure if cold is applied
Cleanse external canal with cotton ball and hydrogen peroxide if needed	Provides drainage removal from ear without introducing pathogens
Place child in lying position on side of affected ear	Promotes drainage from the affected ear

Evaluation
- Complies with medication administration regimen
- Maintains comfort and rest needs for child
- Controls ear pain.

Nursing diagnosis

Knowledge deficit of parent(s) and child related to lack of information about condition (Table 20.3).

Assessment: Request for information about cause of condition, prevention of reinfection, postoperative care for myringotomy and tube insertion.

Evaluation
- Prevents reinfection of middle ear with compliance with medical regimen
- Avoids activities that expose infected middle ear or ear with tube placement to risk of infection
- Complies with postoperative care for tube insertion as instructed
- Takes measures to prevent reinfection
- Verbalizes surgical procedure and postoperative care for tube insertion (myringotomy).

Strabismus

Strabismus, sometimes known as "cross eye," is non-binocular vision in which one eye deviated from the point of fixation. The weaker eye becomes lazy, and the brain eventually suppresses the image in the eye. Strabismus is caused by muscle paralysis or imbalance, poor vision, or congenital factors. Correction may be nonsurgical, or if that is unsuccessful, surgical, to align

Table 20.3: Nursing interventions for knowledge deficit of parent(s) and child.

Interventions	Rationales
Assess past infections, knowledge of ear condition and treatments to prevent complications; knowledge of surgical procedure to insert tubes that provide drainage of middle ear	Provides information needed by parent(s) about infection
Inform parent(s) of causes of otitis media in infant and child and of tendency of repeated infections depending on age group	Provides information about physiological aspects of the ear canal and frequent upper respiratory infections that lead to ear obstruction and infection
Inform parent(s) to feed infant in upright position, to discourage forceful blowing of nose in child, and to encourage gum chewing and blowing games	Preventive measures to control ear infections and promote aeration of the middle ear
Reinforce teaching of antibiotic therapy for 10 days to 2 weeks	Ensures that infection has been eradicated
Inform parent(s) that hearing acuity is lost temporarily during acute stage, and to face child and speak loudly at close proximity	Reduces anxiety of parent(s) when child does not respond to words spoken to them
Inform of surgical procedure to place tubes in the middle ear that drain area in back of tympanic membrane and equalize pressure; that tubes remain for 6 months to 1 year, eventually falling out without further intervention	Inform parent(s) of procedure to promote continuous drainage, ventilation of ear and prevent further infections if condition is chronic or does not respond to traditional therapy
Instruct parent(s) and child in care of tubes following surgery, including avoiding use of shampoo; keeping bath, swimming, or other water out of ear; maintaining dry ear wick that is placed in ear; cleansing area and applying zinc oxide or vaseline to the area if draining and excoriating skin	Prevents entry of water or contaminated substances into ear canal or via tubes, and maintains skin integrity of the area by removing normal drainage for 1–2 days following surgery
Report any hearing impairment, pain behind ear, lethargy, increasing temperature, purulent drainage	Allows for immediate interventions to prevent hearing loss, mastoid infection, or reinfection
Instruct child to avoid noseblowing, swimming, diving, or any activities that allow water to enter ear for 10 days; use ear plug if practical for bathing or swimming	Informs child of actions to take to prevent disruption

the eyes. Left undiagnosed and treated, strabismus may lead to amblyopia and vision loss (**Fig. 20.3**).

Esotropia

Esotropia describes an inward turning of your eye and is the most common type of strabismus in infants. Young children with esotropia do not use their eyes together.

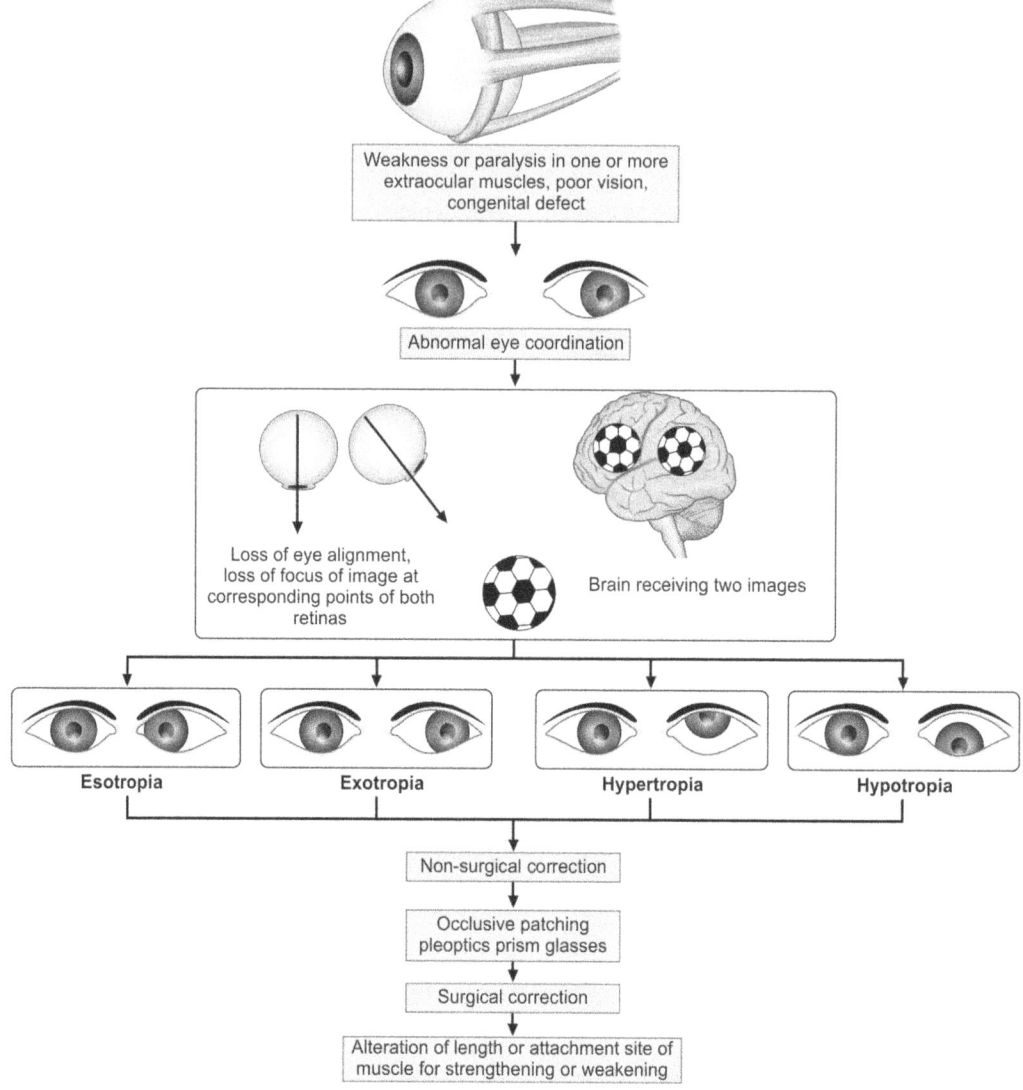

Fig. 20.3: Pathophysiology of strabismus.

"Accommodative esotropia" is a common form of esotropia that is first seen in farsighted children, usually 1–4 years of age or older. When children are young, they can focus their eyes to adjust for farsightedness, a common condition in children. However, the focusing effort (accommodation) required to see clearly stimulates the eyes to converge, or cross.

"Sensory esotropia" is the crossing of an eye with poor vision.

Symptoms
- Decreased vision
- Decreased depth perception
- Crossing or inward deviation of the eyes, often intermittently at first.

Exotropia

Exotropia—or an outward turning of the eyes—is a common type of strabismus accounting for up to 25 percent of all ocular misalignment in early childhood. Transient intermittent exotropia is sometimes seen in the first 4–6 weeks of life and, if mild, can resolve spontaneously by 6–8 weeks of age. Constant exotropia is only rarely present at birth (congenital). More commonly, exotropia develops between 1–4 years of age, first seen only intermittently, particularly when the child is daydreaming, ill, tired, or when a child is focusing on distant objects.

Symptoms
- Decreased vision
- Decreased depth perception
- Outward deviation of the eyes, often intermittently at first
- Sensitivity (closing one eye) in bright light

Hypertropia

Hypertropia is characterized by the misalignment of the eyes, in which the visual axis of one eye is higher than the other.

Hypotropia

In which there is permanent downward deviation of the visual axis of one eye.

Nursing Management

A. Essential Nursing Diagnoses and Nursing Process Associated with this Condition

Nursing diagnosis

Altered growth and development related to perceptual impairment (vision).

Assessment: Reported, measured, or observed impairment of visual acuity, change in behavior pattern, change in response to stimuli; visual distortions.

(Refer Table 14.4 from chapter 14)

B. Specific Nursing Diagnoses and Nursing Process

Nursing diagnosis

Knowledge deficit related to lack of information about condition and treatment **(Table 20.4)**.

Assessment: Request for information about abnormal eye deviation and treatments to prevent complication and preserve vision.

Evaluation
- Complies with prescribed therapy and procedures
- Administers medications correctly
- Performs proper use and care of glasses, patching of eye
- Verbalizes surgical procedure and responsibilities for cooperation
- Prevents complication from strabismus
- Adapts to body image change caused by eye appearance until eye is corrected
- Complies with ongoing follow-up physician visits and eye examinations.

Nursing Process for the Child with Disorder of Eyes, Ears, Nose and Throat

Table 20.4: Nursing interventions for knowledge deficit.

Interventions	Rationales
Assess visual acuity using Snellen chart, cover test, or Hirschberg test depending on age of child; note obvious deviations and direction of deviation	Provides screening for visual deficit and muscle balance or deviation
Inform child to note diplopia, headache, photophobia, inability to see clearly or focus from one distance to another; parent(s) to note frowning or squinting eyes together, tilting head to one side, closing one eye to see	Indicates strabismus and behavior changes associated with it
Inform parent(s) that the condition results from a weakness or paralysis of the eye muscle(s) or that the child may have been born with the defect; that condition Is treated with prescription glasses, occlusion patching of the good eye, or surgery to prevent amblyopia, which leads to vision loss	Identifies cause of the disorder for the parent(s) and suggests possible treatments to correct the condition
Instruct parent(s) and child in eye-patching treatment to improve use and function of the affected eye; apply patch to good eye for 8 weeks, or 1 week for each year of child's age, and do not remove it except to stimulate good eye	Promotes use of the deviated eye by patching good eye
Instruct parent(s) and child about wearing glasses and caring for the glasses, including cleansing with soft cloth or tissue, keeping the glasses in a case when not wearing them, handling the glasses on the frame part when putting on or taking off and cleaning, using straps to keep glasses form falling off; allow child to assist in the selection of the glasses	Promotes correction with proper use of glasses
Instruct the child in eye exercises if ordered	Promotes muscle use and corrects deviation
Inform parent(s) and child of surgical procedure to preserve vision and improve appearance of the deviated eye, that medication will be given for pain, that eyes will be patched following surgery and restraints may be needed temporarily to prevent touching or rubbing eye, that some eye drainage will be present for 24 to 48 hours; use a doll and allow the child to play the situation to expect before and after surgery	Provides information, if surgery is proposed to correct deviation rather than restore vision; therapeutic play informs the child of procedures to expect from surgery
Instruct parent(s) in administration of eye drops and/or application of ophthalmic ointment as ordered	Provides information and procedure for correct administration of medications
Inform parent(s) and child of importance of performing procedures and therapies as instructed and of making follow-up visits to ophthalmologist	Promotes compliance of corrective therapy

Tonsillitis/Tonsillectomy and Adenoidectomy

Tonsillitis is the infection of the tonsils, which are lymphoid organs located in the pharynx. The tonsils are thought to filter pathogens from the air and food entering the respiratory and gastrointestinal tracts. The palatine tonsils appear on both sides of the oropharynx, and the pharyngeal tonsils (adenoid) appear on the posterior wall of the nasopharynx above the palatine tonsils. The inflammation of these organs usually occurs with pharyngitis and may be caused by viral or bacterial pathogens. A viral cause is more common in children under 3 years of age, and a bacterial cause (B hemolytic streptococci, group A) is more common in children over 6 years of age. The swelling associated with the inflammation causes difficulty in breathing and swallowing and may result in mouth breathing which, if chronic, affects taste and smell.

Tonsillectomy and adenoidectomy are the surgical removal of these organs and are usually reserved for hypertrophy and obstruction of air flow. They are usually performed after 4 years of age, although an adenoidectomy may be indicated earlier if the child is suffering from recurrent otitis media, hearing loss, and obstructed nasal breathing **(Fig. 20.4)**.

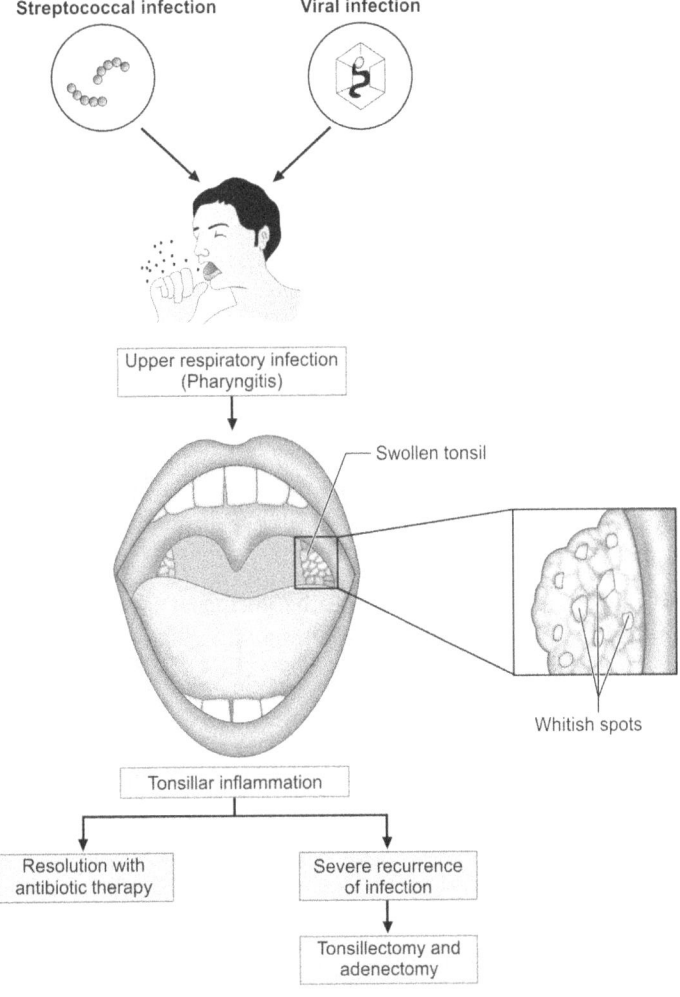

Fig. 20.4: Pathophysiology of tonsillitis.

Symptoms of Tonsillitis

Tonsillitis most commonly affects children between preschool ages and the mid-teenage years. Common signs and symptoms of tonsillitis include:
- Red, swollen tonsils
- White or yellow coating or patches on the tonsils
- Sore throat
- Difficult or painful swallowing
- Fever
- Enlarged, tender glands (lymph nodes) in the neck
- A scratchy, muffled or throaty voice
- Bad breath
- Stomachache, particularly in younger children
- Stiff neck
- Headache.

In young children who are unable to describe how they feel, signs of tonsillitis may include:
- Drooling due to difficult or painful swallowing
- Refusal to eat
- Unusual fussiness.

Nursing Management

A. Essential Nursing Diagnoses and Nursing Process Associated with these Conditions

Nursing diagnosis

Ineffective breathing pattern
1. Related to inflammatory process

    Assessment: Temperature elevation, throat pain, malaise, pharyngeal and tonsillar edema, head congestion, swallowing difficulty, enlarged cervical nodes, red throat with white or yellow exudates, lethargy, hearing difficulty, nasal speech, positive culture of infectious agent.
2. Related to tracheobronchial obstruction

    Assessment: Cough, nasal stuffiness and discharge, throat edema, mouth breathing, rapid respirations, respiratory depth changes, breathing difficulty.

    (Refer Table 14.2 from chapter 14)

Nursing diagnosis

High-risk for fluid volume deficit related to excessive losses through normal routes; deviations affecting fluid intake.

Assessment: Dry skin and mucous membranes, thirst, decreased skin turgor, increased body temperature, increased pulse rate, dysphagia, throat pain and edema, blood loss following surgery, NPO status, vomiting, dysphasia.

(Refer Table 14.11 from chapter 14)

Nursing diagnosis

Hyperthermia related to upper respiratory inflammation/infection illness.

Assessment: Increase of body temperature above normal range, increased respiratory and pulse rates, flushed, hot skin, low grade fever in nasopharyngitis, higher temperature of 100°F or more in streptococcal pharyngitis and tonsillitis.

(Refer Table 14.18 from chapter 14)

B. Specific Nursing Diagnoses and Nursing Process

Nursing diagnosis

Pain related to injuring biological agent (inflammation/infection) **(Table 20.5)**.

Table 20.5: Nursing interventions for pain.

Interventions	Rationales
Assess site of pain, verbal or non-verbal responses of holding or rubbing site of pain, irritability, pointing to site, restlessness, dependent behaviors, crying, groaning, whining, stating of general location and severity of pain	Expression of pain varies with age, developmental level, and is unique to particular child and learned emotional responses; degree of pain, fatigue influences ability of child to perceive and identify discomfort
Inspect throat for redness, swelling, presence of mucus or pus, examine dry, irritated oropharynx with a penlight; note mouth breathing, lethargy, halitosis, nasal speech, or hearing difficulty	Provides clues to source of pain and manifestations of tonsils and adenoids inflammation causing changes in breathing, taste, and smell perception as the enlarged adenoids block the air from passing behind the nares. This results In mouth breathing, dry mouth, and changes in voice sounds as the air is not able to be trapped for speech resulting in a nasal or muffled sound
Assess postoperative pain in throat for severity, associated bleeding, and difficulty in swallowing	Provides information which forms basis for analgesic therapy, to treat pain caused by raw surfaces left by tonsillectomy
Assess effect on food and fluid intake, and effect on rest and sleep patterns as a result of throat pain and/or obstruction of passage of food, fluids, and air	Provides information about pain resulting from tonsillitis or tonsillectomy and associated manifestations of impaired swallowing and restlessness
Administer analgesic and/or antibiotic; for tonsillitis, inject IM antibiotic deeply into large muscle (vastus lateralis in young child, and gluteus in older child)	Analgesic relieves pain, and antibiotic destroys *Streptococcus* by interfering with cell wall synthesis
Provide analgesic for postoperative pain; non-pharmacologic pain-reduction interventions including ice collar, relaxation techniques, music therapy	Promotes continuous comfort and pain relief PO, IV, or rectally for about 24 hours postoperatively, and provides diversion from pain stimuli; ice promotes vasoconstriction, which reduces edema and pain

Contd...

Nursing Process for the Child with Disorder of Eyes, Ears, Nose and Throat

Contd...

Interventions	Rationales
Provide cool, mild fluids to drink, ice chips q2h, and soft foods to eat if child accepts food; hard candies to suck on or gum to chew; warm gargle for older child or throat irrigation for younger child; throat lozenges, if appropriate, for tonsillitis	Promotes comfort and maintain fluids, moistens and soothes throat by increasing saliva production; warm throat irrigation reduces inflammation in the younger child, and the older child may be able to gargle
Postoperatively provide cool, bland fluids for 24 hours, followed by soft, bland foods; avoid irritating, highly seasoned, rough, solid foods or acidic or irritating fluids	Provides fluids and nutrients that do not irritate sore throat or aggravate surgical site and cause bleeding
Place on abdomen or side in position of comfort	Promotes comfort and rest, which reduce pain and allow for drainage

Assessment: Complaints of throat soreness, difficulty in swallowing, headache and muscle aches, crying, restlessness, listless, drooling, edema, bright red pus on tonsillar tissue, enlarged cervical nodes, postoperative pain in throat.

Evaluation
- Verbalizes that pain is reduced or controlled
- Swallows allowed fluids and foods without discomfort
- Provides both pharmacologic and non-pharmacologic relief measures to reduce pain
- Promotes rest and diversional activities
- Avoids fluids and foods that increase throat pain.

Nursing diagnosis

Knowledge deficit of parent(s) and child related to lack of information about condition (Table 20.6).

Table 20.6: Nursing interventions for knowledge deficit of parent(s) and child.

Interventions	Rationales
Assess frequency of tonsillitis, knowledge of treatment; knowledge of surgical procedure to remove tonsils and adenoids and prognosis	Provides information about infection and surgery if contemplated
Inform parent(s) of causes of recurrent infections, need for surgery, procedure performed, and preoperative preparation	Reduces anxiety caused by lack of information and not knowing what to expect
Explain importance of having throat culture done if sore throat and temperature present; instruct in administration of analgesic, antipyretic, and antibiotic as prescribed, all of medication should be taken, even though child feels better in 24–48 hours	Identifies bacterial infection of throat that will respond to antibiotic therapy

Contd...

Contd...

Interventions	Rationales
Inform parent(s) and child that medication will be given for pain; that IV will be given for pain fluid maintenance, as needed, for 24 hours; that throat will be observed for bleeding; and that some secretions, bleeding, and possibly vomiting is usual	Provides information about postoperative treatments
Inform parent(s) and child that coughing, clearing throat, placing hard objects in mouth, brushing teeth, or gargling should be avoided, and that drainage should be expectorated and not swallowed	Prevents irritation of operative site of throat
Reinforce instruction in which type of foods and fluid to take and which to avoid, and to position on side when asleep and upright when eating or drinking; instruct in diet progression as pain and discomfort subside	Prevents irritation to throat and aspiration of drainage, food or fluids
Inform parent(s) and child that ear pain, slight temperature, and mouth odor may occur postoperatively; and to report persistent temperature and bleeding that is bright red and occurs a week after surgery	Assures parent(s) that these occur as a result of surgery and only need reporting if they persist
Inform parent(s) and child that limited activities and school attendance are usually resumed 2 weeks after surgery but that child should be kept quiet and indoors for 2 days following surgery operation	Provides information about return to normal parameters by 3 weeks postoperatively

Assessment: Request for information about prevention and treatment for tonsillitis, and about pre and postoperative care for tonsillectomy/adenoidectomy.

Evaluation
- Prevents reinfection of throat with correct compliance with medication regimen
- Avoids activities that irritate or cause risk of complication following surgery
- Complies with postoperative care for fluid, food, rest, activity regimen
- Verbalizes surgical procedure and postoperative measures
- Reports severe and/or persistent symptoms of tonsillitis or postoperative complications
- Secures throat culture if ordered.

PRACTICE QUESTIONS

1. Baby Laya is admitted in pediatric surgical ward with the diagnosis of tonsillitis. Write the pre and postoperative management for baby Laya.
2. Draw a nursing care plan for the child diagnosed with otitis media.

CHAPTER 21

Nursing Process for the Child with Integumentary Disorder

LEARNING OBJECTIVES
- To understand the age specific needs of the preschool child.
- To establish nursing diagnosis based on the needs of the preschool child.
- To plan the nursing interventions for a preschool child.
- To evaluate the nursing interventions.

INTRODUCTION

The integumentary system includes the skin and associated structures or appendages, which are hair, nails, and sensory skin receptors. Skin acts as a barrier to retain body fluids and electrolytes, a regulator of body heat, and a receptor of sensory stimuli (tactile, pain, heat and cold). It is made up of three layers including the epidermis (outer layer), and the dermis (thicker layer directly under the epidermis), and the subcutaneous (fat and connective tissue under the dermis). Its appearance reflects the general health of an infant or child. Changes in the skin that alter appearance are a source of psychological stress and embarrassment to children. Common integumentary conditions of childhood are infections, lesions, wounds, and dermatitis disorders.

NURSING PROCESS FOR THE CHILD WITH INTEGUMENTARY DISORDER (IN GENERAL)

1. **Nursing diagnosis:** Impaired skin integrity related to infectious process, hypersensitivity reaction, injury or mechanical factors as evidenced by rash, inflammation, abrasion, laceration or disrupted epidermis.
   Goal: Child will be able to restore integrity of skin surface.
   Interventions: Restoring skin integrity.
   - Assess site of skin impairment to determine extent of involvement and plan care
   - Monitor skin impairment every shift for changes in color, warmth, redness, or other signs of infection to identify problems early
   - Determine the child's and family's skincare practices to determine need for education related to skin care
   - Individualize the child's skin care regimen depending on the child's particular skin condition to most appropriately care for skin in light of the child's disorder
   - In the immobile child, use a risk assessment tool (such as a modified Norton or Braden scale) to identify risk for skin breakdown
   - Position the child on the opposite side of the skin impairment to avoid further skin breakdown
   - Encourage appropriate nutritional intake as adequate nutrients are necessary for appropriate immune function and skin healing

- Consult the wound and ostomy care nurse specialist to determine best approach for individualized wound care
- Provide dressing change and wound care as prescribed to promote wound or burn healing.

Evaluation: Attained healing of rash, abrasion, laceration or other skin disruption.

2. **Nursing diagnosis:** Risk for infection related to disruption in protective skin barrier.
   Goal: Child will be able to remain free of local or systemic infection.
   Interventions: Preventing infection.
   - Use appropriate hand hygiene to decrease transmission of infectious organisms
   - Assess the skin impairment site for increased warmth, redness, discharge, or new purulence to identify infection early
   - Assess temperature every 4 hours or more frequently if needed, as children develop fever quickly in response to infection
   - Note white blood cell and culture results, reporting unexpected values to the primary care provider, so that appropriate treatment may be started
   - Follow prescribed therapies for skin alteration to maintain skin moisture and prevent further breakdown, which may lead to infection
   - Encourage appropriate nutritional intake as adequate nutrients are necessary for appropriate immune function and skin healing.

   Evaluation: Child remains afebrile, without additional redness or warmth at skin disruption site.

3. **Nursing diagnosis:** Disturbed body image related to chronic skin changes caused by disease process, burns, or other skin alteration as evidenced by child's verbalization, reluctance to participate in activities or social withdrawal.
   Goal: Child will be able to verbalize or demonstrate.
   Interventions: Promoting appropriate body image.
   - Assess child or teen for feelings about alteration in skin to determine baseline
   - Acknowledge feelings of anger or depression related to skin changes to provide an outlet for feelings
   - Encourage the child or teen to participate in skin care to give some sense of control over what is occurring
   - Help the child or teen to accept self as the perception of self is tied to knowing oneself and identifying what the self-values.

   Evaluation: Child returns to previous level of social involvement.

4. **Nursing diagnosis:** Risk for deficient fluid volume related to burns.
   Goal: Child will be able to maintain balanced fluid volume.
   Interventions: Promoting fluid balance.
   - Assess fluid volume status at least every shift, more frequently if disrupted, to obtain baseline for comparison
   - Strictly monitor intake and output to detect imbalance or need for additional fluid intake
   - Weigh the child daily on the same scale, at the same time, in the same amount of clothing as changes in weight are an accurate indicator of fluid volume status in children
   - Provide intravenous fluid resuscitation in initial period, followed by encouragement of oral fluid intake in the burned patient, to compensate for fluid loss through burned areas.

   Evaluation: Urine output 1–2 mL/kg/h. Oral mucosa moist and pink.

5. **Nursing diagnosis:** Imbalanced nutrition, less than body requirements, related to increase metabolic state (burns) as evidenced by poor wound healing, difficulty gaining or maintaining bodyweight.
   Goal: Child will be able to demonstrate balanced nutritional state.
   Interventions: Promoting nutrition.
   - Assess the child's food preferences and ability to eat provides a baseline for planning nursing care
   - Consult the nutritionist because nutritional needs are increased related to altered metabolic state as a result of burns
   - Collaborate with the nutritionist, child, and parents to plan meals that appeal to the child to increase the child's intake
   - Administer vitamin and mineral preparations as prescribed to supplements nutrients
   - Provide smaller, more frequent meals and snacks to promote increased intake
   - Weigh the child daily to determine progress.

   Evaluation: Child maintains or gain weight as appropriate for situation, will demonstrate improvement.

NURSING PROCESS FOR SPECIFIC INTEGUMENTARY DISORDERS

Burns/Skin Graft

Burns, which are injuries to the skin and underlying tissues caused by flames, electricity, contact with hot articles or water, or radiation therapy affect children of all ages. They are classified according to severity, source, and extent of surface involved. Most burn injuries occur in children under 5 years of age. Severe burns affect all systems with local responses that include edema, circulatory stasis, and fluid loss. Systemic responses include circulation alteration, anemia, fluid loss, metabolic alteration, acidosis, and stress response. Burns that involve over 10% of body surface require hospitalization with management of ventilation, fluid and electrolyte imbalance, pain control, nutrition, wound care, infection prevention, skin grafting, and rehabilitation **(Fig. 21.1)**.

Symptoms of Burns

First-degree Burns

First-degree burns, the mildest of the three, are limited to the top layer of skin:
- *Signs and symptoms:* These burns produce redness, pain, and minor swelling. The skin is dry without blisters.
- *Healing time:* Healing time is about 3 to 6 days; the superficial skin layer over the burn may peel off in 1 or 2 days.

Second-degree Burns

Second-degree burns are more serious and involve the skin layers beneath the top layer:
- *Signs and symptoms:* These burns produce blister, severe pain, and redness. The blisters sometimes break open and the area is wet looking with a bright pink to cherry red color.
- *Healing time:* Healing time varies depending on the severity of the burn. It can take up to 3 weeks or more.

Nursing Process for the Child with Integumentary Disorder

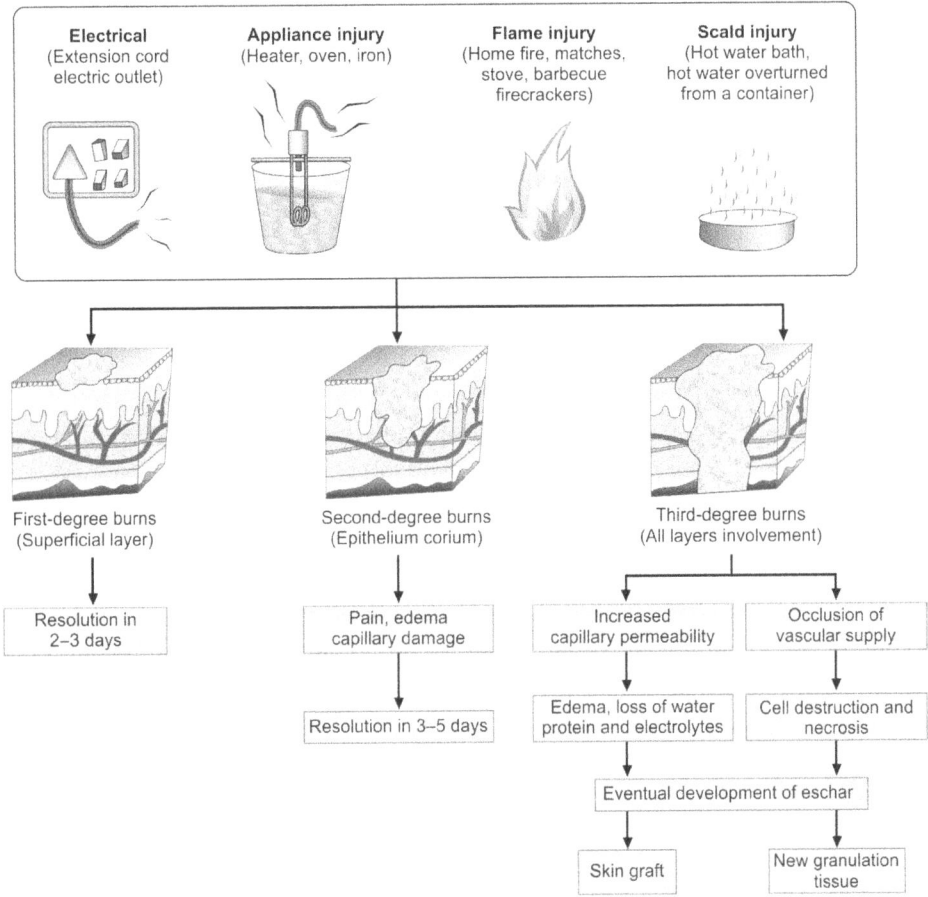

Fig. 21.1: Pathophysiology of burns.

Third-degree Burns

Third-degree burns are the most serious type of burn and involve all the layers of the skin and underlying tissue:
- *Signs and symptoms:* The surface appears dry and can look waxy white, leathery, brown, or charred. There may be little or no pain or the area may feel numb at first because of nerve damage.
- *Healing time:* Healing time depends on the severity of the burn. Deep second- and third-degree burns (called full-thickness burns) will likely need to be treated with skin grafts, in which healthy skin is taken from another part of the body and surgically placed over the burn wound to help the area heal.

Nursing Management

A. Essential Nursing Diagnosis and Nursing Process Associated with this Condition

Nursing diagnosis

High-risk for impaired skin integrity related to external of burn.

Nursing Process for the Child with Integumentary Disorder

Assessment: Disruption of skin surface or layers, destruction of skin layers, edema, altered circulation, altered nutritional state, altered metabolic state.

(Refer Table 12.1 from chapter 12)

Nursing diagnosis

Altered nutrition: Less than body requirements related to inability to ingest, metabolize nutrients.

Assessment: Catabolism, protein and fat wasting, anorexia, diarrhea, weight loss.

(Refer Table 14.3 from chapter 14)

Nursing diagnosis

Impaired physical mobility related to pain and discomfort, musculoskeletal impairment.

Assessment: Limited range of motion, impaired joint flexibility, scar formation, contracture of joints, skin, tendons and ligaments, reluctance to attempt movement.

(Refer Table 14.19 from chapter 14)

Nursing diagnosis

Ineffective breathing pattern related to musculoskeletal impairment.

Assessment: Trauma/edema of airway, oral or nasal membranes, restlessness, tachypnea, dyspnea.

(Refer Table 14.2 from chapter 14)

Nursing diagnosis

High-risk for fluid volume deficit related to excessive losses through normal routes (wound).

Assessment: Loss of protective skin, blood loss from stress ulcer, electrolyte imbalance, reduced cardiac output with reduced plasma and blood volume.

(Refer Table 14.11 from chapter 14)

Nursing diagnosis

Altered growth and development related to effects of long-term disability.

Assessment: Altered physical growth, inability to perform self-care of self-control activities appropriate for age.

(Refer Table 14.4 from chapter 14)

B. Specific Nursing Diagnoses and Nursing Process

7. Nursing diagnosis

Pain related to injuring biological, chemical, physical agents (burn injury) **(Table 21.1)**.

Assessment: Communication (verbal or nonverbal) of pain descriptors depending on severity and type of burn, moaning, crying, restlessness, guarding of injured area.

Nursing Process for the Child with Integumentary Disorder

Table 21.1: Nursing interventions for pain.

Interventions	Rationales
Assess pain in burned area for severity and degree of burn	Provides information about pain that varies in severity with extent and depth of burn, cause of burn injury (chemical, electrical, thermal)
Administer analgesics PO or IV as ordered depending on severity of pain and status of other systems; administer before procedures and care are performed; anticipate need before pain becomes severe	Relieves and controls pain response caused by injury to superficial nerve endings
Provide relaxation, diversional activities	Provides nonpharmacologic relief of pain
Place in position of comfort, change q2h, and handle injured part(s) gently	Promotes comfort and prevents additional pain caused by rough handling or pressure on injured body parts
Avoid touching painful parts, use bed cradle over injured, painful parts	Prevents contact with linens or hard surfaces that cause pain
Apply ointment to healing skin that is itchy and flaking	Provides relief from discomfort of itching with use of an antihistamine cream

(PO: per os or by mouth; IV: intravenous)

Evaluation
- Pain absent or controlled
- Utilizes nonpharmacologic measures to control pain
- Protects injured and healing areas from stimuli that cause pain
- Absence of complaints of pain or discomfort.

Nursing diagnosis

High-risk for infection related to inadequate primary defenses **(Table 21.2)**.

Assessment: Broken skin, traumatized tissue, new skin graft, fever, purulent drainage from open wound or under eschar, positive wound culture.

Evaluation
- Controls contact with infectious agents
- Protects wound site(s) from infectious agents
- Absence of evidence of signs and symptoms of wound infection
- Administers antibiotic therapy via appropriate route
- Eliminates sources of transmission of microorganisms to the child.

Nursing diagnosis

Body image disturbance related to biophysical and psychosocial factors **(Table 21.3)**.

Assessment: Verbal and nonverbal responses to change in body appearance (scarring, deformity), loss of control, dependence, negative feelings about body, multiple stressors and change in daily living limitations and social relationships.

Nursing Process for the Child with Integumentary Disorder

Table 21.2: Nursing interventions for high-risk for infection.

Interventions	Rationales
Assess healing wounds for changes in color, odor and drainage, and temperature elevation	Provides information indicating infection of wound or skin graft area
Administer antibiotics PO or IV based on positive culture results and physician's order	Prevents or treats infection with antibiotic specific to microorganism; destroys infectious agent by preventing cell wall synthesis
Perform protective isolation as appropriate including mask, gown, gloves; perform handwash before giving any care; discourage visits from those who are suffering from an infection or who are ill	Protects child from exposure to infectious organisms
Apply antimicrobial wet dressings to wound or antimicrobial ointment as ordered when performing a dressing change	Destroys infectious agents and protects wound from infection
Use sterile technique to perform all dressing changes and wound care	Protects wound from pathogens and reduces risk of infection

(PO: per os or by mouth; IV: intravenous)

Evaluation
- Verbalizes improved body image and sense of well-being
- Participates in family, school, and social activities as appropriate

Table 21.3: Nursing interventions for body image disturbance.

Interventions	Rationales
Assess child for feelings about multiple restrictions in lifestyle, change in appearance, difficulty in school and social situations, inability to keep up with peers and participate in activities	Provides information about status of self-concept and body image that require special attention
Encourage expression of feelings and concerns and support communications with parent(s), teachers, and peers	Provides opportunity to vent feelings and reduce negative feelings about changes in appearance
Avoid negative comments and stress positive aspects of activities and accomplishments	Enhances body image and confidence
Note withdrawal behavior and signs of depression	Reveals responses to body image changes and possible poor adjustment to changes
Show support and acceptance of changes in appearance of child; provide privacy as needed	Promotes trust and demonstrates respect for child
Allow as much control and decision making by child as possible	Promotes independence and gives child some control over the situation
Allow and encourage parental and peer visits when possible	Promotes social acceptance by peers and support by parents

- Verbalizes feelings about special long-term needs in positive terms
- Supports positive body image and promotes adjustment to change in appearance
- Identifies need for and seeks out social services, psychological counseling as appropriate.

Cellulitis

Cellulitis is an infection of the skin and underlying subcutaneous tissue affecting the lymph nodes within the area of inflammation. It may follow an upper respiratory infection and become systemic in its symptomology. The most common areas affected are the face, periorbital area and extremities. Treatment includes antibiotic therapy **(Fig. 21.2)**.

Symptoms of Cellulitis
- Swelling of the skin
- Tenderness

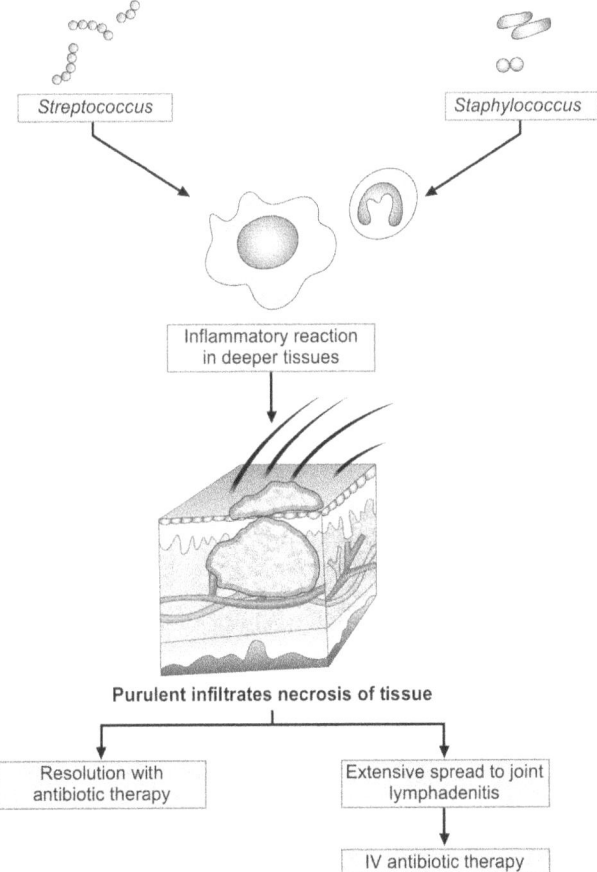

Fig. 21.2: Pathophysiology of cellulitis.

- Warm skin
- Pain
- Bruising
- Blisters
- Fever
- Headache
- Chills
- Weakness
- Red streaks from the original site of cellulitis
- Local lymph node swelling.

Nursing Management

A. Essential Nursing Diagnoses and Nursing Process Associated with this Condition

Nursing diagnosis

Hyperthermia related to illness (infection).

Assessment: Increase in body temperature above normal range, flushed skin which is warm to touch, increased pulse and respiration rate.

(Refer Table 14.18 from chapter 14)

Nursing diagnosis

High-risk for fluid volume deficit related to excessive losses through normal routes.

Assessment: Temperature elevation, diaphoresis, insensible losses.

(Refer Table 14.11 from chapter 14)

Nursing diagnosis

High-risk for impaired skin integrity related to internal factor of infection of skin layers.

Assessment: Redness, swelling, induration, warmth, pain at affected areas, destruction of skin layers.

(Refer Table 12.1 from chapter 12)

B. Specific Nursing Diagnosis and Nursing Process Associated with this Condition

Nursing diagnosis

Knowledge deficit related to lack of information about condition **(Table 21.4)**.

Assessment: Request for information about cause and treatment of the condition, measures to prevent spread of the infection.

Evaluation
- Progressive resolution on the infectious process
- Administers antibiotic therapy correctly
- Reports persistent signs and symptoms and those indicating spread of infection
- Promotes comfort and measures to enhance healing
- Performs treatments to resolve infection.

Nursing Process for the Child with Integumentary Disorder

Table 21.4: Nursing interventions for knowledge deficit.

Interventions	Rationales
Assess knowledge of treatment of an infection, possible complications, extent of infection, and risk of spread	Provides information needed to plan teaching that will assist parent(s) in caring for child with an infection involving skin layers
Inform parent(s) of cause of the infection and manifestations to note including pain, redness, swelling warmth of a localized infection and to report increasing temperature, enlarged lymph nodes in the region, and a red streak along the lymph pathway in a systemic infection	Provides information indicating cellulitis and spreading of infection systemically
Administer antibiotics PO or IV and instruct in oral administration with dose, time, frequency, side effects, and instruct to take until entire prescription is ingested	Provides treatment to destroy causative agent by inhibiting cell wall synthesis; route is dependent upon site and severity of the infection
Inform parent(s) that culture is done to determine treatment	Provides identification of microorganisms and sensitivity to specific antibiotic

(PO: per os or by mouth; IV: intravenous)

Dermatitis

Dermatitis is an inflammatory condition of the superficial layer of the skin. It may be caused by contact with an allergen, urine, or feces, and it may cause irritation characterized by erythema, papules, or vesicles. Treatment includes actions to prevent infection and skin breakdown **(Fig. 21.3)**.

Symptoms of Dermatitis
- Red, dry, itchy patches on the skin that result from inflammation.
- Itching may be severe and constant.
- With frequent scratching, the skin may develop blisters, oozing, crusting, or sores from infection.
- Sometimes, if the child scratches for many weeks to months, the skin may start to become very rough, leathery and darker in color.

In infants
- Eczema commonly affects the face, scalp, arms and legs.

In older children
- Eczema may involve only the insides of the elbows and backs of the knees.
- Some children with severe eczema may have involvement of their entire body.
- Eczema is very itchy.

Nursing Management

A. Essential Nursing Diagnoses and Nursing Process Associated with these Conditions

Nursing diagnosis

High-risk for impaired skin integrity related to external factors of excretions and secretions, contact with allergens or irritants.

Assessment: Rash, erythema, papule, vesicle, lesions, disruptions of skin surface, itching.

(Refer Table 12.1 from chapter 12)

Nursing Process for the Child with Integumentary Disorder

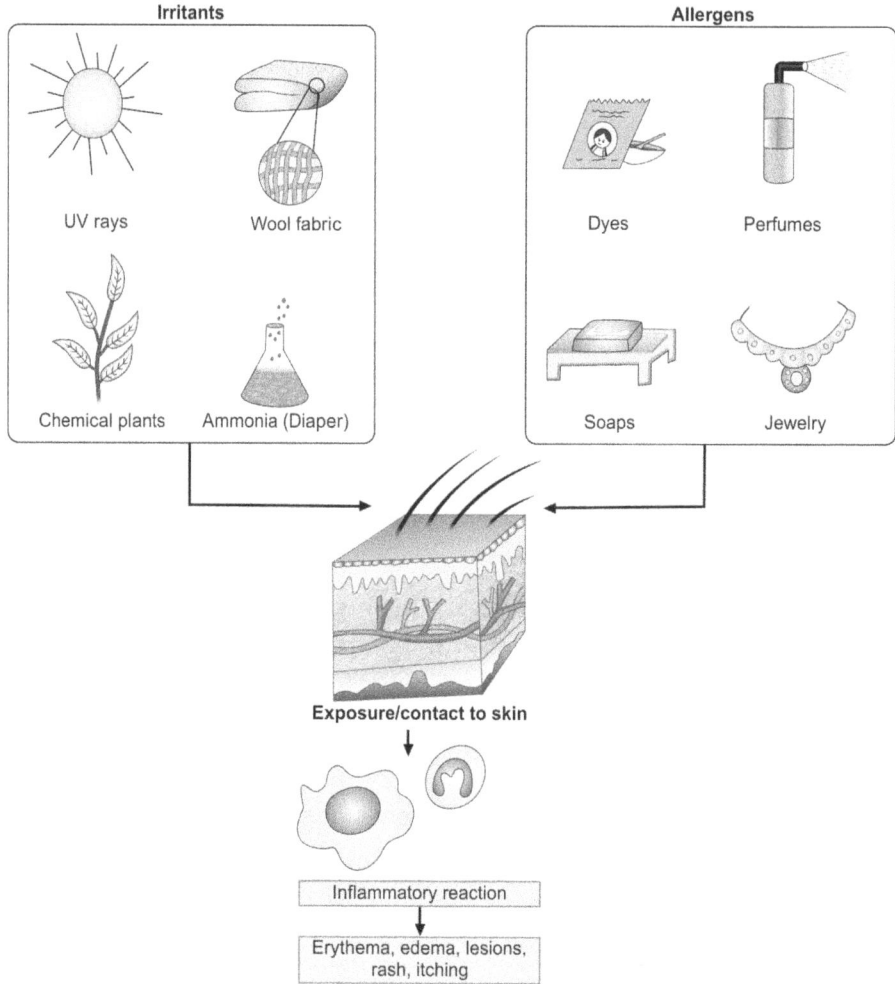

Fig. 21.3: Pathophysiology of dermatitis.

B. Specific Nursing Diagnoses and Nursing Process

Nursing diagnosis

Knowledge deficit related to lack of information about disorder **(Table 21.5)**.

Assessment: Request for information about cause and treatments of dermatitis and measures to prevent recurrence.

Evaluation
- Resolves dermatitis condition
- Prevents recurrence of contact dermatitis by removing or controlling offending agents
- Promotes comfort with palliative measures
- Administers medications correctly with desired effects.

Table 21.5: Nursing interventions for knowledge deficit.

Interventions	Rationales
Assess type and extent of dermatitis including site and offending irritant, presence of redness, papules, vesicles, breaks in skin, excoriation, itching	Provides information about rash resulting from contact which may be chemical or physical and most commonly is caused by ammonia from diaper, plant, animal, cloth, soap, or sun exposure
Inform of potential violators causing eruptions/dermatitis and how to avoid contact with offending agents (clothing, covering all parts of body, to wash after contact with substance, to use hypo-allergic soaps, proper use of skin applications, and proper changing and laundering of diapers)	Provides information to assist in avoiding contact with substances that cause dermatitis
Instruct in application of ointment or lotion (Vaseline, Desitin) to treat diaper rash, to cleanse and dry area well during diaper change, to expose irritated area to the air; laundering diapers by soaking, using mild soap, and double rinsing and drying well in clothes dryer or in sun	Promotes healing of skin irritation caused by ammonia in diapers
Instruct parent(s) in palliative treatments, such as application of warm, wet compresses and lotion or paste to the affected areas, and baths; discourage child from scratching the areas	Promotes comfort and healing, allays pruritus, and prevents infection if skin is broken down
Instruct parent(s) in administration of antibiotics anti-inflammatory, antihistamines as ordered	Reduces allergic reactions and prevents complications associated with dermatitis

PRACTICE QUESTIONS

1. Write the nursing management for the child with 60% of burns by applying nursing process.
2. Draw a nursing care plan for a 10-years child with acute allergic dermatitis.

CHAPTER 22

Nursing Process for the Child with Musculoskeletal Disorder

LEARNING OBJECTIVES
- To identify the signs and symptoms of a child with musculoskeletal disorder.
- To frame nursing diagnosis based on the needs of the child.
- To plan nursing interventions and outcome identification.

INTRODUCTION

The musculoskeletal system includes components that are needed for supportive and protective framework for the body. The system functions to provide the movement that is essential for interacting and adapting to the child's environment and is especially vulnerable to forces in the environment. The system includes bones which compose the skeletal system, muscles which compose the muscular system, joints which compose the articular system, tendons and ligaments. Tendons and ligaments with muscle attach to the surfaces of bones and the combination of all of the components allows for ambulation, personal care, and play. The problems encountered in these systems are classified as traumatic (most common) and long-term disability (degenerative disease), and any problem and abnormality that affects this system commonly affects the function of one or more other organ systems. The functional disruption that occurs as a result of a musculoskeletal problem that requires immobilization leads to physical and emotional alterations in a child who is usually active and curious. With growth and development of the system structures and gross and fine motor development, the child progressively functions within adult parameters for movements and activities of daily living.

NURSING PROCESS FOR THE CHILD WITH MUSCULOSKELETAL DISORDER (IN GENERAL)

1. **Nursing diagnosis:** Impaired physical mobility related to injury, pain or weakness as evidenced by inability to move an extremity, to ambulate or to move without limitations.
   Goal: Child will be able to engage in physical activities within limits of injury or disease.
   Intervention: Maximizing physical mobility.
   - Assess child's ability to move based upon injury or disease and within limits of prescribed treatment to determine baseline
   - Prior to prescribed exercise or major position changes, ensure that pain medication is given: relief of pain increases child's ability to tolerate and participate in activity
   - Use passive and active range-of-motion exercises and teach child and family how to perform them to facilitate joint mobility and muscle development (active range of motion [ROM] and to help increase mobility (within limits of restrictions related to injury or prescribed treatment)
   - Praise accomplishments and emphasize child's abilities to improve self-esteem and encourage feelings of confidence and competence

- Teach child and family necessary care related to mobility issues, so the family can continue with these measures at home.

   Evaluation: Child assists with transfers and positioning in bed and/or participates in prescribed bed exercises.

2. **Nursing diagnosis:** Risk for constipation related to immobility and/or use of narcotic analgesics.

   Goal: Child will be able to demonstrate adequate stool passage.

   Intervention: Promoting appropriate bowel elimination.
   - Assess usual pattern of stooling to determine baseline and identify potential problems with elimination palpate for abdominal fullness and auscultate for bowel sounds to assess for bowel function and presence of constipation
   - Encourage fiber intake to increase frequency of stools. Ensure adequate fluid intake to prevent formation of hard, dry stools
   - Encourage activity within child's limits or restrictions as even minimal activity increases peristalsis.

   Evaluation: Child pass soft, formed stool every day without straining or other adverse effects.

3. **Nursing diagnosis:** Self-care deficit related to immobility as evidenced by inability to perform hygiene care and transfer self independently.

   Goal: Child will be able to demonstrate ability to care for self within age parameters and limits of disease.

   Intervention: Maximizing self-care.
   - Introduce child and family to self help methods as soon as possible promote independence from the beginning
   - Encourage family and staff to allow child to do as much as possible to allow child to gain confidence and independence
   - Collaborate with physical therapy and occupational therapy as needed to provide child and family with appropriate tools to modify environment and methods to promote transferring and self-care to allow for maximum functioning
   - Praise accomplishments and emphasize child's abilities to improve self-esteem and encourage feelings of confidence and competence
   - Balance activity with periods to rest to reduce fatigue and increase energy available for self-care.

   Evaluation: Child is able to feed, dress and manage elimination within limits of injury or disease and age.

4. **Nursing diagnosis:** Risk for impaired skin integrity related to immobility, casting, traction, use of braces or adaptive devices.

   Goal: Child's skin will be able to remain intact.

   Intervention: Promoting skin integrity.
   - Monitor condition of entire skin surface at least daily to provide baseline and allow for early identification of areas at risk
   - Avoid excessive friction or harsh cleaning products that may increase risk of breakdown in child with susceptible skin
   - Keep child's skin free from stool and urine to decrease risk of breakdown
   - Keep linen free from food crumbs and wrinkles to prevent pressure areas from forming

- Change child's position frequently to decrease pressure on susceptible areas
- Monitor condition of skin affected by braces or adaptive equipment frequently to prevent skin breakdown related to poor fit.

For the child in traction:
- Pad bony prominences with cotton padding before applying traction to protect skin from injury
- Gently massage child's back and sacrum with lotion to stimulate circulation.

For the child in spica cast:
- Apply plastic wrap to the perineal edges of the cast to prevent soiling of cast edges, which can contribute to cast breakdown
- Use a fracture bedpan to facilitate toileting without soiling cast
- For the child still in diapers, tuck a smaller diaper under the perineal edges of cast and cover with a larger diaper to prevent cast soiling.

Evaluation: No evidence of redness or breakdown.

5. **Nursing diagnosis:** Deficient knowledge related to cast care, activity restrictions or other prescribed treatment as evidenced by verbalization, questions or actions demonstrating lack of understanding regarding child's condition or care.
   Goal: Child and family will be able to verbalize about disease condition.
   Intervention: Providing patient and family teaching.
   - Assess child's and family's willingness to learn: child and family must be willing to learn for teaching to be effective
   - Provide teaching at an appropriate level for the child and family (depends on age of child, physical condition, memory) to ensure understanding
   - Teach in short sessions: many short sessions are more helpful than one long session
   - Repeat information to give family and child time to learn and understand
   - Provide reinforcement and rewards to facilitate the teaching/learning process
   - Use multiple modes of learning involving many senses (provide written, verbal, demonstration, and videos) when possible: child and family are more likely to retain information when presented in different ways using many senses.

   Evaluation: Child and family will demonstrate accurate understanding about condition and course of treatment through verbalization and return demonstration.

6. **Nursing diagnosis:** Risk for delayed development related to immobility, alterations in extremities.
   Goal: Development will be enhanced.
   Intervention: Promoting development.
   - Screen for developmental capabilities to determine child's current level of functioning
   - Offer age-appropriate toys, play, and activities (including gross motor) to encourage further development
   - Perform exercises or interventions as prescribed by physical or occupational therapist: repeat participation in those activities helps to promote function and acquisition of developmental skills
   - Provide support to families: immobility and extremity deficits may lead to slow progress in achieving developmental milestones, so ongoing motivation is needed.

   Evaluation: Child demonstrated continued progress toward developmental milestones and will not show regression in abilities.

NURSING PROCESS FOR SPECIFIC MUSCULOSKELETAL DISORDERS

Fractures

A fracture is a break in a bone which is usually caused by a fall or injury. Fractures are common in children because of their gross motor function. Injury of this type in an infant or very small child is usually the result of physical abuse. The most common type of fracture in children under 3 years of age is the greenstick which is an incomplete fracture and results in a compression of one side causing it to bend and the other side to fail. A bend fracture is the result of the bone bending and straightening on its own because of the flexibility of the bone at a young age. A buckle fracture is a raised bulging of the bone resulting from compression of the bone near its most porous part. A complete fracture is a division in the bone with or without attachment of a periosteal hinge remaining. The most common sites of fractures in children are the femur, humerus, clavicle, ulna, radius, tibia, and fibula. Treatment includes reduction (open or closed), and immobilization by casting and/or traction depending on the type and severity of the fracture. Healing is faster in the child and takes place within 3-4 weeks. Remodeling is usually completed within 9 months depending on the type and site of the fracture, amount of fragmentation, and the age of the child (**Fig. 22.1**).

Symptoms of Fractures

Types of Bone Fracture

There are many types of fractures, but the main categories are complete, incomplete, compound and simple. Complete and incomplete fractures refer to the way the bone breaks. In a complete fracture, the bone snaps into two or more parts; in an incomplete fracture, the bone cracks but does not break all the way through.

In a compound fracture, also called an open fracture, the bone breaks through the skin. It may then recede back into the wound, so it is no longer visible through the skin. In a simple fracture, also called a closed fracture, the bone breaks but there is no open wound in the skin.

Simple fractures include

Greenstick fracture: An incomplete fracture in which the bone is bent. This type of fracture occurs most often in children.

Transverse fracture: A fracture at a right angle to the bone's axis.

Oblique fracture: A fracture in which the break is at an angle to the bone's axis.

Comminuted fracture: A fracture in which the bone fragments into several pieces.

An impacted fracture: Is one whose ends are driven into each other. This commonly occurs with arm fractures in children and is sometimes known as a buckle fracture.

Among other types of fracture are: A pathological fracture, caused by a disease that weakens the bones; and a stress fracture, which is a hairline crack.

General Signs and Symptoms of a Fracture

- Swelling or bruising over a bone.
- Deformity of an arm of leg.
- Pain in the injured area that gets worse when the area is moved or pressure is applied.
- Loss of function in the injured area.

In compound fractures, bone protruding from the skin.

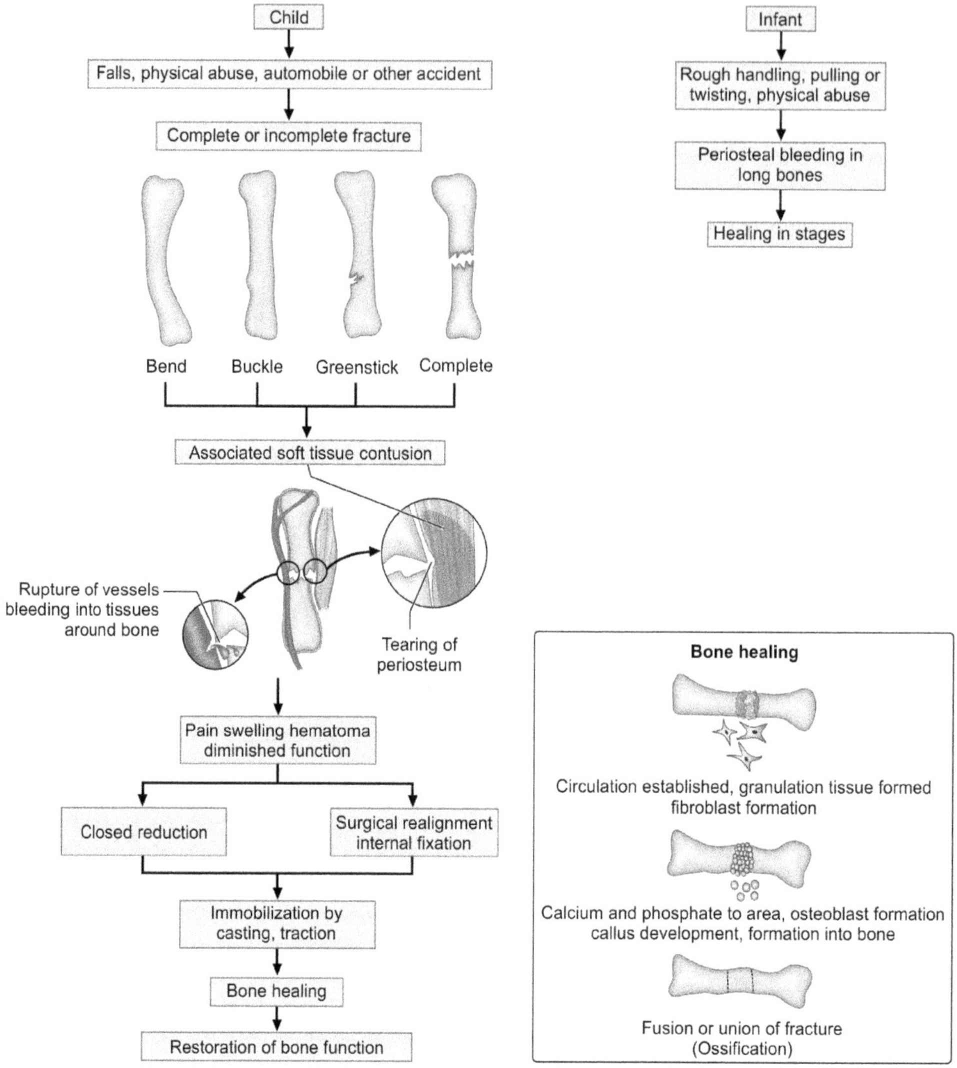

Nursing Process for the Child with Musculoskeletal Disorder

Fig. 22.1: Pathophysiology of fractures.

Nursing Management

A. Essential Nursing Diagnoses and Nursing Process Associated with this Condition

Nursing diagnosis

Impaired physical mobility related to pain and discomfort, musculoskeletal impairment (fracture).

Assessment: Intolerance to activity, decreased strength and endurance, inability to purposefully move within physical environment including bed mobility, transfer and ambulation, reluctance to attempt movement, imposed restrictions of movement including mechanical medical protocol (cast, traction), inability to participate in activities and socializing.

(Refer Table 14.19 from chapter 14)

Nursing Process for the Child with Musculoskeletal Disorder

Nursing diagnosis

Altered tissue perfusion, peripheral related to interruption in arterial and venous flow.

Assessment: Cold, pallor or blue color of extremity, decreased peripheral pulse, cast tightness.

(Refer Table 14.12 from chapter 14)

Nursing diagnosis

High-risk for impaired skin integrity related to external factors of physical immobilization, pressure of cast, traction apparatus, presence of surgical incision from open reduction; internal factors of altered circulation and sensation.

Assessment: Disruption of skin surface, invasion of bony structures, redness, irritation of skin at cast edges or pressure areas, numbness or tingling of casted extremities.

(Refer Table 12.1 from chapter 12)

Nursing diagnosis

Constipation related to inadequate physical activity or immobility.

Assessment: Frequency less than usual, hard formed stool, decreased bowel sounds, straining at defecation.

(Refer Table 12.9 from chapter 12)

B. Specific Nursing Diagnoses and Nursing Process

Nursing diagnosis

Pain related to physical injuring agents (bone fracture); surgery to realign fracture **(Table 22.1)**.

Assessment: Communication of pain descriptors, guarding and protective behavior to injured part, crying, irritability, restlessness, swelling of part, muscle spasms.

Evaluation
- Absence of pain and associated responses
- Pain-provoking actions controlled when giving care or changing positions
- Administration of analgesics/muscle relaxants, then monitor responses.

Nursing diagnosis

High-risk for injury related to internal factors of sensory dysfunction, tissue hypoxia, altered mobility resulting from cast application **(Table 22.2)**.

Assessment: Change in color, temperature, edema, movement of fingers/toes; tingling of numbness of fingers/toes; drainage or musty odor from under cast; skin irritation at cast edges; moist, wet, or broken cast, foreign objects inserted between cast and skin.

Evaluation
- Maintains immobilization by casting
- Maintains neurovascular competency during immobilization by cast
- Verbalizes and provides appropriate cast care
- Avoids activities that damages cast and affects immobilization of casted part

Table 22.1: Nursing interventions for pain.

Interventions	Rationales
Assess site for pain including type, severity, and duration using a pain scale if appropriate: pain as a result of surgical open reduction	Provides information about pain as a basis for analgesic and muscle relaxant therapy
Administer analgesic, muscle relaxant, or both; IV initially and wean to PO administration when appropriate and note response	Reduces pain and promotes rest following injury or surgery
Apply ice to fracture if ordered	Treats pain and edema by vasoconstriction
Apply splint	Relieves pain and prevents further damage by protecting and immobilizing limb
Elevate limb above and below injured area when moving and positioning	Promotes venous return to relieve edema which causes pain and prevents contractures
Support limb above and below injured area when moving and positioning; use smooth movements and avoid abrupt movement of limb	Prevents pain caused by movement

(PO: per os or by mouth; IV: intravenous)

Table 22.2: Nursing interventions for high-risk for injury related to internal factors of sensory dysfunction, tissue hypoxia, altered mobility resulting from cast application.

Interventions	Rationales
Assess pulses in casted upper or lower extremity, swelling, coolness, inability to move digits, pallor or cyanosis, numbness of areas distal to the cast q2h	Provides information about the neurovascular status of an extremity following cast application as swelling continues causing the cast to become tight and compromise circulation; a bivalve cast treats excessive edema to prevent tissue damage
Allow cast to dry thoroughly using a fan, turning q2h, support on pillows and use palm of hands to lift or handle cast exposing as much of the cast to the air as possible	Prevents indentations in the cast which may cause pressure areas, allows cast to dry from inside out for 30 minutes or more depending on substance used for cast and type of cast
Elevate casted part on pillow until completely dry and when at rest for a few days	Promotes venous return to reduce swelling
Provide quiet play for a few days and exercise muscles and joints above and below cast	Maintains muscle and joint function
Remove small articles or food that may be put into the cast	Prevents pressure to injury and infection if skin is broken under the cast
Clean plaster cast with vinegar and water; fiberglass casts are cleaned with mild soap and water	Maintains cleanliness of the cast
Petal cast if rough edges are present; massage skin near cast edges and note any reddened or abrasive areas	Protects skin from irritation and breakdown
Outline area of drainage on cast with pen; and include date and time	Monitors increase in drainage under the cast
Provide muscle strengthening exercises, ROM of unaffected parts, isometric exercises if appropriate	Prepares for crutch walking if appropriate and maintains joint and muscle mobility

(ROM: range of motion)

- Protects skin, tissue, and joints from impairment caused by cast and immobilization
- Participates in activities with proper protection to cast and extremity.

Nursing diagnosis

High-risk for injury related to internal factors of sensory dysfunction, altered mobility resulting from skin or skeletal traction **(Table 22.3)**.

Assessment: Redness, swelling, pain at pin site, change in neurovascular status of extremity, malfunction of traction apparatus, ineffective traction, contractures or weakness of joint and muscles.

Evaluation
- Verbalizes type of traction and purpose
- Maintains maximum effect of traction
- Prevents malfunction or complications of traction apparatus
- Provides pin site care, ROM and exercises to muscles and joints
- Promotes independence in self-care activities and social interaction.

Hip Dysplasia

Hip dysplasia is a congenital disorder of hip development involving the femoral head, acetabulum, or both. It may involve one or both hips and responds to treatment if started early with the most success achieved if initiated before 2 months of age. The degree of severity is classified as preluxation the femoral head is in place in the acetabulum; subluxation in which an incomplete dislocation or a hip that is dislocatable is present; or dislocation (luxation) in which the femoral head is out of the acetabulum and displaced above and in back of the acetabulum rim. Treatment is dependent on age that the abnormality is detected and ranges from application of a reduction device to traction and casting to surgical open reduction. Casting and splinting with correction is usually impossible after 6 years of age **(Fig. 22.2)**.

Symptoms of Hip Dislocation

- Having DDH does not cause pain. A baby with DDH may have
- A hip joint that feels loose or slips out of place when examined
- One leg that seems shorter than the other
- Extra folds of skin on the inside of the thigh(s)
- A hip joint that moves differently than the other.

A child who is walking may:
- Walk on the toes of one foot with the heel up off the floor
- Walk with a limp (or waddling gait if both hips are affected).

Nursing Management

A. Essential Nursing Diagnoses and Nursing Process Associated with this Condition

Nursing diagnosis

Impaired physical mobility related to musculoskeletal impairment (hip defect).

Nursing Process for the Child with Musculoskeletal Disorder

Table 22.3: Nursing interventions for high-risk for injury related to internal factors of sensory dysfunction, altered mobility resulting from skin or skeletal traction.

Interventions	Rationales
Assess type and purpose of traction, extremity or body part involved	Provides information about use of traction to realign bone ends, provide immobilization of a part, reduce muscle spasms, correct a deformity provide rest for an extremity; traction may be manual traction as in cast application, skin traction in which the pull is attached to the skin with bandages or straps, or skeletal traction in which the pull is attached to a pin, wire, or tongs inserted into the bone at a distal position to the fracture
Assess functioning part of the traction apparatus including correct weight amount and hanging, ropes in tract with secure knots, pulleys in original site with movable wheels, position of frames, splints	Provides information needed to ensure correct traction applied to body part
Assess skin color, pulses, numbness, or changes in movement of body part; weakness or contractures of uninvolved muscles and joints; q24H	Indicates muscular changes resulting from immobilization
Assess pressure points noting any redness or breakdown and reposition if possible; massage uninjured skin areas	Prevents prolonged pressure on skin that results in breakdown and decreased blood flow to area
Maintain bed position as ordered with head or foot elevated	Provides desired amount of pull and counter traction
Maintain correct body alignment especially in hips, legs, arms, and shoulders; realign after the child has moved or changed position	Promotes comfort and prevents deformity
Perform ROM to unaffected joints, apply foot plate if appropriate	Prevents contractures and foot drop
Maintain nonadhesive straps or bandages used; do not remove or change unless permitted while someone maintains traction; note tightness or looseness that may cause ineffective traction	Supplies attachment for pull in skin traction
Cleanse and dress pin site daily; apply antiseptic ointment if ordered; check skin for infection at site; examine screws within metal clamp for proper attachment of clamp to traction; do not remove traction	Supplies attachment for pull in skeletal traction and treats pin site to prevent infection
Assist child to perform ADL activities independently as much as possible; facilitate self-care with assistive aids	Promotes independence in self-care within limitations of age and immobilization
Provide diversional activities and encourage visits from family and friends, move bed to area of activity with peers	Provides and promotes social interactions

(ROM: range of motion; ADL: activities of daily living)

Nursing Process for the Child with Musculoskeletal Disorder

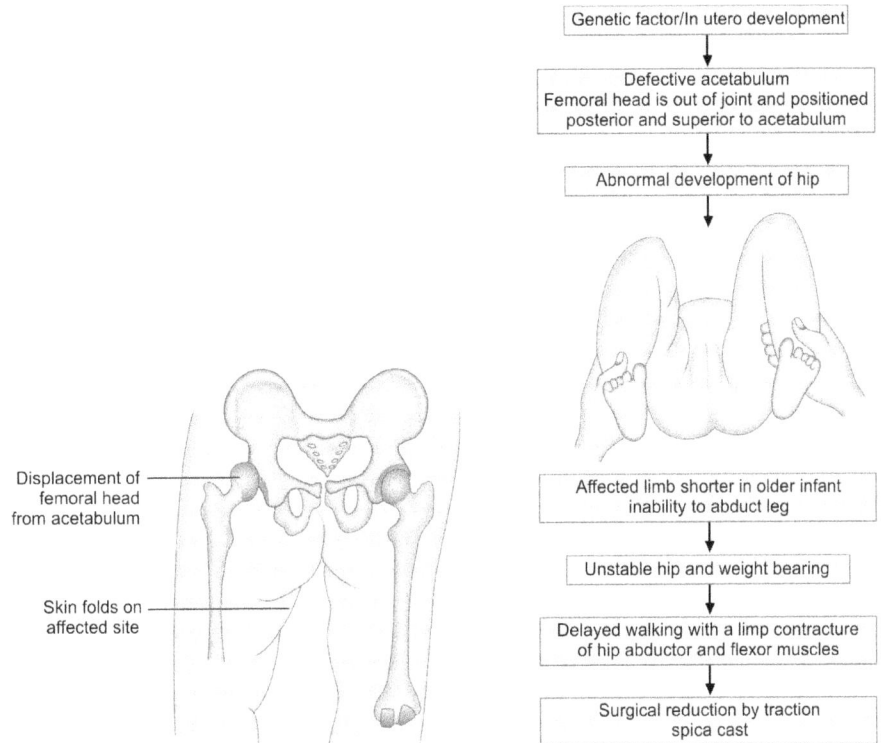

Fig. 22.2: Pathophysiology of hip dysplasia.

Assessment: Imposed restriction of movement by harness, cast, traction, or splint; inability to purposefully move within physical environment including bed mobility; ambulation.

(Refer Table 14.19 from chapter 14)

Nursing diagnosis

High-risk for impaired skin integrity related to external factor of physical immobilization; internal factor of altered circulation; sensation by pressure of device, cast, traction.

Assessment: Edema, tight appliance or cast, change in skin color and temperature proximal to spica cast or device or pin site, skin irritation at pin site or cast edges, numbness proximal to cast.

(Refer Table 12.1 from chapter 12)

Nursing diagnosis

Constipation related to musculoskeletal impairment, inadequate physical activity or immobility.

Assessment: Frequency less than usual, hard formed stool, decreased bowel sounds, straining at defecation.

(Refer Table 12.9 from chapter 12)

Nursing Process for the Child with Musculoskeletal Disorder

Nursing diagnosis

Altered growth and development related to effects of physical disability (immobilization).

Assessment: Environmental and stimulation deficiencies, inability to perform self-care activities appropriate for age, isolation with long-term immobilization.

(Refer Table 14.4 from chapter 14)

B. Specific Nursing Diagnoses and Nursing Process

Nursing diagnosis

High-risk for injury related to internal physiological factor of untreated or improper treatment for dislocation **(Table 22.4)**.

Assessment: Late onset dislocation, absence of early recognition and intervention for correction, muscle contracture, muscle shortening, femoral and acetabulum deformity, tight spica cast, inappropriate traction or malfunctioning traction.

Evaluation
- Early detection of defect note, and treatments begun
- Applies diapers, pillow splint, and harness correctly and maintains correct reduction of hip over prescribed periods of time
- Provides effective traction and/or cast care as appropriate over prescribed periods of time
- Verbalizes causes of deformity, reason and purpose of treatment, prognosis of condition
- Verbalizes knowledge of deformity and promotes corrective therapy
- Controls possible complications of traction or cast application
- Complies with follow-up supervision of medical regimen to correct deformity
- Absence of cast syndrome and traction functioning correctly.

Nursing diagnosis

Impaired social interaction related to limited physical mobility **(Table 22.5)**.

Assessment: Change in pattern of interaction, lengthy treatment and immobilization, boredom, inability to engage in usual activities for age group, environment that lacks diversion.

Table 22.4: Nursing interventions for high-risk for injury related to internal physiological factor of untreated or improper treatment for dislocation.

Interventions	Rationales
Assess infant up to 2 months of age for frank breech birth, cesarean birth, hip joint laxity or dislocation (Ortolani or Barlow test), degree of dysplasia or dislocation, shortened limb on the affected side (telescoping), broadened perineum, asymmetry of thigh and gluteal folds with increased number of folds and flattened buttocks	Provides information about the presence and degree of dysplasia; may be preluxation, subluxation, or dislocation (luxation) and involve a laxity of the capsule or an abnormal acetabulum; identification of the presence of the deformity at this age results in the highest success rate in complete correction

Contd...

Contd...

Interventions	Rationales
Assess child's shortened leg affected with telescoping; palpation of femur when thigh is extended and pushed toward the head and puled in distal direction; delayed walking and a limp that causes lurching toward affected side; downward tilt of pelvis toward unaffected side if weight bearing on affected side when standing; lordosis and waddling gait if both hips affected	Provides information about the presence of deformity in one or both hips in the older infant or toddler and preschool age group; usually identified when the child begins to walk or stand, and limb is shortened and adductor and flexor muscle contracture has occurred; requires closed reduction (traction and cats) or open reduction (surgery, cast, splint) to correct
Apply Pavlik harness splinting device to infant up to 6 months of age to be worn continuously for 3–6 months to ensure hip stability	Maintains abducted, reduced position for maintaining the femur in the acetabulum
Maintain skin traction in presence of abduction contracture in the infant up to 6 months of age and spica cast if applied following the traction; maintain skin traction for gradual reduction of the hip adductor and flexor muscles with a spica cast application for immobilization in child 6–18 months of age	Promotes hip abduction until stable; applied with a spica cast if unable to maintain stable reduction of the hip for 3–6 months; removal of the spica cast is followed by an abduction brace for protection
Provide traction care including correct alignment of extremity, correct amount of weights, free hang of weights, correctly functioning pulleys with secure knots neurologic and circulatory checks q4y for color, warmth, sensation	Maintains safe, effective traction to affected hip(s) with child's response to traction monitored
Provide spica cast care including support of cast when moving, removing crumbs and small articles that may get into cast, petal cast edges, avoiding insertion of anything into cast to scratch, clean cast when needed, allow to dry completely, protect cast from soiling and dampness from elimination or bathing; neurologic and circulatory checks q4h for color, peripheral pulse, warmth, capillary refill, sensation; nausea and vomiting resulting from cast syndrome	Maintains safe, effective immobilization to ensure permanent stability of hip with child's response to cast monitored for cast syndrome caused by tight spica cast compressing the superior mesenteric artery of the duodenum
Provide diaper change frequently and as needed; use disposable diapers or plastic protection over diaper	Maintains clean harness, brace, or cast

Evaluation
- Participates in positive interaction with peers and family members
- Maintains age appropriate stimulation and play activities
- Participates in family activities
- Promotes a variety of activities contributing to growth and development needs.

Lupus Erythematosus

Lupus erythematosus is a chronic systemic inflammatory disease of the collagen or supporting tissues and affecting any organ in the body.

Table 22.5: Nursing interventions for impaired social interaction.

Interventions	Rationales
Provide age appropriate toys to be used in bed while in a prone or sitting position depending on type of treatment and degree of immobilization	Promotes social and developmental activities and reduces boredom during long-term treatment
Provide exposure to other children by moving bed near areas of activity or near a window; wheel on a stretcher, wheelchair, or stroller; allow to walk with cast or brace if permitted	Provides environmental stimulation and social interaction
Encourage family and friends to visit or stay with child	Promotes social interaction with others during long-term treatment and reduces boredom
Place toys and other articles within reach	Provides access to diversion activities when needed

It is classified into a transient type affecting neonates and a type with an onset after infancy that is the same as systemic lupus erythematosus affecting adults. The disease is characterized by remission and exacerbations and may appear in children as young as 6 years of age but is most commonly seen in those 10 years of age and older. Disease manifestations include lesions or rash on face, neck, trunk and extremities; pleurisy; pericarditis; kidney failure; arthritis; anemia; gastrointestinal abnormalities; and enlarged lymph nodes. Prognosis is dependent on the response to the medical regimen and prevention of exacerbations and severe complications of the renal system **(Fig. 22.3)**.

Symptoms of Systemic Lupus Erythematosus

- Fever
- Fatigue
- Weight loss
- Hair loss
- Stomach pain
- Rashes on the face or upper body
- Headaches
- Easy bruising
- Painful joints
- Seizures or psychosis
- Decline in school performance
- Symptoms of anxiety or depression.

Nursing Management

A. Essential Nursing Diagnoses and Nursing Process Associated with this Condition

Nursing diagnosis

High-risk for impaired skin integrity related to internal factors of altered pigmentation, circulation, immunological.

Nursing Process for the Child with Musculoskeletal Disorder

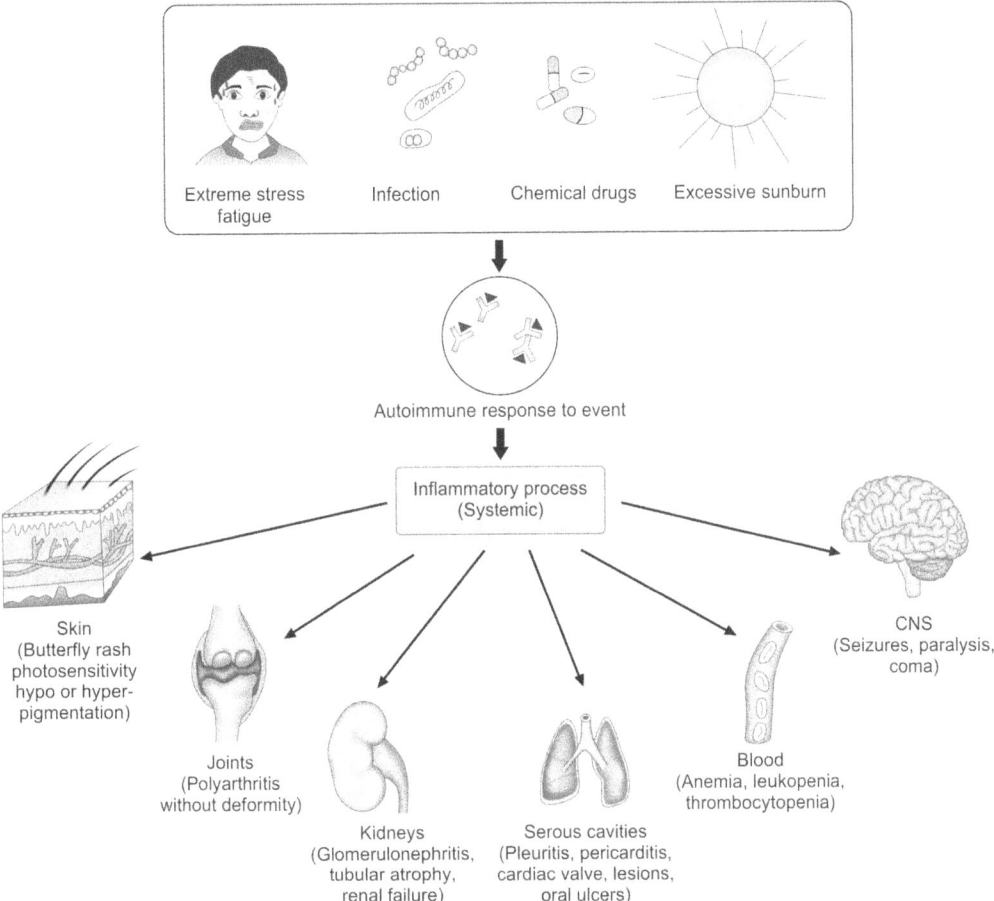

Fig. 22.3: Pathophysiology of lupus erythematosus.

Assessment: Disruption in skin surface; scaly erythematous blush or patchy area over nose and cheeks in the shape of a butterfly; sensitivity to cold in hands and feet with or without cyanosis; dry, cracked skin; alopecia.

(Refer Table 12.1 from chapter 12)

Nursing diagnosis

Impaired physical mobility related to intolerance to activity, decreased strength and endurance, pain and discomfort.

Assessment: Generalized weakness; joint swelling, stiffness, and pain; limited range of motion; generalized aching; arthralgia; fatigue.

(Refer Table 14.19 from chapter 14)

Nursing diagnosis

Hyperthermia related to illness (inflammation).

Assessment: Increase in body temperature above normal range, low grade elevation.

(Refer Table 14.18 from chapter 14)

Nursing diagnosis

Altered thought process related to physiological changes.

Assessment: Forgetfulness, changes in consciousness, excitability, seizures, psychosis, irritability, nystagmus, diplopia, disorientation.

(Refer Table 12.14 from chapter 12)

Nursing diagnosis

High-risk for fluid volume deficit related to failure of regulatory mechanisms (renal failure).

Assessment: Increased urine output, altered intake, weight loss or gain, edema, dry skin and mucous membranes, thirst, hypotension, increased pulse rate, proteinuria.

(Refer Table 14.11 from chapter 14)

Nursing diagnosis

Decreased cardiac output related to mechanical factor of alteration in preload, electrical factor of altered conduction.

Assessment: Variations in hemodynamic readings, arrhythmias, ECG changes, cyanosis, skin and mucous membrane pallor, decreased peripheral pulses, rales, dyspnea, orthopnea, restlessness.

(Refer Table 14.1 from chapter 14)

Nursing diagnosis

Altered nutrition: Less than body requirements related to inability to ingest, digest, and absorb nutrients.

Assessment: Anorexia, nausea, vomiting, diarrhea, abdominal discomfort.

(Refer Table 14.3 from chapter 14)

B. Specific Nursing Diagnoses and Nursing Process

Nursing diagnosis

Body image disturbance related to biophysical and psychosocial factors **(Table 22.6)**.

Assessment: Verbal and nonverbal responses to change in body appearance (alopecia, skin rashes, steroid side effects), negative feelings about body, multiple stressors and change in daily living limitations and social relationships.

Evaluation
- Verbalizes improved body image and sense of well-being
- Participates in family, school, and social activities as appropriate
- Verbalizes feelings about special needs in positive terms
- Supports positive body image and promotes adjustment to chronic illness
- Modifies appearance with special clothing, wig, cosmetics to cover and/or protect skin; alopecia; weight gain.

Table 22.6: Nursing interventions for body image disturbance.

Interventions	Rationales
Assess child for feelings about multiple restrictions in lifestyle, chronic illness, difficulty in school and social situations, inability to keep up with peers and participate in activities	Provides information about status of self-concept and body image that require special attention
Encourage expression of feelings and concerns and support communications with parent(s), teachers, and peers	Provides opportunity to vent feelings and reduce negative feelings about changes in appearance
Avoid negative comments and stress positive activities and accomplishments	Enhances body image and confidence
Note withdrawal behavior and signs of depression	Reveals responses to body image changes and possible poor adjustment to changes
Note hair loss, skin rashes or changes, weight gain and shift in body fat distribution, hirsutism, edema and effect on child	Reveals side effects of steroid therapy and disease manifestations that affect body image
Show support and acceptance of changes in appearance of child; provide privacy as needed	Promotes trust and demonstrates respect for child

Table 22.7: Nursing interventions for pain.

Interventions	Rationales
Assess severity of joint pain, location, duration, remissions, and exacerbations and what precipitates pain such as weight gain, activity; affect on mobility and participation in ADL; presence of joint deformity	Provides information symptomatic of the effect of the disease on the musculoskeletal system; allows for analgesic selection and better management of activity involvement
Administer analgesic and anti-inflammatory and assess effect of medications in relieving pain	Relieves pain and the inflammatory process associated with the pain
Apply warm compresses or packs to painful areas	Promotes circulation to the area by vasodilatation to relieve pain
Provide 1–2 rest periods during day and quiet environment for sleep	Decreases stimulation that increases pain, and it promotes rest
Allow to assume position of comfort	Promotes comfort and rest for joints to reduce pain
Provide toys, TV, books, games, for quiet play during painful episodes	Promotes diversional activity to detract from pain

(ADL: activities of daily living)

Nursing diagnosis

Pain related to biological injuring agents (inflammatory process) **(Table 22.7)**.

Assessment: Communication of pain descriptors, joint pain achiness, joint swelling and stiffness.

Evaluation
- Pain relieved or controlled
- Limits or avoids factors that initiate or increase pain

Nursing Process for the Child with Musculoskeletal Disorder

Table 22.8: Nursing interventions for knowledge deficit of parent(s) and child.

Interventions	Rationales
Assess knowledge of disease, type of treatments, effect on all systems, importance of compliance with medical regimen	Provides information needed to understand this complex disease and adjust long-term treatment and restrictions
Inform parent(s) and child of the disease process, effect on connective tissue and all systems, and treatment regimen needed to maintain remission	Provides information about known facts related to the disease to enhance knowledge of potential for exacerbations which may lead to early death
Instruct parent(s) and child in the administration and side effects of anti-inflammatories and immunosuppressant drugs, the importance of strict compliance to the medication protocol without decreasing or skipping the dose if side effects appear, and the need to adjust dosage during stressful situations	Promotes compliance to long-term medication regimen even when affected by undesirable side effects; an abrupt withdrawal of the medication may cause a serious physiological complication
Instruct parent(s) and child in activity restrictions or moderate activities allowed and how to weigh one activity against another as appropriate for the child	Prevents exacerbation of the symptoms while considering the long-term difficulty the child faces when activities are restricted
Instruct parent(s) and child to avoid sun exposure directly	Prevents skin eruptions/reactions common to this disease when exposed to the sun
Inform parent(s) and child of child's need to take naps and have 8 hours of sleep/night; avoid fatigue or stressful situations; avoid medications such as sulfonamides, tetracyclines, anticonvulsants, and others that cause an exacerbation	Prevents exacerbations of the disease symptoms
Inform parent(s) and child to report bruising, petechiae, elevated temperature, blood in urine or stool, increased irritability, vomiting, inability or remission in taking medications, respiratory or urinary changes	Provides for early interventions if complications occur

- Analgesic therapy based on severity of pain and age with desired results
- Decreasing need for analgesics administration
- Complies with long-term anti-inflammatory therapy.

Nursing diagnosis

Knowledge deficit of parent(s) child related to lack of information about chronic illness (Table 22.8).

Assessment: Request for information about disease and the special needs associated with the disease; prevention of exacerbation and complications of the disease; risk of noncompliance with multiple preventive precautions.

Evaluation
- Complies with lifelong medical regimen to prevent exacerbations and complications
- Verbalized disease process, affects to each system, treatments and limitations imposed by the disease

- Complies strictly to medication and activity protocols
- Prevents risk of exacerbations by avoiding factors that precipitate signs and symptoms
- Utilizes community agencies for assistance, information, and support
- Reports untoward signs and symptoms to physician
- Monitors vital signs, weight, urine and fecal testing as instructed.

Nursing diagnosis

Ineffective individual coping related to multiple life changes, personal vulnerability (Table 22.9).

Assessment: Alteration in social participation, inappropriate use of defense mechanisms (denial, regression, projection), withdrawal, intolerance of new experiences, lifelong hardships of medical regimen and limitations.

Evaluation
- Identifies and uses positive coping mechanisms
- Engages in decision making and expression feelings about illness
- Participates in therapeutic play and other activities that allow expression of frustration
- Verbalizes meaning of behaviors and factors that contribute to them
- Develops new coping mechanisms that are acceptable for age and level of development
- Initiates counseling services when needed.

Table 22.9: Nursing interventions for ineffective individual coping.

Interventions	Rationales
Assess coping behaviors of child and factors that induce use of defense mechanisms, response to stressful situations (avoidance behavior, cooperation or resistance, aggression, regression, delaying tactics, inappropriate humor)	Provides information about child's coping mechanisms and pattern and use of coping strategies
Allow child to express feelings and provide outlet for release of feelings in an accepting environment	Promotes independence and control over a situation
Provide therapeutic play including throwing ball or balloons, pounding board, hand painting, water play	Provides expression of feelings and outlet to release aggression
Involve child in care decisions and encourage independence in as much of the care as possible	Promotes active participation in care with assistance as needed
Identify and support coping mechanisms during play, social interactions, painful procedures, restrictions and bed rest	Allows for experiences which gives the child an opportunity to practice successful coping behaviors which enhance development of one's self-esteem
Encourage parent(s) to participate in child's care and support	Increases feelings of security when the child must deal with new situations

Osteochondritis Deformans

Osteochondritis deformans (Legg-Calve-Perthes disease) is a disease of the femoral head occurring in children between 3–12 years of age. Its cause is unknown but the disease is characterized by a necrosis of the femoral head resulting from an impaired circulation of the femoral epiphysis extending to the acetabulum. Joint dysfunction with hip pain or ache and a limp that is continuous or intermittent are common signs and symptoms of the condition. Early treatment to maintain the femoral head in the acetabulum determines the prognosis. The disease progression and resolution is classified into four stages: stage I is the necrosis and degeneration of the femoral head (avascular); stage II is the bone absorption and vascularization (revascularization); stage III is the new bone formation with ossification (reparative); and stage IV is the reformation of the femoral head to a sphere (regenerative) **(Fig. 22.4)**.

Symptoms of Osteochondritis Deformans

- Hip pain
- Limited leg motion
- Limp
- Tender hip muscles
- Hip muscle spasm
- Degeneration of the femoral head.

Fig. 22.4: Pathophysiology of osteochondritis deformans.

Nursing Management

A. Essential Nursing Diagnoses and Nursing Process Associated with this Condition

Nursing diagnosis

Impaired physical mobility related to musculoskeletal impairment (femoral head).

Assessment: Imposed restrictions of movement by medical protocol of corrective device (cast, brace, sling, traction), reluctance to attempt movement, restriction in weight bearing, limited ROM, bed rest.

(Refer Table 14.19 from chapter 14)

Nursing diagnosis

High-risk for impaired skin integrity related to external factor of physical immobilization, pressure of cast or appliance and altered circulation, sensation.

Assessment: Change in skin color and temperature proximately to cast, skin irritation at cast edges, numbness or tingling proximal to cast, redness on skin from prolonged pressure, break in skin from surgical correction.

(Refer Table 12.1 from chapter 12)

Nursing diagnosis

Altered growth and development related to effects of immobilization.

Assessment: Environmental and stimulation deficiencies, inability to perform self-care activities appropriate for age, inability to participate in school and social activities.

(Refer Table 14.4 from chapter 14)

B. Specific Nursing Diagnoses and Nursing Process

Nursing diagnosis

Knowledge deficit of parent(s) and child related to lack of information about the disease (Table 22.10).

Assessment: Request for information about initial and long-term treatment, management of the therapy, and modification of activities.

Evaluation
- Complies with long-term medical regimen to correct disorder
- Maintains correct position of hip joint; applies brace, belt, or harness correctly
- Prevents complications resulting from cast or appliance
- Verbalizes signs and symptoms of disease, cause of disease, length of treatment, type of treatment, prognosis, and projected outcome
- Complies with follow-up care requirements to monitor healing
- Prevents risk of degeneration by weight bearing or noncompliance of medical regimen
- Allows for continuing school and activities adapted to appliance within disease limitations
- Include in family activities with necessary preparations made to accommodate restrictions of disease/appliance
- Devises new activities and interests within restrictions of mobility.

Nursing Process for the Child with Musculoskeletal Disorder

Table 22.10: Nursing interventions for knowledge deficit of parent(s) and child.

Interventions	Rationales
Assess knowledge of pathology of the disease and its four stages, treatment and prognosis, signs and symptoms	Provides information needed to develop a plan of instruction to ensure compliance of the medical regimen for correction; usually lasts 2–3 years and affects children 3–12 years of age with each stage lasting approximately 9–12 months; the younger the child at the time of diagnosis, the more positive the results and prognosis
Inform parent(s) and child that hip pain or stiffness that is constant or intermittent with involvement of the knee or thigh, may be limited ROM of the hip joint, a limp on the affected side may indicate aseptic necrosis of the femoral capital epiphysis with degenerative changes in the femoral head	Reveals signs and symptoms of the disease usually noted in the second stage
Inform parent(s) and child of the need for bed rest and avoidance of weight bearing activities for several weeks	Prevents weight bearing to reduce inflammation and ultimately restore motion and function by maintaining the femur in the acetabulum and increasing the blood supply to the area
Inform parent(s) and child of use and purpose of traction if used	Applied to stretch adductor muscles before abduction brace, cast, or harness is used
Inform and instruct parent(s) in purpose and application of an abduction brace, leather harness sling, abduction-ambulation brace; after ROM achieved, demonstrate and allow for return demonstration of application	Provides containment of the position of the femur by preventing weight bearing on the affected limb until ossification is completed; cast or brace use is continued for 2–4 years following traction and bed rest; braces made from lightweight materials allow for near normal activity for the child
Inform parent(s) and child of importance of avoiding weight bearing on the affected limb and need to be relatively inactive, and advise activities suitable to stage of condition such as hobbies, crafts, games museums, events of interest	Prevents degeneration of the hip joint caused by femoral damage resulting from weight bearing activities
Inform parent(s) to advise school of activities that are allowed for learning and peer interactions	Provides special needs of child in order to continue school attendance and activities that may be adapted to appliance to promote feeling of acceptance
Instruct parent(s) in care of cast or brace including cleaning, tightness, alignment with joints	Promotes proper function of appliance used and prevents complications associated with its use
Instruct parent(s) and child in use and care of crutches if used including swing through gait; monitor for repair needs as presence of loose screws and worn tips	Promotes safe use of crutches for mobility
Inform parent(s) to maintain pathways clear of clutter or toys	Prevents falls and injury
Inform parent(s) to prepare for attendance at special activities by calling in advance for special transportation, use of wheelchairs or other aids	Provides for participation in outside activities to enhance growth and development needs in long-term therapy

(ROM: range of motion)

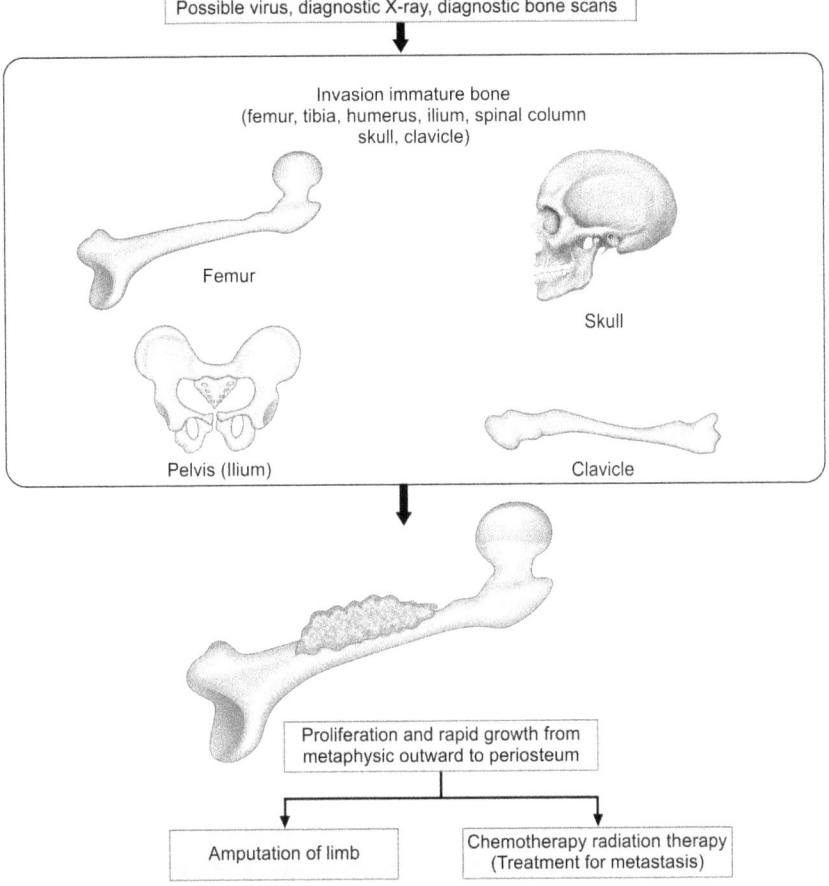

Fig. 22.5: Pathophysiology of osteogenic sarcoma.

Osteogenic Sarcoma

Osteogenic sarcoma is a primary malignancy of the bone with the metaphysic of the long bones most commonly affected. These include the femur, humerus, and tibia. Metastasis most commonly affects the lungs but may involve other organs. The disease most commonly occurs in children over 10 years of age. Treatment consists of amputation of the limb with chemotherapy before and/or following surgery, or a bone and joint replacement in selected children to salvage the limb with chemotherapy before the surgery **(Fig. 22.5)**.

Symptoms of Osteogenic Sarcoma

- Pain in the affected bone is the most common system. This pain may initially come and go and then gradually become more severe and constant
- As the tumor grows, there may be visible swelling and limitation of motion
- Tumors in the legs cause limping, while those in the arms cause pain on lifting
- Swelling over the tumor may be warm and slightly reddened

Nursing Process for the Child with Musculoskeletal Disorder

- Sometimes, the first sign may be a bone fracture
- The tumor may cause weakness in the affected area of the bone
- A fracture at the site of the tumor is called a "pathological fracture", which occurs after what often seems like a routine movement. For example, a young athlete who breaks an arm during a routine throw should be tested to ensure there is no underlying bone problem, such as a tumor or cyst.

Nursing Management

A. Essential Nursing Diagnoses and Nursing Process Associated with this Condition

Nursing diagnosis

Altered nutrition: Less than body requirements related to inability to ingest and digest food, chemotherapy.

Assessment: Anorexia, nausea, vomiting from chemotherapy, anxiety, grieving, weight loss, NPO status before and after surgery.

(Refer Table 14.3 from chapter 14)

Nursing diagnosis

High-risk for fluid volume deficit related to altered intake; excessive losses through normal routes.

Assessment: Diarrhea, vomiting from chemotherapy, NPO status before and after surgery.

(Refer Table 14.11 from chapter 14)

Nursing diagnosis

High-risk for impaired skin integrity related to external factors of chemotherapy IV, surgical site, and use of prosthesis.

Assessment: Disruption of skin surfaces, destruction of skin surfaces, redness, edema, excoriation of stump site, improper fit or application of prosthesis, extravasations of IV site with swelling pain, redness, and tissue necrosis.

(Refer Table 12.1 from chapter 12)

Nursing diagnosis

Impaired physical mobility related to musculoskeletal impairment (amputation).

Assessment: Inability to move within physical environment, reluctance to attempt movement, imposed restrictions of movement with loss of limb, inability to adapt to prosthesis or brace, use of crutches or wheelchair.

(Refer Table 14.19 from chapter 14)

Nursing diagnosis

Diarrhea related to chemotherapy.

Assessment: Increased frequency of bowel sounds and loose, liquid stools.

(Refer Table 13.8 from chapter 13)

Table 22.11: Nursing interventions for anxiety of parent(s) and child.

Interventions	Rationales
Assess level of anxiety of parent(s) and child and how it is manifested; the need for information that will relieve anxiety	Provides information about source and level of anxiety and need for interventions to relieve it; sources for the child may be procedures, fear of mutilation or death, unfamiliar environment of hospital and may be manifested by restlessness, inability to play or sleep or eat
Assess possible need for special counseling services for child	Reduces anxiety and supports child dealing with illness and promotes adjustment to lifestyle changes
Allow open expression of concerns about illness, procedures treatments, and possible consequences of surgery and prognosis	Provides opportunity to vent feelings and fears to reduce anxiety
Communicate with child at appropriate age level and answer questions calmly and honestly; use pictures, models, and drawings for explanations	Promotes understanding and trust
Allow child as much input in decisions about care and routines as possible	Allows for more control and independence in situations
Allow parent(s) to stay visitation; provide a telephone number to call for information	Promotes care and support by parent(s)
Orient child to surgical and ICU unit, equipment, noises, and staff	Reduces anxiety caused by fear of unknown

B. Specific Nursing Diagnoses and Nursing Process

Nursing diagnosis

Anxiety of parent(s) and child related to change in health status, threat of death, threat to self-concept **(Table 22.11)**.

Assessment: Increased apprehension and fear of diagnosis; expressed concern and worry about preoperative procedures and preparation, postoperative effects of therapy on physical and emotional status, possible metastasis of disease, loss of limb and use of prosthesis.

Evaluation
- Expresses reduction in anxiety as information and explanations are given
- States concerns and reason for anxiety and behavior
- Verbalizes and participates in preoperative and postoperative procedures
- Explores and notes anger about diagnosis and proposed change in body structure and function
- Utilizes existing and new support systems
- Participates in decision making regarding care and postoperative rehabilitation.

Nursing diagnosis

Altered oral mucous membrane related to medication (chemotherapy) **(Table 22.12)**.

Assessment: Stomatitis, oral ulcers, hyperemia, oral pain or discomfort, oral plaque.

Nursing Process for the Child with Musculoskeletal Disorder

Table 22.12: Nursing interventions for altered mucous membrane.

Interventions	Rationales
Assess oral cavity for pain, ulcers, lesions, gingivitis, mucositis or stomatitis and effect on ability to ingest food and fluids	Provides information about effect of chemotherapy
Provide mouth rinses, cleansing with swabs or soft toothbrush	Provides mouth care without irritating oral mucosa
Administer medication topically (xylocaine) before meals and offer bland, smooth foods that are not hot or spicy	Permits eating with more comfort
Administer an antiseptic mouth rinse (nystatin) 30 minutes before any food or fluid intake	Promotes comfort of oral mucosa and maintains integrity
Encourage child to select foods that are allowable and that they prefer	Allows for independence and control over situation to reduce helplessness and increase nutrition

Evaluation
- Oral mucous membranes intact and reduced inflammation present
- Complies with measures to prevent trauma breakdown of mucosa
- Control discomfort associated with impaired oral mucosa
- Progressive return of oral mucous membranes baseline following chemotherapy protocol.

Nursing diagnosis

Altered protection related to drug therapy (antineoplastics): abnormal blood profile (leucopenia, thrombocytopenia, anemia, coagulation) **(Table 22.13)**.

Assessment: Altered clotting, bone marrow suppression, deficient immunity against infection, hematoma, petechiae, bleeding from nose or gums, hematemesis, blood in stool.

Evaluation
- Absence of excessive bleeding or infection during chemotherapy
- Complies with measures to prevent excessive bleeding or infection based on blood profile
- Reports signs and symptoms of complication to physician
- Complies with laboratory blood testing and follow-up visits to physician.

Table 22.13: Nursing interventions for altered protection.

Interventions	Rationales
Assess for bleeding from any site, WBC, platelet count, HCT, absolute neutrophil count, and febrile episodes	Provides information about frank bleeding or blood profile abnormalities that predispose to bleeding caused by bone marrow suppression and immunosuppression resulting from chemotherapy
Avoid trauma by use of hard toothbrush or dental floss, taking rectal temperatures, performing unnecessary invasive procedures	Prevents bleeding caused by trauma during chemotherapy which alters platelet and clotting factors
Carry out handwashing technique before giving care, use mask and gown when appropriate, provide a private room, monitor for any signs and symptoms of infections especially pulmonary	Prevents transmission of pathogens to a compromised immune system during chemotherapy if neutrophil count is less than 1,000/cm mm

(HCT: hematocrit; WBC: white blood cell)

Table 22.14: Nursing interventions for high-risk for injury related to internal physical factor of broken skin and altered mobility, external physical factor of prosthesis use.

Interventions	Rationales
Assess child for type of surgery and condition and healing of the stump, type of bandaging or cast, presence of drains, type of prosthetic device and fit	Provides information about amputation needed to provide specific care of stump and rehabilitation
Assess dressing for bleeding, redness, pain, drainage at stump area q24h; maintain dressing (pressure) or wrapping of stump as ordered; change dressing only if ordered	Indicates infection or risk of hemorrhage at amputation
Maintain trendelenburg and prone position; avoid elevation (with pillow), external rotation, or abduction of stump	Prevents deformities and contractures caused by hip flexion
Perform ROM daily and exercises recommended by physical therapist	Promotes mobility and healing of the stump and prevents contractures
Cleanse stump and socket daily with mild soap and warm water, rinse and pat dry	Promotes adaptation to device and prevents infection caused by pathogens transmitted via the prosthetic device
Support expressions about of loss of lifestyle and permanent disability adjustment difficulties (age appropriate)	Promotes venting of feelings and assists to cope with change in body image

(ROM: range of motion)

Nursing diagnosis

High-risk for injury related to internal physical factor of broken skin and altered mobility; external physical factor of prosthesis use **(Table 22.14)**.

Assessment: Amputation of a limb, changes in stump incision (redness, irritation, swelling, drainage), improper fit of prosthesis and failure to adapt to it, improper positioning and alignment of the stump, psychosocial maladaption to prosthesis.

Evaluation
- Maintains appropriate and effective care of stump and prosthetic device
- Complies with exercise and physical therapy regimen
- Surgical site is healing and free of infection
- Proper fit and use of prosthesis with progressive mobility
- Adapts daily to loss of limb and dependence on prosthesis
- Provides changes in lifestyle and appearance necessary to preserve body image
- Resumes preoperative activities gradually
- Utilizes aids (crutches, wheelchair) until healing and prosthesis use and competency realized.

Osteomyelitis

Osteomyelitis is an infection of the bone caused by any infectious agent through an exogenous or hematogenous (most common) route. It may involve one or more bones or joints with the femur and tibia the most common sites in children and the skull the most common site in infants. Osteomyelitis most commonly occurs in children 5–14 years of age. It may be acute with the child suffering severe symptoms and appearing irritable and restless requiring immediate,

Nursing Process for the Child with Musculoskeletal Disorder

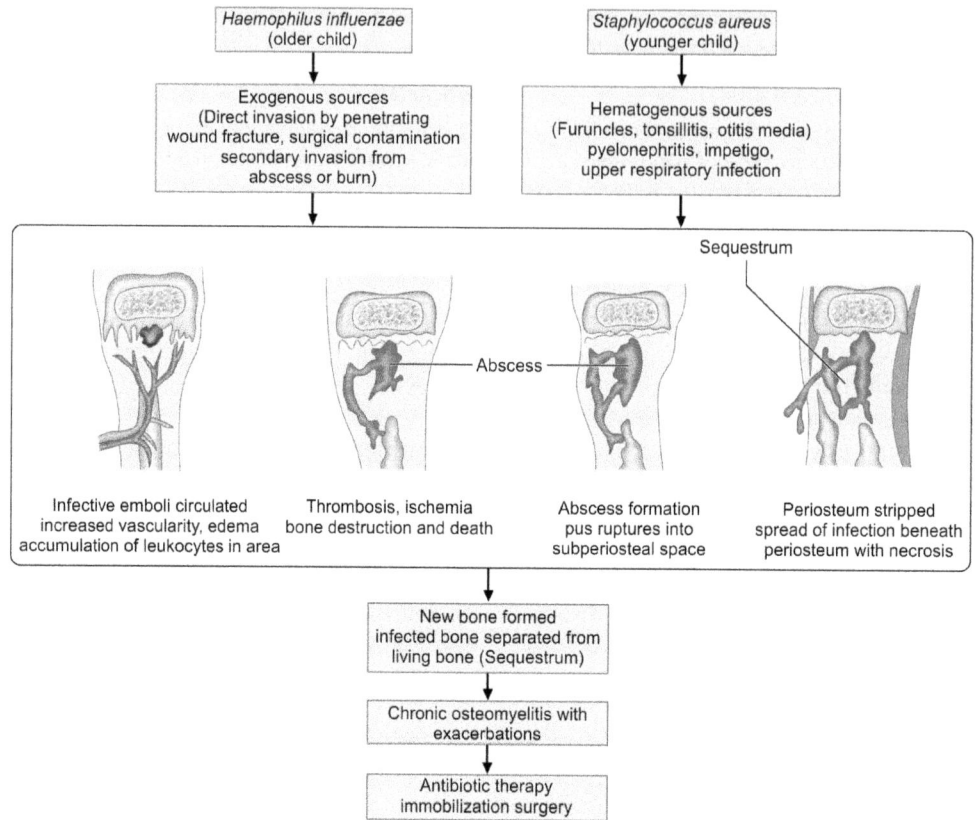

Fig. 22.6: Pathophysiology of osteomyelitis.

long-term treatment with antibiotics. A subacute osteomyelitis occurs when the symptoms are relieved by antibiotic therapy given for other infections in the presence of the disease. Physical therapy completes the medical regimen to restore or rehabilitate the affected area **(Fig. 22.6)**.

Symptoms of Osteomyelitis

- Fever of chills
- Irritability or lethargy in young children
- Pain in the area of the infection
- Swelling, warmth and redness over the area of the infection.

Nursing Management

A. Essential Nursing Diagnosis and Nursing Process Associated with this Condition

Nursing diagnosis

Hyperthermia related to illness (infection).

Assessment: Increase in body temperature above normal range, warm to touch, increased respiratory and pulse rate.

(Refer Table 14.18 from chapter 14)

Nursing diagnosis

High-risk for fluid volume deficit related to excessive losses through normal routes.

Assessment: Elevated temperature, diaphoresis, thirst, altered intake, insensitive losses.

(Refer Table 14.11 from chapter 14)

Nursing diagnosis

Impaired physical immobility related to pain and discomfort, musculoskeletal impairment.

Assessment: Reluctance to attempt movement, imposed restrictions of movement by immobilization of part by cast and/or bed rest, restriction in weight-bearing.

(Refer Table 14.19 from chapter 14)

Nursing diagnosis

Altered nutrition: Less than body requirements related to inability to ingest food.

Assessment: Anorexia, irritability, restlessness, weight loss, inadequate food intake.

(Refer Table 14.3 from chapter 14)

Nursing diagnosis

High-risk for impaired skin integrity related to external factor of physical immobilization, pressure of cast and altered circulation, sensation.

Assessment: Change in color and temperature of skin proximal to cast or device, skin irritation at cast edges, numbness proximal cast, prolonged pressure on an area with redness present, break in skin from surgical wound.

(Refer Table 12.1 from chapter 12)

B. Specific Nursing Diagnoses and Nursing Process

Nursing diagnosis

Anxiety of parent(s) and child related to change in health status, change in environment (hospitalization) **(Table 22.15)**.

Assessment: Expressed apprehension and concern about prolonged hospitalization resulting from spread of infection, possible surgical drainage of infected area.

Evaluation
- Verbalizes reduction in anxiety about disease, diagnostic procedures, and treatments
- Verbalizes positive effects of surgical intervention and postoperative treatments
- Participates in care and support of child and decision making during hospitalization.

Nursing diagnosis

Pain related to physical injuring agent (inflammation/infection) **(Table 22.16)**.

Assessment: Communication of pain descriptors, crying, irritability, restlessness, withdrawal, reluctance to use or move affected limb, tenderness.

Nursing Process for the Child with Musculoskeletal Disorder

Table 22.15: Nursing interventions for anxiety of parent(s) and child.

Interventions	Rationales
Assess source and level of anxiety and need for information that will relieve anxiety	Provides information about anxiety, its effect and need to relieve it; sources may include prolonged immobilization and hospitalization, long-term antibiotic instillation into wound, risk of complications from disease and high dose medication therapy
Allow expression of concerns and time to ask questions about condition, procedures, prognosis, recovery time by parent(s) or child	Provides opportunity to vent feelings and fears to reduce anxiety
Answer questions calmly and honestly; use pictures, drawings, and models for information and demonstrations	Promotes trust and a secure, supportive environment
Encourage parent(s) to stay with child during hospitalization, and encourage to assist in care; encourage visits from friends and relatives	Allows parent(s) to care for and support child, continue parental role and promote security for the child
Give parent(s) and child as much input into decisions about care and usual routines as possible	Allows for more control over situations and maintains familiar routines for care

Table 22.16: Nursing interventions for pain.

Interventions	Rationales
Assess site for pain on movement of extremity; resistance of muscles to passive movement, holding extremity in semiflexion; severity, type, and duration of pain using a pain scale if appropriate	Provides information about pain as a basis for analgesic therapy
Administer analgesic and sedative as ordered and note response	Reduces pain and promotes rest to reduce stimuli that causes pain
Place extremity in position of comfort and support with pillows at 30° elevation	Promotes comfort and reduce or prevents pain by reducing edema when venous return is enhanced
Move extremity with smoothness and care	Prevents pain caused by careless handling or abrupt movement of affected part
Provide diversional activities and quiet play during acute stage	Diverts attention from the pain

Evaluation
- Absence of pain and associated responses
- Controls pain provoking actions when giving care or changing position
- Administer analgesics and sedatives correctly and monitor responses.

Nursing diagnosis

High-risk for injury related to internal factors of infection spread, immobilization, effects of cast application **(Table 22.17)**.

Table 22.17: Nursing interventions for high-risk for injury related to internal factors of infection spread, immobilization, effects of cast application.

Interventions	Rationales
Assess presence of localized pain, swelling, and warmth over the affected bone; purulent drainage with a musty odor from open wound, under cast, or over the infected area that is left open for observation	Provides information about site of infection(s) which may be open wound, bone, or surgical drainage wound; inadequate treatment may result in chronic osteomyelitis or persistence and spread of infection
Administer antibiotics IV based on culture and sensitivity results and physician orders; administer antibiotics	Treats infectious process and prevents spread of infection by preventing cell wall synthesis of the invading bacteria
PO following acute phase of the disease; administer via IV heparin lock if therapy is long-term	IV therapy may last for 3–4 weeks or longer depending on the response to treatment
Administer antibiotic solution into the wound, if present, via an IV administration set at a regulated rate; provide wound drainage by connecting tubes from wound to low suction	Treats open wound infections and ensures continuous wound drainage
Place in isolation or maintain universal body fluid precautions	Prevents wound contamination or spread of infection
Maintain sterile technique for all procedures and dressing changes; cleanse, pack wound as ordered	Prevents introduction of infectious organisms
Measure limb circumference when assessing infectious process	Reveals changes caused by edema
Monitor WBC, ESR, and antibiotic levels as appropriate	Increases in WBC and ESR found in infections and antibiotic levels reveal if therapeutic levels are maintained for effective treatment
Provide immobilization of limb by maintaining cast, splint, and bed rest status, monitor color, temperature, sensation, and motion of digits	Maintains limb alignment, limits spread of infection, and prevents possible complications

(IV: intravenous; PO: per os or by mouth; WBC: white blood cell; ESR: erythrocyte sedimentation rate)

Assessment: Changes in color and temperature, tactile perception of casted extremity increased body temperature, purulent drainage, edema, erythematous infection site, musty odor under cast, increased WBC, positive wound culture.

Evaluation
- Absence of infection spread
- Administers antibiotic therapy correctly; IV, PO, or wound instillation as appropriate
- Maintains isolation or wound and skin precautions
- Performs hand wash and proper technique during care and procedures
- Maintains safe, effective cast or splint care for immobilization
- Reports and prevents complications of immobilization or medication administration.

Nursing diagnosis

Impaired social interaction related to limited physical mobility, therapeutic isolation (**Table 22.18**).

Nursing Process for the Child with Musculoskeletal Disorder

Table 22.18: Nursing interventions for impaired social interaction.

Interventions	Rationales
Provide age-appropriate toys that can be used in bed while in a prone or sitting position depending on type of treatment and degree of immobilization	Promotes social and developmental activities and reduces boredom during long-term treatment
Provide exposure to other children by moving bed near areas of activity or near a window; wheel on a stretcher or in a wheelchair or stroller, allow to walk with cast or splint when permitted	Provides environmental stimulation and social interaction
Encourage family and friends to visit or stay with child; if in isolation provide frequent interactions or someone to stay with child	Promotes social interaction with others during long-term treatment and reduces boredom
Place toys and other articles within reach	Provides access to diversion activities when needed

Assessment: Change in pattern of interaction, lengthy treatment and immobilization boredom, inability to engage in usual activities for age group, environment that lacks diversion.

Evaluation
- Participates in positive interaction with peers and family members
- Maintains age appropriate stimulation and play activities
- Participates in family activities
- Promotes a variety of activities contributing to growth and development needs.

Rheumatoid Arthritis (Juvenile)

Rheumatoid arthritis of the juvenile type is a chronic inflammatory disease that involves the synovium of the joints resulting in effusion and eventual erosion and destruction of the joint cartilage. It is classified into different types and characterized by remissions and exacerbations with the onset most common between 2–5 and 9–12 years of age. Pauciarticular type of arthritis involves only a few joints, usually under four; polyarticular type of arthritis involves many joints, usually more than five; and systemic arthritis involves the presence of arthritis and associated high temperature, rash, and other organs such as the heart, lungs, eyes, and those located in the abdominal cavity. Prognosis is based on the severity of the disease, type of arthritis, and response to treatment with the most severe complications of the permanent deformity, hip disease, and iridocyclitis with visual loss **(Fig. 22.7)**.

Symptoms of Rheumatoid Arthritis (Juvenile)
- Persistent joint swelling, pain, and stiffness that juvenile idiopathic typically is worse in the morning of after a nap
- Intermittent fever
- Loss of appetite
- Weight loss
- Anemia, of a blotchy rash on a child's arms and legs may also signal juvenile rheumatoid arthritis

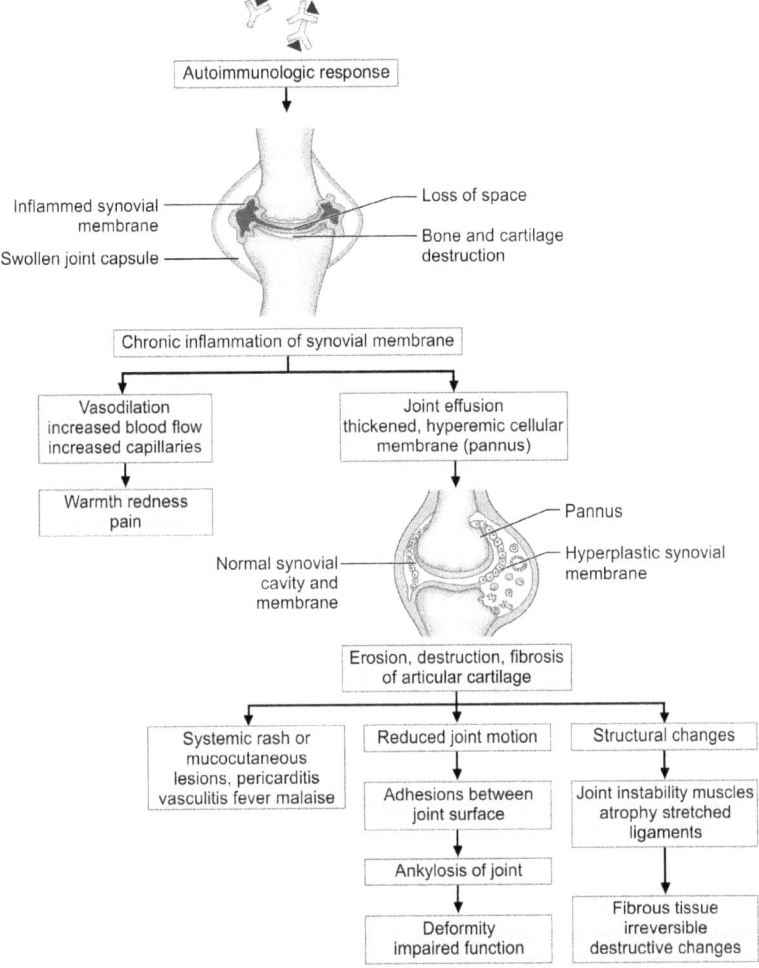

Fig. 22.7: Pathophysiology of rheumatoid arthritis (juvenile).

- The pain may limit movement of the affected joint, although many children, especially younger ones, do not complain of pain
- One of the earliest signs of JRA may be limping in the morning because of a stiff knee.

Nursing Management

A. Essential Nursing Diagnoses and Nursing Process Associated with this Condition

Nursing diagnosis

Impaired physical mobility related to musculoskeletal impairment, pain, and discomfort.

Assessment: Reluctance to attempt movement, limited range of motion, imposed restrictions of movement by medical protocol, resting or immobilization of joint(s) by splinting and positioning, fatigue, malaise.

(Refer Table 14.19 from chapter 14)

Nursing diagnosis

High-risk for impaired skin integrity related to external factor or physical immobilization.

Assessment: Skin irritation under splint(s), redness from prolonged pressure, break in skin from surgery if done, macular rash on extremities and trunk areas.

(Refer Table 12.1 from chapter 12)

Nursing diagnosis

Altered growth and development related to effects of physical disability.

Assessment: Environmental and stimulation deficiencies, inability to perform self-care activities appropriate for age, growth retardation during active disease, reduced peer relationships.

(Refer Table 14.4 from chapter 14)

Nursing diagnosis

Hyperthermia related to illness of inflammation.

Assessment: Increase in body temperature above normal range, chills, low grade temperature or high elevations late in day or twice a day.

(Refer Table 14.18 from chapter 14)

Nursing diagnosis

Altered nutrition: Less than body requirements related to inability to ingest food.

Assessment: Anorexia, weight loss or poor gain, weakness, fatigue, irritability.

(Refer Table 14.3 from chapter 14)

B. Specific Nursing Diagnoses and Nursing Process

Nursing diagnosis

Chronic pain related to chronic physical disability **(Table 22.19)**.

Assessment: Verbalization or observed evidence of pain experienced for more than 6 months, guarded movement, fear of reinjury, altered ability to continue activities, physical and social withdrawal, single or multiple joint involvement, joint stiffness, loss of motion, edema, and warmth in joint(s) and painful to touch.

Evaluation
- Pain and inflammation relieved or controlled
- Limits or a voids factors that initiate or increase pain
- Complies with long-term medication protocol
- Minimal discomfort during movement or activity
- Administers medications properly with meals, reports side effects, complies with laboratory testing as ordered.

Nursing diagnosis

Body image disturbance related to biophysical and psychosocial factors **(Table 22.20)**.

Assessment: Verbal and nonverbal responses to change in body appearance (joint deformity, steroid side effects), negative feelings about body, multiple stressors and change in daily living limitations and social relationships.

Nursing Process for the Child with Musculoskeletal Disorder

Table 22.19: Nursing interventions for chronic pain.

Interventions	Rationales
Assess severity of joint(s) pain, location, duration, remissions and exacerbations, stiffness and what precipitates pain, activity, fatigue; effect on mobility and participation and ADL; presence of joint deformity	Provides information symptomatic of the effects of the disease on the musculoskeletal system: allows for analgesic/anti-inflammatory selection and better management of activity involvement; inflammatory process causes pain with the edema resulting from joint effusion and synovial thickening and limited motion resulting from muscle spasms; joint deformity resulting from joint destruction
Administer steroid or nonsteroid anti-inflammatories as ordered and assess effect of medications in relieving pain	Relieves pain and the inflammatory process associated with the pain; drugs may be administered alone or in combination including the nonsteroidal anti-inflammatory drugs which act as analgesic, antipyretic and anti-inflammatory; sloweracting antirheumatic drugs which may be added for optimal effect if NSAIDs are ineffective; corticosteroid drugs in lowest effective dose for short period of time especially in the presence of a life-threatening situation
Apply warm compresses, packs, or soaks to painful areas; paraffin baths and whirlpool as ordered	Promotes circulation to the area by vasodilation to relieve pain; moist heat relieves painful, stiff joints
Provide 1–2 rest periods during day and quiet environment for sleep	Decreases stimulation that increases pain, and it promotes rest, especially during acute episodes
Allow to assume position of comfort, elevate and support painful joints when changing position	Provides comfort and rest for joints to reduce pain
Apply splints if ordered for night use	Provides immobilization of joints to ease pain during movement

(ADL: activities of daily living; NSAIDs: non-steroidal anti-inflammatory drugs)

Table 22.20: Nursing interventions for body image disturbance.

Interventions	Rationales
Assess child for feelings about multiple restrictions in lifestyle, chronic illness, difficulty in school and social situations, inability to keep up with peers and participate in activities	Provides information about status of self-concept and body image than require special attention
Encourage expression of feelings and concerns, and support communications with parent(s), teachers, and peers	Provides opportunity to vent feelings and reduce negative feelings about changes in appearance
Avoid negative comments and stress positive activities and accomplishments	Enhances body image and confidence
Note withdrawal behavior and signs of depression	Reveals response to body image changes and possible poor adjustment to changes
Note presence of joint deformities, need to use splints, weight gain, shift in fat distribution, edema, and effect on child	Reveals side effects of steroid therapy and disease manifestations that affect body image
Show support and acceptance of changes in appearance of child; provide privacy as needed	Promotes trust and demonstrates respect for child

Nursing Process for the Child with Musculoskeletal Disorder

Table 22.21: Nursing interventions for self-care deficit (bathing/hygiene, dressing/grooming, feeding, toileting).

Interventions	Rationales
Assess abilities and level of care and assistance needed	Provides information about child's ability to perform self-care and to monitor progress
Allow as much independence in ADL as possible but assist when needed	Promotes independence and control over daily personal care needs without damage to joints
Encourage to perform own care and praise all accomplishments	Promotes sense of accomplishment and independence; motivates to continue progress in ADL
Position article needed for care within reach; provide physical aids/devices to assist in performance of ADL (crutches, wheelchair, utensils that are easy to handle, hand bard, handles that are easy to open, clothing that is easy to put on and take off with zippers	Promotes independence and allows child access to aids to enhance independence
Assist parent(s) and child to develop plan and goals for daily ADL and suggest inclusions of actions taught by physical and occupational therapist	Promotes independence and compliance in self-care

(ADL: activities of daily living)

Evaluation
- Verbalizes improved body image and sense of well-being
- Participates in family, school, and social activities as appropriate
- Verbalizes feelings about special long-term needs in positive terms
- Supports positive body image and promotes adjustment to chronic illness.

Nursing diagnosis

Self-care deficit (bathing/hygiene, dressing/grooming, feeding, toileting) related to pain, discomfort, and musculoskeletal impairment **(Table 22.21)**.

Assessment: Impaired ability in performance of ADL and maintenance of complete physical care; pain and weakness of joints and intolerance to activity; immobility status; joint deformity and/or contractures.

Evaluation
- Performs ADL within physical abilities without fatigue or injury to joints
- Maximizes capabilities for self-care with use of aids/devices as appropriate
- Plans and schedules ADL with daily progression in independence
- Avoids activities that cause pain or injury to joints.

Nursing diagnosis

Ineffective family coping: Compromised related to inadequate or incorrect information or understanding, prolonged disease or disability progression that exhausts the physical and emotional supportive capacity of caretakers **(Table 22.22)**.

Assessment: Expression and/or confirmation of concern and inadequate knowledge about long-term care needs, problems and complications, anxiety and guilt, overprotection of child.

Table 22.22: Nursing interventions for ineffective family coping.

Interventions	Rationales
Assess family coping methods used and effectiveness, family interactions and expectations related to long-term care, developmental level of family, response of siblings, knowledge and use of support systems and resources, presence of guilt and anxiety, overprotection and/or overindulgence behaviors	Provides information identifying coping methods that work and the need to develop new coping skills and behaviors, family attitudes; child with special long-term needs may strengthen or strain family relationships and an undue degree of over protection may be detrimental to child's growth and development (disallow school attendance and peer activities, avoiding discipline of child, and not allowing child to assume responsibilities for ADL)
Encourage family members to express problem areas and explore solutions responsibly	Reduces anxiety and enhances understanding; provides family an opportunity to identify problems and develop problem solving strategies
Assist family to establish short and long-term goals for child and to integrate child into family activities include participation of all family members in care routines	Promotes involvement and control over situations and maintains role of family members and parent(s)
Provide assistance of social worker, counselor, clergy, or other as needed	Provides support to the family faced with long-term care of child with a chronic illness
Allow family members to express feelings, how they deal with the chronic needs of family member and coping patterns that help or hinder adjustment to the problems	Allows for venting of feelings to determine need for information and support, and to relieve guilt and anxiety

(ADL: activities of daily living)

Evaluation
- Verbalizes and clarifies child's and family's knowledge about long-term needs and care
- Develops and uses coping skills and problem solving techniques effectively
- Supports and cares for child by family members while meeting own needs
- Preserves family relationships and minimizes family stressors with differences resolved
- Progressive adaptation and acceptance of long-term condition and therapy by family
- Implements preventive measures of follow-up care to ensure optimal function and health of child.

Scoliosis

Scoliosis is a lateral curvature of the spine with the thoracic area being the most commonly affected. It is classified as either structural, which is the result of a congenital defect, or functional which results from an underlying problem of posture or another deformity. Structural scoliosis is more progressive and causes changes in supporting structures such as the ribs, and correction includes electrical stimulation, brace, and/or surgical instrumentation and bone graft. Functional scoliosis disappears when the child lies down, and correction includes exercises, use of shoe lifts and correction of visual defects. The deformity may occur at any age from infancy through adolescence with the best prognosis related to those with less growth remaining and when the curvature is of a mild degree **(Fig. 22.8)**.

Nursing Process for the Child with Musculoskeletal Disorder

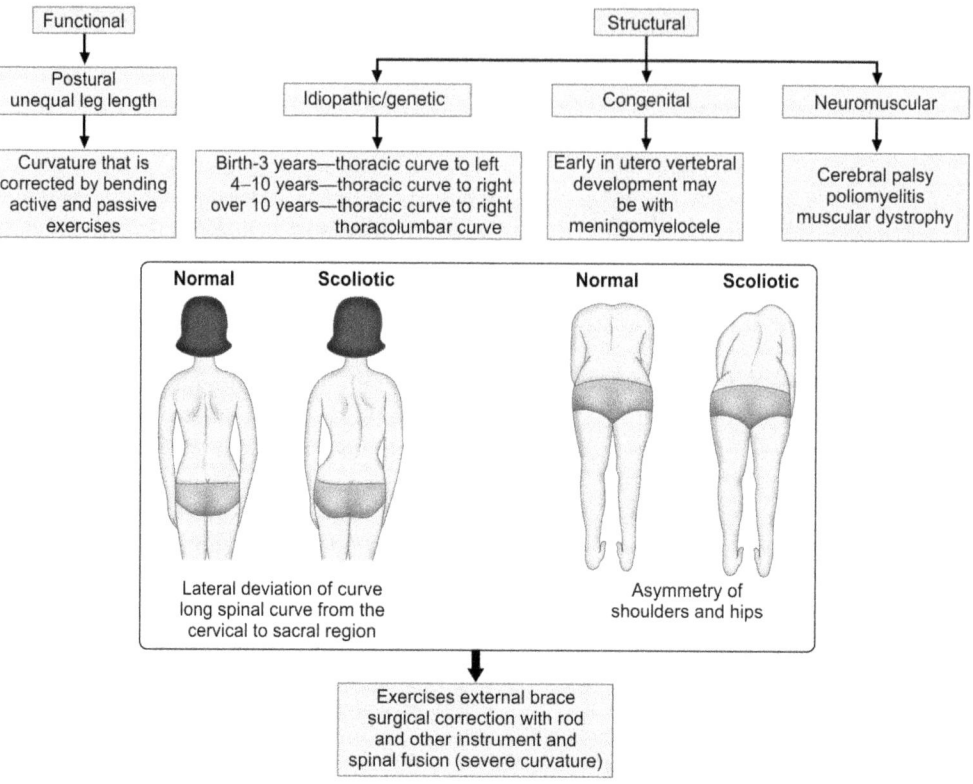

Fig. 22.8: Pathophysiology of scoliosis.

Symptoms of Scoliosis

- Uneven shoulders
- One shoulder blade that appears more prominent than the other
- Uneven waist
- One hip higher than the other

If a scoliosis curve gets worse, the spine will also rotate or twist, in addition to curving side to side. This causes the ribs on one side of the body to stick out farther on the other side.

- Severe scoliosis can cause back pain and difficulty breathing.

Nursing Management

A. Essential Nursing Diagnoses and Nursing Process Associated with this Condition

Nursing diagnosis

Impaired physical mobility related to musculoskeletal impairment (curvature of spine).

Assessment: Imposed restrictions of movement by medical protocol of corrective device (brace, cast following surgery, traction), bed rest and inability to purposefully move with in the physical environment following surgery or with halo traction or cast.

(Refer Table 14.19 from chapter 14)

Nursing diagnosis

High-risk for impaired skin integrity related to external factors of physical immobilization, pressure of cast, traction, or brace and altered sensation and circulation, surface electrical stimulation.

Assessment: Change in skin color and temperature, skin irritation at simulation, brace, cast sites, redness on areas from prolonged pressure, break in skin from surgical correction or implantation of stimulator, numbness or tingling proximal to cast.

(Refer Table 12.1 from chapter 12)

Nursing diagnosis

Altered growth and development related to effects on immobilization and restricted movement from spinal curvature.

Assessment: Environmental and stimulation deficiencies, inability to participate in self-care and social activities with long-term continuous brace use.

(Refer Table 14.4 from chapter 14)

B. Specific Nursing Diagnoses and Nursing Process

Nursing diagnosis

Knowledge deficit of parent(s) and child related to lack of information about correction of functional or structural scoliosis **(Table 22.23)**.

Assessment: Request for information about treatments for scoliosis, application of brace of jacket, surgical procedure to correct scoliosis.

Evaluation
- Verbalizes knowledge of spinal defect, cause and treatment
- Compliance and adjustment to long-term therapy regimen
- Appropriate application, removal, and care of brace of jacket
- Performs daily exercises appropriate to specific child
- Performs electrical stimulation without complications
- Verbalizes understanding of need for surgical interventions and potential for positive outcome for child
- Absence of accidents or injury with use of brace or during ambulation following surgery
- Complies with physiotherapy until independent in activities
- Absence of complications from cast application, use of brace, or surgical alignment of spine.

Nursing diagnosis

Body image disturbance related to biophysical and psychosocial factors of spinal deformity **(Table 22.24)**.

Assessment: Verbal response to actual change in structure of spine, negative feelings about body, dependence on long-term use of brace, feeling of rejection by peers, inability to participate in some activities.

Evaluation
- Verbalizes improved body image and sense of well-being
- Participates in family, school, and social activities as appropriate

Nursing Process for the Child with Musculoskeletal Disorder

Table 22.23: Nursing interventions for knowledge deficit of parent(s) and child.

Interventions	Rationales
Assess knowledge of deformity, cause, and treatments	Provides information about teaching needs
Inform parent(s) and child of presence of functional or structural defect and methods of treatment modalities specific to age of child and severity of the deformity	Promotes understanding of type of defect and treatment protocol to relieve anxiety; functional scoliosis is corrected by treating the underlying problem, and structural scoliosis is treated with long-term bracing and exercising or surgical fixation to straighten and realign spine
Instruct parent(s) and child in application, care, and removal of brace or orthoplast jacket, and inform that appliance must be worn for 23 hours/day and may be removed for bathing	Provides nonoperative bracing to prevent progressive curvatures; curves 30–60 degrees are treated with Milwaukee brace until growth has been completed; low curvatures are treated with the orthoplast jacket that is molded to treat specific corrections needed
Instruct child in exercises performed in and out of the brace or other appliance and to perform them daily	Prevents atrophy of muscles of spine and abdomen
Instruct child in maintaining proper posture, use of shoe lifts, exercises, and other prescribed treatments for functional scoliosis	Corrects functional scoliosis which is usually caused by poor posture or unequal length of legs
Instruct parent(s) and child in use of electrical stimulation, application of electrodes, skin protection, connection of leads, operation of machine to be used at night	Provides stimulation to the muscles to treat curves of under 4° to prevent progression of curvature
Inform parent(s) and child of operative procedure planned and preoperative preparation required; reinforce physician information and use pictures, models and drawings to aid in teaching	Provides information about option for internal surgical instrumentation.

Table 22.24: Nursing interventions for body image disturbance.

Interventions	Rationales
Assess child for feelings about wearing brace, long-term treatments, restrictions in lifestyle, inability to keep up with peers and participate in activities	Provides information about status of self-concept and changes in appearance
Encourage expression of feelings and concerns and support child's communications with parent(s), peers and teachers	Provides opportunity to vent and reduce negative feelings about changes in appearance and continuing wearing of an appliance
Maintain positive environment and promote activities that are allowed (sports, play, games)	Enhances body image and confidence, and promotes trust and respect of child
Assist with plan for independence in ADL, application and removal of appliance, selection of shoes and clothing to wear such as T-shirt	Promotes independence and adjustment to appliance
Assist child to adjust to self-perception of short leg, use of appliance and effect on appearance	Promotes positive self-image and realistic view of appearance

(ADL: activities of daily living)

- Verbalized feelings about special long-term needs in positive terms
- Supports positive body image and prompt adjustment to restrictions caused by use of appliance of surgery
- Avoids activities potentially injurious for spinal correction
- Promotes independence and decision making in ADL.

Talipes

Talipes (clubfoot) is a congenital disorder of the foot usually with ankle involvement characterized by a twisting out of a normal position that is unable to be manipulated into a different position. The deformity is typed and named according to the position of the foot and include talipes varus (foot inversion), talipes valgus (foot eversion), talipes equinus (plantar flexion), and talipes calcaneus (dorsiflexion). Most are a combination of these with the most common deformity known as talipes equinovarus (inversion and plantar flexion of the foot). The defect may occur alone or in association with other congenital syndromes or defects **(Fig. 22.9)**.

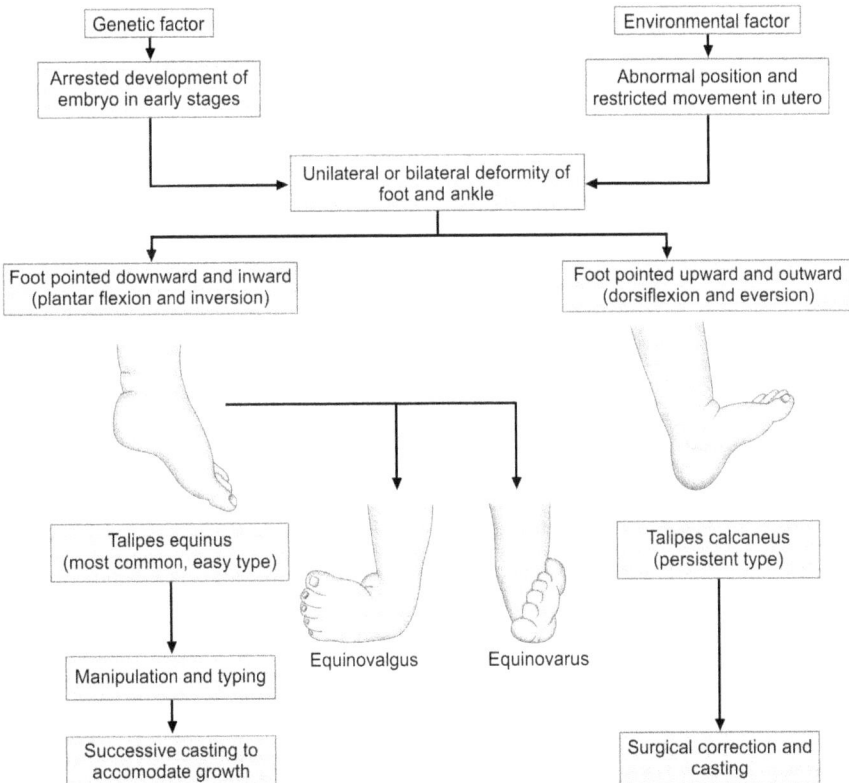

Fig. 22.9: Pathophysiology of talipes (club foot).

Symptoms of Talipes (Clubfoot)
- The top of the foot is usually twisted downward and inward, increasing the arch and turning the heel inward.
- The foot may be turned so severely that it actually looks as if it's upside down.
- The calf muscles in the affected leg are usually underdeveloped.
- The affected foot may be up to 1/2 inch (about 1 centimeter) shorter than the other foot.

Nursing Management

A. Essential Nursing Diagnoses and Nursing Process Associated with this Condition

Nursing diagnosis

Impaired physical mobility related to musculoskeletal impairment (talipes deformity).

Assessment: Imposed restrictions of movement by medical protocol of corrective device, serial cast application.

(Refer Table 14.19 from chapter 19)

Nursing diagnosis

High-risk for impaired skin integrity related to external factor of physical immobilization by cast(s); internal factors of altered circulation, sensation by cast pressure.

Assessment: Edema, rapid growth rate, tight cast or appliance, color change and cool skin proximal to cast.

(Refer Table 12.1 from chapter 12)

Nursing diagnosis

Altered growth and development related to effects of physical disability (immobilization).

Assessment: Delay in performing motor skills typical of age group during cast applications, lack of stimulation while cast is present.

(Refer Table 14.4 from chapter 14)

B. Specific Nursing Diagnoses and Nursing Process

Nursing diagnosis

Knowledge deficit of parent(s) related to lack of information about condition **(Table 22.25)**.

Assessment: Request for information about disorder, its cause and treatment for correction, follow-up care.

Evaluation
- Complies with long-term medical regimen to correct deformity
- Maintains correct position of feet, applies strapping or splint correctly and in appropriate frequency
- Prevents circulatory complications of cast application
- Verbalizes type of deformity, cause, length, and projected outcome of treatment

Table 22.25: Nursing interventions for knowledge deficit of parent(s).

Interventions	Rationales
Assess knowledge of disorder, type of deformity, and if one or both feet are involved; type of immobilization and application and/or care; presence of associated congenital disorders or syndromes	Provides information needed to develop plan of instruction to ensure compliance to medical regimen for correction; usually begins in infancy and lasts for 3–5 months, and most commonly occurs in males
Inform parent(s) of type of talipes deformity and describe the position of the foot and ankle and the stages of corrective treatment	Provides information about how the correction is accomplished, maintained, and re-evaluated to ensure the correction and prevent recurrence of the deformity
Instruct parent(s) in manipulation of feet in one smooth motion, demonstrate and allow for return demonstration	Ensures correct positioning of the feet in preparation for immobilization
Instruct parent(s) in application of Denis Browne splints including applying socks and then shoes attached to the bar, tightening shoes against bar with a key, and maintaining shoe placement on the bar; protect feet with socks; change position q2h and note edema, color change of feet	Ensures correct splinting of deformity for one method that immobilizes feet in high shoes placed on bar to maintain rotation of the ankle

- Protects casts from damage
- Complies with follow-up care requirements of cast changes
- Prevents risk of recurrence of deformity by prolonged overcorrection of deformity.

PRACTICE QUESTIONS

1. Baby Rakshitha age 5-years accidentally had right ulnar fracture and admitted in pediatric surgical ward. Draw a nursing care plan in order to meet the major needs of baby Rakshitha.
2. Write nursing care plan for a child with hip dysplasia.

CHAPTER 23

Nursing Management of Child with Mental Health Disorders (Including Behavioral Disorders)

> **LEARNING OBJECTIVES**
> - To identify the signs and symptoms of a child with physiosocial and psychosocial disorders.
> - To frame nursing diagnosis based on the needs of the child.
> - To plan nursing interventions and outcome identification.

INTRODUCTION

The physical, mental, and social considerations of children's health problems do not lend themselves to specific conditions. These considerations include the child's ability to deal with hospitalization, abuse, and death. They require special empathy and sensitivity to the needs and feelings of children based on age and related growth and development parameters.

NURSING MANAGEMENT OF CHILD WITH MENTAL HEALTH DISORDERS (INCLUDING BEHAVIORAL DISORDERS) IN GENERAL

1. **Nursing diagnosis:** Impaired social interaction related to altered social skills as evidenced by impulsivity, intrusive behavior, inability to follow through, anxiety, depressed mood and feelings of unattractiveness or unworthiness.
   Interventions: Promoting appropriate social interaction.
   - Identify factors that may aggravate the child's performance to minimize stimuli that exacerbate the child's undesired behaviors
   - Modify the environment to decrease distracting stimuli as child's ability to deal with external stimuli may be impaired
   - Ensure that the child hears his name and makes eye contact prior to conversing or instructions, so that child is engaged and has increased ability to follow through
   - State expectations for tasks or behaviors clearly as understanding are necessary to ensure completion
   - Provide positive feedback for appropriate behaviors or task completion, encouraging the child to adopt expectations into his behaviors and routine.

   Outcome identification and evaluation: The child will demonstrate socially acceptable skills, interacting successfully with peers and in the educational setting, completing tasks as required.

2. **Nursing diagnosis:** Ineffective individual coping related to inability to deal with life stressors as evidenced by few or no meaningful friendships, inability to empathize or give/receive affection, low self-esteem or maladaptive coping behaviors such as substance abuse.
   Interventions: Promoting coping skills.
   - Encourage discussion of thoughts and feelings, as this is an initial step toward learning to deal with them appropriately.

- Provide positive feedback for appropriate discussion, as this increases the likelihood of continuing performance
- Demonstrate unconditional acceptance of the child as a person to increase self-esteem in the child who has been feeling rejection
- Set clear limits on behavior as needed, so the child has a structure to adhere to
- Teach the child problem-solving skills as an alternative to acting-out behaviors
- Role-model appropriate social and conversation skills, so the child can see what's expected in a non-threatening manner.

Outcome identification and evaluation: The child will demonstrate improved coping, verbalize feelings, socially engage and demonstrate problem-solving skills.

3. **Nursing diagnosis:** Imbalanced nutrition less than body requirements related to intake, insufficient to meet metabolic needs as evidenced by weight loss, failure to gain weight, less than expected increases in stature and weight, loss of appetite or refusal to eat.

    Interventions: Improving nutritional intake.
    - Provide favorite foods to encourage the child with poor appetite to eat more
    - Assist families to choose nutrient-rich foods, so that the food the child does eat is most beneficial.

    For the child with an eating disorder:
    - Mutually establish a contract related to treatment to promote the child's sense of control
    - Provide mealtime structure as clear limits, let the child known what the expectations are
    - Encourage the child to choose foods and timing of meals to develop independence
    - Ensure the eating environment is pleasant and relaxed, with minimal distractions, to minimize the child's anxiety and guilt about not eating
    - Withdraw attention if child refuses to eat (secondary gain is minimized if refusal to eat is ignored)
    - Provide continuous supervision during the meal and for 30 minutes following it, so that the child cannot conceal or dispose of food or induce vomiting.

4. **Nursing diagnosis:** Delayed growth and development related to disability, behavioral disorder or altered nutrition as evidenced by lack of attainment of age-appropriate skills, regression in skills or altered intellectual functioning.

    Interventions: Promoting development.
    - Use therapeutic play and adaptive toys to facilitate developmental functioning
    - Provide stimulating environment when possible to maximize potential for growth and development
    - Praise accomplishments and emphasize child's abilities to improve self-esteem and encourage feeling of confidence and competence
    - Follow through with physical, occupational and speech therapist's recommendations to maximize exposure to exercises designed to increase the child's skills
    - Determine parent's expectations of child's future achievement to help them work toward these goals.

    Outcome identification and evaluation: Child will demonstrate progress toward developmental milestones; child expresses interest in the environment and people around him/her, interacts with environment in an age-appropriate way.

5. **Nursing diagnosis:** Disturbed thought processes related to behavioral disorder, depression, anxiety, abusive situation or substance abuse as evidenced by distractibility, non-reality based thinking, hyper vigilance, or inaccurate interpretation of interactions of others.
   Interventions: Improving thought processes.
   - Observe for causes of altered thought processes to provide a baseline for assessment and intervention
   - Perform an age-appropriate mental status examination to determine extent of altered thinking
   - Adjust communication style based on child's cues to improve communication
   - Listen carefully and seek clarification to determine basis for child's agitation or other behaviors
   - Provide validation of the child's thoughts and feelings to improve trust in the relationship
   - Establish a daily routine to provide the child with a sense of security.

   Outcome identification and evaluation: Child's thought processes will improve; child will demonstrate appropriate orientation, remain free from physical harm and perform activities of daily living as able.

6. **Nursing diagnosis:** Hopelessness related to child's perception of his/her life situation, negative life view or alteration in mental well-being as evidenced by passivity, verbalization, alterations in sleep, or lack of initiative.
   Interventions: Promoting hope.
   - Monitor and document potential for suicide, as hopelessness often leads to suicidal ideation
   - Assist the child to identify reasons for hope and for living, so the nurse is aware or the child's values
   - Help the child to set goals that are important to him to allow the child to see possibilities
   - Encourage simple decision making on a daily basis, as hopelessness often occurs as a response to loss of control
   - Assist the child to identify positive qualities in himself herself and his/her life to facilitate the development of involve parents or others the child loves in the child's care as social support is critical to the development of hope.

   Outcome identification and evaluation: Child will display a sense of hope, will verbalize feelings, participate in care and make positive statements.

7. **Nursing diagnosis:** Caregiver role strain related to long-term care of the child with a chronic mental health disorder as evidenced by fatigue, inattention to own needs, conflict or ambivalence.
   Interventions: Decreasing role strain.
   - Teach the parent or caregiver about the child's illness, treatments and medications to clarify expectations for the child and parent
   - Role model appropriate interaction behaviors with the child, so the parent can learn these techniques by watching
   - Encourage structure in daily routines to allow the parent to meet own needs and allow for adequate rest
   - Gradually increase the parent's responsibility related to care of the child to help the parent feel less overwhelmed

- Allow the parent to move at his/her own pace in assuming care to enhance the chances for success
- Help the parent to identify a back-up caregiver, so the parent has times of respite from constant involvement with the child.

Outcome identification and evaluation: The child's caregiver will participate in the child's care, verbalizing the child's needs and treatment plan and demonstrating skills necessary for care. Involve parents or others the child loves in the child's care as social support is critical to the development of hope.

NURSING PROCESS FOR SPECIFIC MENTAL HEALTH DISORDERS

Abused Child

Child abuse (maltreatment) is defined as an intentional action toward a child that includes the areas of physical abuse or neglect, emotional abuse or neglect, and sexual abuse. The most common form of child abuse is neglect, which may include deprivation of physical and/or emotional needs (food, clothing, shelter, medical care, education, affection, love, nurturing) or aggressive emotional abuse (isolation, terrorizing, rejection). Physical abuse may include burns, bruises, fractures, lacerations, poisoning of the child; sexual abuse may be indicated by bruising and bleeding of anus or genitals; discharge and pain in genitals; sexually transmitted disease; urinary incontinence and infections or odor, swelling, and itching of genitalia. Regardless of the type of abuse, the nurse's responsibilities are to identify the maltreatment and to protect the child from further abuse **(Fig. 23.1)**.

Symptoms of Abused Child

- A child who's being abused may feel guilty, ashamed or confused.
- He or she may be afraid to tell anyone about the abuse, especially if the abuser is a parent, other relative or family friend. In fact, the child may have an apparent fear of parents, adult caregivers or family friends. That's why it is vital to watch for red flags, such as:
  - Withdrawal from friends or usual activities
  - Changes in behavior—such as aggression, anger, hostility or hyperactivity or changes in school performance
  - Depression, anxiety or a sudden loss of self-confidence
  - An apparent lack of supervision
  - Frequent absences from school or reluctance to ride the school bus
  - Reluctance to leave school activities, as if he or she doesn't want to go home
  - Attempts at running away
  - Rebellious or defiant behavior
  - Attempts at suicide

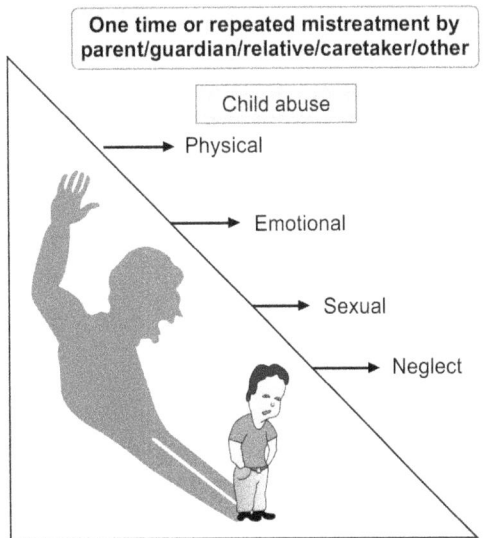

Fig. 23.1: Pathophysiology of abused child.

Specific Signs and Symptoms Depending on the Type of Abuse

Physical Abuse Signs and Symptoms
- Unexplained injuries, such as bruises, fractures or burns
- Injuries that don't match the given explanation
- Untreated medical or dental problems.

Sexual Abuse Signs and Symptoms
- Sexual behavior or knowledge that is inappropriate for the child's age
- Pregnancy or a sexually transmitted infection
- Blood in the child's underwear
- Statements that he or she was sexually abused
- Trouble walking or sitting
- Abuse of other children sexually.

Emotional Abuse Signs and Symptoms
- Delayed or inappropriate emotional development
- Loss of self-confidence or self-esteem
- Social withdrawal
- Depression
- Headaches or stomachaches with no medical cause
- Avoidance of certain situations, such as refusing to go to school or ride the bus
- Desperately seeks affection.

Neglect Signs and Symptoms
- Poor growth or weight gain
- Poor hygiene
- Lack of clothing or supplies to meet physical needs
- Taking food or money without permission
- Eating a lot in one sitting or hiding food for later
- Poor record of school attendance
- Lack of appropriate attention for medical, dental or psychological problems, even though the parents have been notified
- Emotional swings that are inappropriate or out of context to the situation
- Indifference.

Parental Behavior
Sometimes a parent's demeanor or behavior sends red flags about child abuse. Warning signs include a parent who:
- Shows little concern for the child
- Appears unable to recognize physical or emotional distress in the child
- Denies that any problems exist at home or school, or blames the child for the problems
- Consistently blames belittles or berates the child and describes the child with negative terms, such as "worthless" or "evil"

Nursing Management of Child with Mental Health Disorders (Including Behavioral Disorders)

- Expects the child to provide him or her with attention and care and seems jealous of other family members getting attention from the child
- Uses harsh physical discipline or asks teachers to do so
- Demands an inappropriate level of physical or academic performance
- Severely limits the child's contact with others
- Offers conflicting or unconvincing explanations for a child's injuries or no explanation at all.

Nursing Management

A. Essential Nursing Diagnoses and Nursing Process Associated with these Conditions

Nursing diagnosis

Altered nutrition: Less than body requirements related to inability to ingest food.

Assessment: Withholding of food by parent/caretaker, weight loss, malnutrition, lack of subcutaneous fat, failure to thrive.
(Refer Table 14.3 from chapter 14)

Nursing diagnosis

High-risk for impaired skin integrity related to external factor of trauma.

Assessment: Disruption of skin surface (lacerations, burns, abrasion), various skin trauma in different stages of healing, lack of bathing causing unclean skin, teeth, hair.
(Refer Table 12.1 from chapter 12)

Nursing diagnosis

Altered growth and development related to inadequate caretaking, indifference, environmental and stimulation deficiencies.

Assessment: Delay or difficulty in performing skills (motor, social, or expressive) typical of age group, altered physical growth, inability to perform self-care or self-control activities appropriate for age, flat affect, decreased responses, withdrawal, antisocial behavior, fearfulness, poor relationships with peers, regressive behavior, acting out behavior.
(Refer Table 14.4 from chapter 14)

B. Specific Nursing Diagnoses and Nursing Process

Nursing diagnosis

Anxiety of child related to threat to self-concept, change in health status, change in interaction patterns, situational crisis **(Table 23.1)**.

Assessment: Increased apprehension and uncertainty, fearfulness, feeling of powerlessness, fear of consequences, repeated episodes of maltreatment, mistrust, trembling, quivering voice, poor eye contact.

Evaluation
- Reduces anxiety by establishing accepting, safe environment
- Participates in play with others
- Establishes relationships with staff member(s)
- Exhibits reduction in negative behavior, signs and symptoms of anxiety and fear.

Table 23.1: Nursing interventions for anxiety of child.

Interventions	Rationales
Assess level of anxiety and fear in child and how it is manifested; needs of child that are the source of anxiety and reactions to staff and parent(s)	Provides information about the source and level of anxiety and what might relieve it any criteria to judge improvement
Demonstrate affection and acceptance of the child even if not returned or ignored; avoid reinforcing any negative behavior	Promotes trust of staff and positive behavior of the child
Provide a play program with other children; set aside time to be alone with child or quiet time for child as well; praise child or reward with a special treat when appropriate	Modifies negative behavior by promoting interactions with others and regarding desired behaviors; promotes self-esteem
Provide consistent staffing for child, preferably late well to child	Promotes familiarity and trusting relationship with staff
Allow expression of concerns and fears of child about treatments, environment; allow questions and provide honest explanations and communication at child's age level	Provides opportunity to vent feelings, which reduces anxiety
Provide treatment of injuries; avoid treating child as a victim, asking too many questions, or forcing any discussion	Prevents increased anxiety and stress in child by discussion of abuse
Assess possible need for counseling services for the child	Reduces anxiety and supports child in dealing with abuse and negative behavior

Nursing diagnosis

Altered parenting related to unmet social and emotional maturation needs of parental figures, ineffective role modeling, lack of knowledge, situational crisis or incident **(Table 23.2)**.

Assessment: Lack of parental attachment behaviors, verbalization of resentment toward child and of role inadequacy, inattention to needs of child, noncompliance with health practices and medical care, inappropriate discipline practices, frequent accidents and illness of child, growth and development lag in child, history of child abuse or abandonment, multiple caretakers without regard for needs of child, evidence of physical and psychological trauma, actual abandonment of child.

Evaluation
- Participate in child care with increased understanding of child's needs for age and developmental level
- Reduce behaviors that are harmful to child and to relationship between parent and child
- Demonstrate proper parenting behaviors
- Demonstrate improved and positive interaction with child
- Attend parenting classes and support group activities
- Meet own needs for health and optimal functioning
- Secure assistance to solve problems that lead to abusive behavior.

Table 23.2: Nursing intervention for altered parenting.

Interventions	Rationales
Assess parent(s) for achievement of developmental tasks of self and understanding of child's growth and development; how they are bonded and attached to child; how they interpret and respond to child; how they accept and support child; how they meet child's social, psychological and physical needs	Provides information about parent-child relationship and parenting styles that may lead to child abuse; identifies parents at risk for violence or other abusive behavior
Provide a child nurturing role model for parent(s) to emulate, and suggest what they might do to develop parent(s) skills	Promotes development of parenting skills by imitation
Praise parent(s) for their participation in child's care, tell them that they are giving good care to child	Reinforces positive parenting behaviors and increases feeling of adequacy
Include parent(s) in planning care and setting goals	Promotes participation of parent(s) in meeting child's needs
Provide an opportunity for parent(s) to express their feelings, personal needs, and goals; avoid making judgmental remarks or comparing them to other parent(s)	Support parent(s) in meeting their own needs
Initiate referrals to social services, parenting classes, or counseling as appropriate	Provides options if parenting is unsatisfactory or inadequate

Nursing diagnosis

High-risk for other directed violence related to child abuse, maladaptive behavior of parent(s) or other **(Table 23.3)**.

Assessment: Sexual assault of child, evidence of physical abuse of child, history of abuse of abuser, social isolation of family, low self-esteem of caretaker, inadequate support systems, violence against other members of the family.

Evaluation
- Protects child from recurrence of or continuance of abuse
- Protects privacy of child and family
- Complies with laws governing child abuse
- Records all events associated with suspected or actual child abuse
- Absence of trauma or injury to the child
- Identifies abusive behavior and acts to remove child from the abusive environment
- Assists parent(s) in seeking support and self-help groups
- Referral to social worker, nurse, or counselor for economic, social, psychological and physical needs of child and family.

Dying Child

Care of the dying child includes the physical and emotional interventions necessary to support the totally dependent child and grieving family. Nursing considerations involve the dissemination of information to the child, whose perceptions of death and responses to death

Nursing Management of Child with Mental Health Disorders (Including Behavioral Disorders)

Table 23.3: Nursing interventions for high-risk for other directed violence.

Interventions	Rationales
Assess the abuser for violent behavior or other abusive patterns, use of alcohol or drugs, or other psychosocial problems	Provides information to determine warning signs of child abuse
Assess behavior of parent(s) toward child, including response to the child's behavior, ability to comfort the child, feelings and perceptions toward the child, expectations for the child, over protectiveness or concern for the child	Reveals characteristics that may indicate risk for abuse
Protect child and parental privacy by not discussing events with others and preventing others from discussing events with the abused child	Protects the rights of the child and parent(s)
Review laws governing child abuse	Provides information about legal aspects of child abuse and actions to take on behalf of all concerned
Communicate information and needs of child to those on the abuse team or to new caretakers if child being placed with a foster parent or someone other than parents; provide written instruction for care and child's needs	Provides care plan for child based on court decision to caretakers working with the family
Accurately record facts, events, and observations in an objective manner	Provides information that may be used in legal action regarding abuse
Initiate referral to social worker, psychological counselor before discharge to home	Provides support to child and family, and monitors behaviors following discharge

and dying are age-related. The nurse should approach the parent(s) with sensitivity, caring, and honesty. The nurse also helps the child move through the stages of awareness and acceptance, and helps the parent(s) and family move through the stages of grieving **(Flowchart 23.1)**.

Nursing Management

A. Essential Nursing Diagnoses and Nursing Process Associated with this Condition

Nursing diagnosis

Sleep pattern disturbance related to internal factors of illness and stressors.

Flowchart 23.1: Pathophysiology of dying child.

```
Life-threatening illness    Congenital anomaly    Trauma from accident
                                                   or violence
                    ↓              ↓                      ↓
                    └──→ Complete physical dependency ←──┘
                                    ↓
                              Pain relief
                              Airway patency
                              Skin integrity
                              Rest promotion
                              Nutritional maintenance
                              Elimination maintenance
                              Medication administration
```

Nursing Management of Child with Mental Health Disorders (Including Behavioral Disorders)

Assessment: Fatigue, lethargy, irritability, restlessness, pain, psychological stress (anxiety, fear).
(Refer Table 14.10 from chapter 14)

Nursing diagnosis
Impaired physical mobility related to pain and discomfort.
Assessment: Weakness, inability to purposefully move fatigue, limited strength, changes in consciousness.
(Refer Table 14.19 from chapter 14)

Nursing diagnosis
Altered nutrition: Less than body requirements related to inability to ingest food.
Assessment: Weakness, anorexia, poor feeding, lack of interest in food.
(Refer Table 14.3 from chapter 14)

Nursing diagnosis
High-risk for impaired skin integrity related to external factors of immobilization.
Assessment: Redness, disruption of skin surface, prolonged pressure on skin and bony prominences.
(Refer Table 12.1 from chapter 12)

Nursing diagnosis
Altered thought processes related to physiological changes.
Assessment: Disorientation, changes in consciousness.
(Refer Table 12.14 from chapter 12)

Nursing diagnosis
Ineffective airway clearance related to decreased energy and fatigue, tracheobronchial secretions.
Assessment: Increasing secretions, changes in respiratory rate or depth (stridor, irregularity), inability to cough and remove secretions.
(Refer Table 11.1 from chapter 11)

Nursing diagnosis
Constipation related to less than adequate physical activity and intake.
Assessment: Frequency less than usual pattern, hard-formed stool, decreased bowel sounds.
(Refer Table 12.9 from chapter 12)

B. Specific Nursing Diagnoses and Nursing Process

Nursing diagnosis
Pain related to biological, physical, psychological injuring agents **(Table 23.4)**.
Assessment: Communication (verbal or coded) of pain descriptors, guarding, protective behavior, facial mask of pain, crying, moaning, withdrawal, changes in VS, irritability, restlessness.

Nursing Management of Child with Mental Health Disorders (Including Behavioral Disorders)

Table 23.4: Nursing interventions for pain.

Interventions	Rationales
Assess severity of pain, fear of receiving pain medication, anxiety and coping mechanisms associated with pain, ability to rest and sleep	Provides information as a basis for analgesic administration
Administer analgesic intermittently or continuously depending on pain severity over 24 hours via PO, IV, using narcotic and non-narcotic medications; administer before any painful procedure or care is performed	Provides 24 hours coverage of pain medications to ensure freedom from any type of pain and discomfort including administration of analgesic for prompt relief if given intermittently
Provide position changes as tolerated, use pillows to support position, move slowly with gentle handling, give backrub	Reduces pain by nonpharmacologic measures
Provide companionship (family member or customary support person for child, familiar toys	Reduces fear and supports comfort of child
Support coping mechanisms of child and family and adjust analgesic accordingly, with input from child, parent(s), and physician	Promotes child's comfort, supports coping abilities, and includes parent(s) and child in decision making regarding care
Dim lights, avoid noise, maintain clean, comfortable bed with loose sheets and clothing, disturb for care only when needed to promote comfort	Provides environment free of stimuli that increases anxiety and pain

Evaluation
- Controls pain and maintains comfort
- Reduces fear of pain and its consequences
- Administers correct analgesic by correct route based on continuous assessment of pain control
- Administers nonpharmacologic measures to maintain comfort
- Reduces stimuli that trigger or increase pain.

Nursing diagnosis

Anticipatory grieving related to perceived potential loss of significant other **(Table 23.5)**.

Assessment: Expression of distress at potential loss of child, denial of loss, guilt, anger, sorrow, choked feelings, change in need fulfillment, crying, self-blame.

Evaluation
- Verbalizes understanding of grief process and responses
- Shares feelings with professionals and other members of the family
- Performs parental tasks/care to child
- Accepts and uses coping skills that support grieving
- Makes decisions regarding placement and care of dying child
- Contacts and utilizes support services of clergy, social services and hospice as appropriate
- Maintains a presence of parent of family member and privacy to be with child.

Nursing Management of Child with Mental Health Disorders (Including Behavioral Disorders)

Table 23.5: Nursing interventions for anticipatory grieving.

Interventions	Rationales
Assess stage of grief process, problems encountered, feelings regarding terminal nature of illness and potential loss of child	Provides information about need for grieving, which varies with individuals members of a family when child's death is expected
Provide emotional and spiritual comfort in an accepting environment, and avoid conversations that cause guilt or anger	Provides for emotional need of parent(s) and family and helps them to cope with dying child without adding stressors that are difficult to resolve
Provide opportunities for family to express feelings and respond to child commensurate with stage of grieving	Promotes progression through grieving and ability to express desires for themselves and their child
Allow parent(s) and family members to be with child as much as they feel a need to, and help them understand the child's behavior and needs	Promotes feelings that they are helping and supporting their child
Assist family in identifying and use effective coping mechanisms and in understanding situation over which they have no control	Promotes effective coping that is positive for the family
Provide privacy when needed, while being available to the family	Promotes a helping relationship with the family
Arrange for clergy, social services, hospice care, or return to home for dying as appropriate; support choices made by the family	Provides for and assists with alternative care and preferences for that care

Nursing diagnosis

Anxiety of child and parent(s) related to threat of death **(Table 23.6)**.

Table 23.6: Nursing interventions for anxiety of parent(s) and child.

Interventions	Rationales
Assess anxiety level, fears and concerns, ability to express needs, and how anxiety is manifested	Reveals information needed for interventions to relieve anxiety and increase comfort
Allow family member to stay with child or remain with child during stressful periods if family not able to be there	Promotes comfort of child and provides support during anxious and fearful times
Allow expressions of fears and concerns about terminal stage of illness, answer all questions honestly based on what family has been told about prognosis	Provides opportunity to vent feelings and fears to reduce anxiety
Provide necessary procedures; avoid procedures that increase pain or fear	Promotes only palliative treatments, without interventions that increase discomfort and anxiety
Provide calm reassurance and kindness; be available to child at all times as needed for support	Promotes comfort and love of child to reduce anxiety
Involve child and parent(s) in as much planning and care as possible without forcing participation	Promotes interactions and attitude of caring within family

Nursing Management of Child with Mental Health Disorders (Including Behavioral Disorders)

Assessment: Increased apprehension and fear of death, loss of control, loneliness; increased feelings of helplessness and hopelessness; poor prognosis of terminal illness.

Evaluation
- Expresses and exhibits a reduction in anxiety, fear of loneliness
- States sources of anxiety and measures to reduce it
- Utilizes support systems and open visitation, remains with child whether parent or family member
- Promotes accepting, nonjudgmental, calm environment
- Provides comfort measures for child and family to reduce anxiety and concerns.

PRACTICE QUESTIONS

1. Draw a nursing care plan for a dying child by applying nursing process.
2. Write nursing care plan for an adolescent girl undergone physical abuse and admitted in pediatric intensive care.

Index

Page numbers followed by *f* refer to figure, *fc* refer to flowchart, and *t* refer to table.

A
Abdomen 172
Abnormal breath sounds flaring alae nasi 30
Abuse, types of 382
Abused child, pathophysiology of 381*f*
Accommodative esotropia 316
Aches 285
Acquired immunodeficiency syndrome 266, 273
  pathophysiology of 267*f*
  symptoms of 266
Activity intolerance
  high-risk for 75, 76*t*, 161, 162*t*
  nursing interventions for 188*t*, 200*t*, 219*t*, 224*t*, 276*t*
Acute lymphoblastic leukemias 285
Acyanotic defects 182*f*
Adenoidectomy 318, 319
Airway clearance, infective 85
Allergic rhinitis 309
  pathophysiology of 309*f*
  symptoms of 309
Allergy 230
  history of 230
Altered body temperature 259
Altered family process, nursing interventions for 141*t*
Altered growth and development 106, 111, 125, 136, 168, 184, 219, 317, 328, 346, 355, 368, 376
  nursing interventions for 188*t*
Altered mucous membrane, nursing interventions for 251*t*, 290*t*, 360*t*
Altered nutrition 74, 78, 89, 93, 103, 111, 116, 129, 136, 151, 157, 161, 168, 172, 175, 184, 208, 218, 223, 231, 269, 248, 275, 287, 297, 304, 313, 328, 350, 358, 363, 368
  nursing interventions for 186*t*
Altered oral mucous membrane 250, 289, 359
Altered protection, nursing interventions for 251*t*, 281*t*, 285*t*, 290*t*, 360*t*

Altered tissue perfusion 203, 224, 274, 341
  nursing interventions for 198*t*
Altered urinary elimination pattern 117, 139, 229
  nursing interventions for 117*t*, 139*t*, 230*t*
Anemia 273
  pathophysiology of 274*fc*
Anorexia 230
Anticipatory grieving, nursing interventions for 221*t*, 271*t*, 389*t*
Anti-diuretic hormone 231
Antithymocyte globulin 278
Anxiety 52, 56, 75, 79, 83, 86, 89, 106, 112, 118, 122, 142, 148, 152, 168, 176, 199, 227, 238, 244, 249, 270, 288, 359, 363
  nursing interventions for 57*t*, 75*t*, 79*t*, 83*t*, 86*t*, 90*t*, 106*t*, 113*t*, 118*t*, 123*t*, 150*t*, 152*t*, 176*t*, 199*t*, 228*t*, 239*t*, 244*t*, 249*t*, 250*t*, 270*t*, 288*t*, 359*t*, 364*t*, 384*t*, 389*t*
  symptoms of 348
Apnea 78
Appendicitis 146
  pathophysiology of 146*f*
  signs of 146
  symptoms of 146
Appetite 77, 102, 161, 217
  lack of 240
  loss of 93, 146, 248
Arthralgia 207
Aseptic technique 97
Asthma 68
  attack, prevention of 76, 76*t*
  pathophysiology of 69*f*
  symptoms of 69
Ataxia 111
Autonomic nervous system 95

B
Bacteremia 87
Bacteria 87
Bad breath 217
Behavioral disorders 378
Betty Neuman system model 28*f*
  application of 25*t*

Biochemical regulatory function, internal factory of 131*t*
Bladder 213, 239
Blisters 332
Blood
  in urine 248
  pressure 183
    high 222, 248
  stream 87
  urea nitrogen 222
Blurred vision 102, 201, 297
Body image disturbance 139, 220, 329, 350, 368, 373
  nursing interventions for 140*t*, 220*t*, 291*t*, 330*t*, 351, 369*t*, 374*t*
Body mass index 45
Bone
  fracture, types of 339
  pain 217
Bowel incontinence 138
  nursing interventions for 138*t*
Bowel movements 174
Brain 111
  tumor, symptoms of 111
Brassy cough 84
Breath, shortness of 69, 87, 93, 248, 286
Breathing 191
  difficulty 89, 102, 287
  effort 222
  pattern, infective 89
  rate 87
Broken skin 131*t*, 154*t*, 361*t*
Bronchiolitis 77
  symptoms of 77
Bronchopulmonary dysplasia 202
Bruising 332
Burns 326
  first-degree 326
  pathophysiology of 327*f*
  second-degree 326
  symptoms of 326
  third-degree 327

C
Cardiac failure, congestive 201
Cardiac function 110
Cardiac output 114, 181, 183*t*, 193, 350

Index

Cardiovascular disorder 177, 181
Carditis 206
Care planning 7
Cast application, effects of 365t
Cells 263
Cellulitis 331, 332
   pathophysiology of 331f
   symptoms of 331
Central nervous system 95, 119, 129
Cerebellum 111
Cerebrospinal fluid 109
Chest
   congestion 69
   pain 69, 93
   tightness 69
Chills 87, 93, 121, 332
Chronic pain 368
   nursing interventions for 369t
Chronic renal failure 217
   pathophysiology of 218fc
Clay-colored stools 161
Cleft lip 149
   pathophysiology of 151f
   symptoms of 150
Cleft palate 149
   pathophysiology of 151f
   symptoms of 150
Clubfoot 375
   pathophysiology of 375f
   symptoms of 376
Cold intolerance 303
Communicable diseases 259
Confusion 110
Congenital heart defects 181
   pathophysiology of 182, 182f
Congestive cardiac failure 201
Congestive heart failure 191
   pathophysiology of 192fc
   symptoms of 191
Constipation 116, 136, 147, 172, 174, 248, 303, 341, 345
   nursing interventions for 116t
Convulsion 201
Cough 69, 77, 85, 287, 310
Crepitations 85
Crohn's disease 167
Cyanosis 30, 78
Cyanotic defects 182f

D

Dark urine 161
Data
   collection of 2
   documentation of 2
   organization of 2, 3
   recording of 2
   types of 2
   validation of 2
   purposes of 2
Dehydration 78, 99, 174
Depression 110, 168
   symptoms of 348
Dermatitis 333
   symptoms of 333
Diabetes insipidus 99
Diabetes mellitus 110, 294, 297
   pathophysiology of 298f
   symptoms of 297
Diarrhea 147, 157, 161, 168, 172, 230, 232, 240, 248, 269, 287, 358
   nursing interventions for 158t
Diminished urine output 222
Discomfort, abdominal 161, 230
Diversional activity deficit 56
   nursing interventions for 58t
Documentation, purposes of 3
Dorsiflexion 375
Double vision 102, 110
Droopy eyelids 304
Drowsiness 110
Dry hair 303
Dry skin 303
Dull facial expression 303

E

Ear
   disorder of 306, 309
   infections 151
   tubes surgery 313
Edema 223
Elastic skin turgor 99
Electrocardiogram 183
Emotional abuse
   signs of 382
   symptoms of 382
Endocrine disorders 293, 297
Energy, lack of 174
Enlarged lymph nodes 268, 286
Entropy 21
Epiglottis, symptoms of 81
Epiglottitis 81
   pathophysiology of 82f
Epispadias 226
Epispadiasis
   pathophysiology of 226f
   symptoms of 226, 227
Epistaxis 201
Erythema marginatum 207
Erythrocyte 263
   sedimentation rate 365
Esotropia 315
Eustachian tube 309
Exercise intolerance 303
Exotropia 317
Exploitation 17, 21
Extreme hunger 297
Eyes
   disorder of 306, 309
   sun setting of 101
   watery 309

F

Failure to thrive 201
Fatigue 78, 80, 86, 92, 191, 201, 222, 230, 297, 303, 310, 348
   nursing interventions for 80t, 87t, 232t
Feeling sick 191
Femoral head, degeneration of 354
Fever 77, 84, 93, 101, 120, 161, 172, 230, 240, 248, 268, 286, 332, 348, 362
   high 87
   low 146
Fluid
   accumulation 89, 223
   volume deficit, high-risk for 74, 79, 83, 85, 89, 103, 111, 121, 147, 156, 161, 165, 168, 172, 175, 194, 196t, 203, 227, 232, 241, 243, 248, 275, 287, 298, 313, 320, 328, 332, 350, 358, 363
   volume excess 103, 193, 203, 217, 223, 231
      nursing interventions for 194t
Flu-like symptoms 160
Foot
   eversion 375
   inversion 375
Foul-smelling urine 240
Fracture 339
   comminuted 339
   oblique 339
   pathophysiology of 340f
   signs of 339
   simple 339
   symptoms of 339
   transverse 339
Frequent coughing 69
Frequent urination 297

G

Gastroenteritis 155
   pathophysiology of 156f
   symptoms of 156
Gastrointestinal disorder 142, 146
Gastrointestinal tract 142
Genetic disorder 62

Glomerulonephritis 221
  pathophysiology of 223f
  symptoms of 222
Greenstick fracture 339
Growth 151, 168, 191
Grunting 30, 78
Guillain-Barré syndrome 114
  pathophysiology of 115f
  symptoms of 114

H

Haemophilus influenzae 119, 311
Hair loss 348
Headache 95, 101, 103, 109-111,
    201, 217, 222, 268, 286, 310,
    332
  persistent 120
  severe 120
Health 23
  assessment 1
  seeking behaviors 76
    nursing interventions for 76t
Hearing deficit 217
Heart
  defects, congenital 181
  failure, congestive 191
Hematocrit 222, 251, 290
Hematologic disorder 263, 266
Hematologic system 263
Hemoglobin 222
Hemophilia
  A 278
  B 278
  pathophysiology of 280f
  symptoms of 279
Hepatitis 160
  A 160
  B 160
  D 160
  pathophysiology of 160f
  symptoms of 160
Hernia 163
  symptoms of 164
Hip
  dislocation, symptoms of 343
  dysplasia 343
    pathophysiology of 345f
  muscle spasm 354
  pain 354
Hoarse voice 303
Hormone regulation 110
Human immunodeficiency virus 266
Human T-cell lymphotropic virus 266
Hydration status 99
Hydrocephalus 101
  pathophysiology of 102f

signs of 101
  symptoms of 101
Hyperglycemia, internal biochemical
    factors of 299t
Hypertension 200, 230
  pathophysiology of 202fc
  symptoms of 201
Hyperthermia 79, 83, 89, 106, 111,
    117, 121, 147, 157, 207, 219,
    227, 234, 238, 241, 243, 283,
    288, 313, 321, 332, 349, 362,
    368
  nursing interventions for 208t
Hypertropia 317
Hypoglycemia, internal biochemical
    factors of 299t
Hypospadias 226
Hypospadiasis
  pathophysiology of 226f
  symptoms of 226
Hypotension 230
Hypothermia 138
  nursing interventions for 138t
Hypothyroidism 302
  pathophysiology of 303f
  symptoms of 302
Hypotropia 317
Hypoxia 78, 131t

I

Idiopathic thrombocytopenic
    purpura 283
  pathophysiology of 284f
  symptoms of 283
Imbalanced nutrition 214, 215, 255,
    295
Impacted fracture 339
Impaired adjustment, nursing
    interventions for 170t
Impaired gas exchange 73, 78
  nursing interventions for 73t
Impaired physical immobility 363
Impaired physical mobility 111, 117,
    136, 208, 279, 328, 340, 343,
    349, 355, 358, 367, 372, 376
  nursing interventions for 209t
Impaired skin integrity, high-risk for
    103, 104t, 136, 157, 161, 165,
    168, 219, 224, 227, 232, 234,
    238, 243, 249, 275, 280, 283,
    287, 297, 304, 327, 332, 333,
    341, 345, 348, 355, 358, 363,
    368, 373, 376
Impaired social interaction 346, 365
  nursing interventions for 348t,
    366t
Implementation skills 9

Ineffective airway clearance 70, 78,
    82, 115, 151, 269
  nursing interventions for 70t
Ineffective breathing pattern 73, 78,
    82, 85, 114, 129, 164, 184, 193,
    269, 310, 320, 328
  nursing interventions for 185t
Ineffective family coping 155, 190,
    282, 291, 301, 370
  nursing interventions for 132t,
    155t, 190t, 282t, 292t, 302t,
    371t
Infection
  high-risk for 108, 137, 137t, 189,
    210, 219, 224, 228, 233, 238,
    245, 271, 276, 310, 329
  nursing interventions for high-
    risk for 149t, 189t, 211t,
    220t, 225t, 229t, 233t, 239t,
    246t, 272t, 277t, 311t, 330t
  symptoms of 230
Inflammatory bowel disease 167
  pathophysiology of 167f
  symptoms of 167
Inguinal hernia, pathophysiology
    of 164f
Injury
  high-risk for 90, 90t, 107, 108, 112,
    122, 129, 131t, 154, 165, 172,
    175, 189, 203, 221, 225, 245,
    249, 277, 298, 341, 343, 346,
    361, 364
  nursing interventions for high-
    risk for 107t-109t, 113t, 154t,
    165t, 173t, 175t, 190t, 203t,
    222t, 225t, 247t, 278t, 299t,
    342t, 344t, 346t, 361t, 365t
Integumentary disorder 324, 326
Integumentary system 324
Intensive care unit 249
Intermittent coughing 69
Interpersonal theory, application
    of 11
Intestinal obstruction 165t
Intracranial pressure 101, 109-111
Intracranial tumor 109
  pathophysiology of 110f
  symptoms of 109
Intussusception 171
  pathophysiology of 171f
  symptoms of 172
Irritability 101, 102, 110, 201, 217,
    230, 240, 297, 310, 362

J

Jaundice 160, 174
Joint pain 121, 161, 223

Index

K
Katharine Kolcaba comfort theory 11
Kidney 213, 239
Knowledge deficit, nursing
   interventions for 81t, 124t,
   133t, 153t, 159t, 162t, 166t,
   170t, 173t, 201t, 204t, 233t,
   236t, 241t, 243t, 279t, 300t,
   304t, 315t, 318t, 322t, 333t,
   335t, 352t, 356t, 374t, 377t

L
Laryngotracheobronchitis 84
   pathophysiology of 85f
   symptoms of 84
Leg motion 354
Legg-Calve-Perthes disease 354
Lethargy 172, 174, 201, 222, 230, 362
Leukemia 285
   pathophysiology of 286f
   symptoms of 285
Leukocytes 263
Leukocytosis 207
Limp 354
Lobar pneumonia, pathophysiology
   of 88f
Lower bone density 168
Lump 172
Lung abscess 87
Lupus erythematosus 347
   pathophysiology of 349f
Lymph node swelling 332
Lymphoma 285, 287
   pathophysiology of 286f
   symptoms of 287

M
Macrohematuria 230
Malaise 217, 268
Mass, abdominal 217
Meninges, inflammation of 119
Meningitis 119
   pathophysiology of 120f
   signs of 120
   symptoms of 120
Meningocele 135
Meningococcal meningitis
   signs of 121
   symptoms of 121
Menstrual flow 304
Mental alertness 217
Mental health disorders 378, 381
Monitor vital signs 95-97
Mucous membranes 99
Multiple sclerosis 25, 25t
Muscle
   ache 121
   cramps 303
   movements 111
   paralysis of 110
   tone 217
Musculoskeletal disorder 336, 339
Musculoskeletal system 336
Myelomeningocele 135
Myringotomy 311, 313
   pathophysiology of 312f

N
NANDA nursing diagnosis, list of 4t
Nasal congestion 77, 310
Nasal discharge 77
Nasal flaring 78
Nausea 101, 109, 120, 147, 161, 248
Neck stiffness 120
Negentropy 22
Neisseria meningitidis 119
Neoplastic disorder 253
Nephritic syndrome 230
   pathophysiology of 231f
   signs of 230
   symptoms of 230
Nerves, paralysis of 10
Neuman's system model 21, 24
Neurological disorder 95, 101
Neurological impairment 135
Neurosensory deficits 125
   pathophysiology of 126fc
Night sweats 93, 287
Non-steroidal anti-inflammatory
   drugs 369
Nose
   bleeds 283
   disorder of 306, 309
Nursing care 9, 30, 35, 38, 41, 45, 48
   plan 8
Nursing theories, application of 11

O
Orchiopexy 237
Osteochondritis deformans 354
   pathophysiology of 354f
   symptoms of 354
Osteogenic sarcoma 357
   pathophysiology of 357f
   symptoms of 357
Osteomyelitis 361
   pathophysiology of 362f
   symptoms of 362
Otitis media 311
   pathophysiology of 312f
   symptoms of 311

P
Pain 112, 120, 147, 210, 244, 280, 288,
   313, 321, 332, 351, 362, 363
   abdominal 161, 230
   chronic 368
   joint 121, 161, 223
   nursing interventions for 112t,
   118t, 148t, 166t, 169t, 211t,
   228t, 245t, 275t, 281t, 289t,
   314t, 321t, 329t, 342t, 351t,
   364t, 388t
Pale skin 217, 223, 286
Paralysis 110
Parental behavior 382
Peplau's theory application,
   nursing process 17
Peritonitis 230
Personality changes 109, 110
Petechiae 283, 286
Physical abuse
   signs 382
   symptoms 382
Physical trauma 131t
Pitting edema 230
Plantar flexion 375
Plasma 263
Platelets 263
Play 59
   pathophysiology of 60fc
Pleural effusion 89
Pneumonia 87
   pathophysiology of 88f
   signs of 87
   symptoms of 87
Polyarthritis 206
   infectious 114
Powerlessness, nursing
   interventions for 59t
Prematurity 202
Protein 222
Psychosis 348
Puberty, delayed 168
Pulmonary edema 230
Pulmonary tuberculosis,
   pathophysiology
   of 92f
Pyloric obstruction,
   internal factor of 175t
Pyloric stenosis 174
   pathophysiology of 174f
   symptoms of 174

R
Rapid breathing 121
Rash 223, 348
Red blood
   cell 222
   corpuscle 275, 276, 286
Renal disorder 213, 217
Renal failure 217, 222t
Renal function 225t
Respiratory disorder 65
Respiratory distress 201, 230
Respiratory failure 78, 81
Respiratory function 110

Index

Respiratory tract 65
  infection 76, 76t, 230
Rheumatic fever 205
  pathophysiology of 205fc, 206f
  symptoms of 206
Rheumatoid arthritis 366
  pathophysiology of 367f
  symptoms of 366
Rhinorrhea 84
Runny nose 309

S

Scoliosis 371
  pathophysiology of 372f
  symptoms of 372
Seizure 101, 102, 110, 131t, 230, 348
  disorders 129
  pathophysiology of 130fc
Self-care deficit 56, 370
  nursing interventions for 58t, 370t
Sensory dysfunction, internal factors of 342t, 344t
Sensory esotropia 316
Sepsis 230
Sexual abuse
  signs 382
  symptoms 382
Sexually transmitted diseases 234
  pathophysiology of 235fc
Shock, signs of 230
Skeletal traction 344t
Skin
  color, abnormal 121
  graft 326
  rash 121
  swelling of 331
  thickened 303
  warm 332
Sleep pattern disturbance 74, 86, 111, 193, 310
  nursing interventions for 195t
Sleep-disordered breathing 201
Sleepiness 101, 102
Slow pulse 303
Slow speech 304
Slurred speech 110
Smell, sense of 310
Sneezing 309
Social isolation 272
  nursing interventions for 273t
Sore muscles 161
Sore throat 85, 222, 310
Speech difficulties 151
Spina bifida 134
  occulta 134
  pathophysiology of 135f
  symptoms of 134
Staphylococcus aureus 311

Stomach
  cramps 121
  pain 348
Strabismus 314
  pathophysiology of 316f
Streptococcal infection 207
Streptococcus pneumoniae 119, 311
Stressors 22
Stridor 30, 84
Stuffy nose 310
Stunted growth 217
Subcutaneous nodules 207
Suffocation
  high-risk for 84
  nursing interventions for high-risk for 84t
Surgery, internal physical factor of 154t
Surgical trauma 247t
Swelling 331, 362
  abdominal 287
Swollen face 304
Sydenham's chorea 207
Syndrome of inappropriate antidiuretic hormone secretion 99
Systemic lupus erythematosus, symptoms of 348

T

Tachypnea 30, 230
Talipes 375
  calcaneus 375
  equinus 375
  pathophysiology of 375f
  symptoms of 376
  valgus 375
Tender hip muscles 354
Tenderness 331
Therapeutic play 59
  pathophysiology of 60fc
Thoracic compression 230
Throat, disorder of 306, 309
Thrombocytes 263
Thrombocytopenia 278t
Thyrocalcitonin 302
Thyroid-stimulating hormone 302, 303
Thyroxine-binding globulin 302
Tiredness 286
Tissue 131t, 223
  hypoxia 342t
  swelling 217
Tonsillectomy 318, 319
Tonsillitis 318
  pathophysiology of 319f
  symptoms of 320
Trauma
  abdominal 202
  high-risk for 60
  nursing interventions for high-risk for 60t

Tuberculosis 92
  symptoms of 92
Tympanostomy 313
Tympanotomy 313

U

Umbilical catheterization, history of 202
Umbilical hernia, pathophysiology of 163f
Undescended testes 236
  pathophysiology of 237f
  symptoms of 237
Upper urinary tract 239
Ureters 213, 239
Urethra 213, 239
Urinary incontinence 217
Urinary reflux
  signs of 242
  symptoms of 242
Urinary tract 213
  infection 239
    pathophysiology of 240fc
    recurrent 217
    symptoms of 240
  lower 239
Urine
  measure specific gravity of 96
  output 217
    adequate 99

V

Vesicoureteral reflux 242
Visual changes 110
Visual disturbances 95
Voice, hoarseness of 84
Vomiting 95, 101, 111, 120, 147, 161, 172, 217, 240, 286

W

Weakness 110, 332
Weight
  gain 303
  loss 92, 168, 174, 223, 286, 287, 297, 348
Wheezing 69, 85
  sound 69
White blood cell 251, 286, 290, 365
Wilms tumor 246
  pathophysiology of 247fc
  signs of 248
  symptoms of 248
Written plan of care, advantages of 8

Y

Yeast infection 297

EU GSPR Authorised Reprsentative
Logos Europe, 9 rue Nicolas Poussin
1700, La Rochelle, France
Phone: +33 (0) 6 67 93 73 78
E-mail: contact@logoseurope.eu

www.ingramcontent.com/pod-product-compliance
Ingram Content Group UK Ltd.
Pitfield, Milton Keynes, MK11 3LW, UK
UKHW050456150426